T0146066

Achieving Health for All

Achieving Health for All

Primary Health Care in Action

Edited by
DAVID BISHAI, PhD, MD, MPH
MEIKE SCHLEIFF, MSPH, DrPH

Johns Hopkins University Press
Baltimore

This book was brought to publication in part with the generous support of the J. G. Goellner Endowment.

Johns Hopkins University Press
2715 North Charles Street
Baltimore, Maryland 21218-4363
www.press.jhu.edu

Library of Congress Cataloging-in-Publication Data

Names: Bishai, David, editor. | Schleiff, Meike, editor.
Title: Achieving health for all : primary health care in action /
   edited by David Bishai and Meike Schleiff.
Description: Baltimore : Johns Hopkins University Press, 2020. | Includes bibliographical
   references and index.
Identifiers: LCCN 2019036591 | ISBN 9781421438122 (hardcover ; alk. paper) |
   ISBN 9781421438139 (ebook)
Subjects: MESH: Alma-Ata Declaration (1978) | Primary health care | Population health
   management | Quality improvement | Community health services | Developing countries
Classification: LCC RA425 | NLM W 84.61 | DDC 362.1—dc23
LC record available at https://lccn.loc.gov/2019036591

A catalog record for this book is available from the British Library.

*Special discounts are available for bulk purchases of this book. For more information, please
contact Special Sales at specialsales@press.jhu.edu.*

Johns Hopkins University Press uses environmentally friendly book materials, including
recycled text paper that is composed of at least 30 percent post-consumer waste, whenever
possible.

CONTENTS

FOREWORD

In 1978, the Alma-Ata Declaration proposed a forward-thinking vision that has been the foundation of primary health care (PHC) for more than forty years. Moving away from the predominant biomedical focus, the declaration was founded on principles of social justice and equity, acknowledged the importance of addressing the wider determinants of health through preventive measures, emphasized intersectoral action; and placed patient and community engagement and empowerment as key to achieving health for all.

These principles were reiterated at the 2018 Global Conference on Primary Health Care in Astana, Kazakhstan. The Astana Declaration defines PHC as an orientation toward health systems that are integrated, community based, and the product of user engagement and empowerment, thus facilitating the needs of all throughout their life course. PHC in the twenty-first century is conceptualized by the World Health Organization and the United Nations Children's Fund's Operational Framework as health services and essential public health functions at the core of integrated health systems, multisectoral policy and action, and empowered people and communities.

Implementing the Astana vision requires a shift in focus from curative care to health promotion and disease prevention, as well as the development of new models related to service delivery, financing, and governance for PHC. These requirements reflect the need for resilient, adaptive, and comprehensive PHC systems based on local context and codeveloped by empowered people engaged in their own health.

Increasingly, it is recognized that it will not be possible to achieve the health-related Sustainable Development Goals (SDGs), including universal health coverage, without stronger PHC. Universal health coverage means that all people, including those who are marginalized or vulnerable, have access to quality health care services that put their needs at the center without financial hardship. As such, the Astana Declaration identifies PHC as the most effective, efficient, and equitable approach to enhancing health, and foundational to achieving universal health coverage.

Yet, PHC implementation and PHC systems reforms are challenged by the lack of contextualized knowledge and a dearth of research on effective approaches to strengthen PHC, especially in low- and middle-income countries. There is a need to advance the science and practice of PHC, with a forward-looking view of the innovations, challenges, and shared responsibilities in driving PHC forward.

This book contributes to bridging the knowledge gap on contextualized evidence to enhance PHC by providing lessons from successful PHC implementation in low- and middle-income countries, and informing current strategies to operationalize the Astana Declaration.

We believe this publication will provide PHC stakeholders with relevant and useful insights on effective approaches to enhance PHC policy and practice worldwide. These lessons will also provide critical evidence to strengthen PHC systems and position primary health care as the backbone of universal health coverage, with a view of moving toward Health for All in the twenty-first century.

Dr. Soumya Swaminathan, Chief Scientist, World Health Organization

FOREWORD

The 2018 Astana Declaration clearly indicates that research, knowledge, and experience sharing will have a role to play in strengthening capacities to achieve primary health care (PHC). A strong research base is needed to inform action on achieving PHC's three pillars—namely, primary care and essential public health functions, empowered people and communities, and multisectoral policy and action.

In low- and middle-income countries (LMICs) especially, evidence on what works to strengthen PHC is greatly needed to address fragmentation, underresourcing, and governance challenges. Critical knowledge gaps exist on key aspects of PHC systems strengthening, which need to be informed by real-world and policy-relevant evidence. Importantly, more PHC systems research emerging from LMIC stakeholders is needed to provide contextualized understanding to and ownership of PHC systems challenges.

For more than twenty years, the Alliance for Health Policy and Systems Research (the Alliance)—a partnership hosted by the World Health Organization (WHO)—has supported the generation and use of evidence to strengthen LMIC health systems. The Alliance has positioned itself as a leader in supporting research to inform PHC policy decisions and drive PHC reforms. We have achieved this by bringing together researchers and policymakers to identify research priorities that respond to the needs of countries and LMIC stakeholders. The Alliance has spearheaded different initiatives in PHC research, including the Primary Health Care Systems initiative, which supported the development of twenty case studies of PHC systems in selected LMICs. The Alliance has also played a key role in profiling the coproduction approach in PHC research by developing an innovative model of embedding research in PHC policy and systems decision-making.

This collection of case studies from LMICs that have embraced comprehensive PHC as foundational strategies to develop their health systems offers evidence and ideas for current and future PHC systems. It presents research findings from a selection of countries that intentionally undertook systems-level approaches to establish people-centered and comprehensive PHC. Its publication also contributes to bridging the gap in context-sensitive evidence to support PHC policy-making and PHC systems reforms in LMICs.

The Alliance is delighted to support the publication of this volume, building on our commitment to knowledge generation and uptake for LMIC health systems strengthening. It is our hope that the insights collected within these chapters will inspire PHC policymakers and implementers across diverse settings to transform the ideals of the Astana Declaration into action.

Dr. Abdul Ghaffar, Executive Director, Alliance for Health Policy and Systems Research, World Health Organization

ACKNOWLEDGMENTS

First, we wish to thank all of the co-authors of the chapters of this text for sharing their rich experiences from across all countries and other programs and projects. We also wish to thank the Alliance for Health Policy and Systems Research for their financial support as well as close collaboration and guidance throughout this process. In addition, we would like to thank leadership of the Department of International Health and the Health Systems program at Johns Hopkins School of Public Health for supporting and encouraging the initial planning and launch of this project.

Several students, particularly Ria Shah, Navya Ravoori, and Alice Kuan, have provided essential organizational, writing/editing, and other skills to numerous aspects of the editorial process. Finally, we wish to thank Dr. Fran Baum and the late Dr. David Sanders who provided encouragement and willingness to endorse and promote this book and the pragmatic and experiential approach that we have taken to further the dialogue and action related to primary health care.

Why Does Primary Health Care Matter in the Twenty-First Century?

David Bishai

The World's First Global Health Crisis

For the citizens of medieval Caffa on the Crimean Peninsula, 1346 was a very bad year. Generations of Genoese and Venetian traders had managed to prosper in this Italian enclave, trading the bounty of central Asia through the Black Sea and into the Mediterranean. However, 1346 brought siege at the hands of the Mongol Army. The great Mongol khan, Jani Beg, smelled fortune beyond the walls of Caffa and wanted in. The siege was dragging on, so the warriors turned to terror. A rain of bloated black corpses of fallen Mongol comrades was catapulted over the walls and into the city (Wheelis 2002).

Unbeknownst to all, another invader was launching conquest under Jani Beg's feet. Plague bacteria (*Yersinia pestis*) had overgrown and blocked the guts of the fleas living on the rats and men in the Mongol camp. Desperate constipated fleas began a cycle of frenzied biting and vomiting into the wounds they inflicted on both rats and men. The army of the Golden Horde was melting away, and the khan could tell the siege would have to end. Black plague overtook Caffa and devastated Europe, carried by rats and fleas and men in Genoese ships. The world population fell from 440 million to 350 million by 1400 (US Census Bureau 2013).

Black plague was the first documented global health catastrophe.* There were no global conferences, no blue-ribbon scientific committees. Collective

---

*The human genome bears a record of a genetic bottleneck around twenty thousand years ago, suggesting that the world's *Homo sapiens* population was reduced to about one hundred people in Africa. This near-miss extinction would have been a global health event, too.

action in the face of the oncoming plague was futile given the world's state of knowledge. The hopelessness is crystalized in Giovanni Boccaccio's *The Decameron*, set in Florence in 1348. In this frame story, the principals agree that death will find them no matter what, so the best thing to do with a lethal pandemic is to hole up in a villa telling one another tall tales.

Much has changed in global health. Now, there are things that can be done. There has been success, and there has been variation in success. There are good practices and bad practices to learn from. There are nonfiction stories to tell about what cities, districts, states, and countries do in health policy and implementation of programs. These stories are a matter of life and death.

This book examines the lessons that countries drew from the Alma-Ata Conference of 1978, the first global conference to focus on primary health care. This conference articulated a vision of comprehensive primary health care (PHC) that still matters deeply for the health of populations in every community in the world. Comprehensive PHC encompasses both whole population activities and services that reach one person at a time. Whole populations need PHC to improve the safety of air, food, water, roads, homes, and workplaces. Individuals need services to deliver health care at a primary medical care visit or when they open their door to a community health worker. The Alma-Ata Declaration described how comprehensive PHC could be established as a multi-stakeholder partnership among citizens, their government, civil society, and the private sector.

Many retrospective discussions of the conference take a wistful tone, depicting it as a moment of unfounded optimism as though the principles announced in the Alma-Ata Declaration were only aspirational and not practical. It is true that the full agenda set out by conference delegates in 1978 never became mainstream practice by a majority of the world's health systems. However, some health systems did succeed in making the principles of the Alma-Ata Declaration a reality. Moreover, many of the countries where this happened—Bangladesh, Cuba, Nepal, Ghana, and others flagged in chapter 2—turned out to make better than average progress in gaining life expectancy given their economic growth. How they did that matters, and these details are the main point of this book.

Reading a success story can inspire only if there is a sense that the success was neither inevitable nor impossibly accidental. The success stories related in this book occurred in countries that faced substantial obstacles to better health, including wars, revolutions, challenging topography, and poverty. Success was never inevitable. Each success story carries many contextual differences, but the common theme is that they adhered more or less to the principles of comprehensive PHC. This chapter introduces a theme that will recur throughout the book: that the principles of comprehensive PHC announced in the Alma-Ata Declaration remain relevant everywhere and that every community can open a pathway to similar success.

The World's First Global Health Conference: A Miraculous Consensus

From September 6 to September 12, 1978, delegates from 134 countries and representatives from 67 nongovernmental organizations, agencies, and United Nations (UN) organizations gathered in the city of Alma-Ata at the invitation of the USSR under the aegis of the World Health Organization (WHO) and United Nations International Children's Emergency Fund (UNICEF). The purpose of the conference was to exchange experience about something called *primary health care*. The delegates gathered to define PHC, to promote it, and to learn how governments, NGOs, and UN agencies could cooperate and support PHC. The Alma-Ata Conference led to an important consensus about what could be done to make populations healthy (Newell 1975; Litsios 2002).

Getting 134 countries to agree on anything during the height of the Cold War was a miracle. A large part of the miracle was allowing the term *primary health care*, or PHC, to remain loosely defined. Some thought PHC was a code word for social justice, while others thought it referred to the organization of clinical services (Litsios 2008). Planners used a working definition of PHC as the combination of basic health services plus community participation plus intersectoral engagement, and that definition offered something for everyone.

Parallel camps on either side of the Cold War spent the early 1970s with convergent dissatisfaction about the vertical approach to single diseases that dominated US agencies and the WHO since the 1950s. A big push from the United States to eradicate malaria had failed, and leading Western voices in global health had to concede as much (Litsios 2002). A 1973 WHO report saw the failure to eradicate malaria as symptomatic of "widespread dissatisfaction of populations about their health services." Failures included a lack of citizen inclusion, a feeling of helplessness on the part of citizens, and widening health disparities (Newell 1988). Physician groups began dominating health budgets in low-income countries to construct expensive hospitals and to pay for drugs that served the more well-off and not the poor. In the words of Jack Bryant, writing in 1969: "Large numbers of the world's people, perhaps more than half, have no access to health care at all, and for many of the rest, the care they receive does not answer the problems they have. . . . The most serious needs cannot be met by teams with spray guns and vaccinating syringes" (Bryant 1969, ix–x). The Christian Medical Commission helped feed both UNICEF and WHO case studies of successful bottom-up approaches from China, Cuba, Tanzania, Bangladesh, Iran, and the Jamkhed project in India. American public health leaders Ruth and Victor Sidel described amazing progress by the barefoot doctors of China (Newell 1975). Carl Taylor described community participatory approaches in India (Cueto 2004). These success stories were disseminated and influential throughout UNICEF, the WHO, and regional offices (Djukanovic and Mach 1975; Newell 1975). Soviet representatives of the WHO saw an opening to make political gains inside the UN in the wake of Western failure and campaigned to sponsor an international conference hosted on Soviet soil to discuss the concept of PHC. It could not have escaped the Soviets' notice that many of the best practices promoted by the WHO, UNICEF, and Western scholars were from either Communist-orbit or nonaligned countries.

Given years of planning and skillful diplomacy by the WHO, the Alma-Ata Conference managed to avoid explicit political confrontation between Western and Soviet ideology. However, Chinese–Soviet tensions in the 1970s led to China not attending the conference (Cueto 2004). US Senator Ted Kennedy gave a keynote address. Leonid Brezhnev sent welcoming remarks read by a member of the Presidium of the Supreme Soviet. But overt Cold War politics did not get in the way of consensus. The text of the Alma-Ata Declaration had been previewed by delegates and was adopted by acclamation on September 12, 1978. Dr. Marcella Davies of Sierra Leone came to the podium to read the text aloud to the hall of three thousand in one of the most uplifting and sublime moments of unity of the twentieth century.

Prior to the Alma-Ata Conference of 1978, there had been countless international scientific conferences for extensive international sharing of biomedical and public health knowledge. The Alma-Ata Conference was different because it focused on the application of that knowledge into collective human action. The conference was not about one disease or one disease determinant. What was global at the Alma-Ata Conference was a recognition of an approach to tackling the root causes of ill health that could be universalized, in any place, at any time.

The conference brought together medical scientists, heads of national health ministries, and policymakers. Most remarkably, the participants achieved consensus around seven simple principles in the declaration that distill truths about what makes people healthy and that delegates acclaimed to be relevant everywhere and for all health threats.

Like most historical documents, it used words from its era that have shifted in their meaning. At the time, the term *primary health care* meant different things to different parties, but most understood the emphasis on *primary* as referring to the first thing to do about the health of people. Today, because *primary care doctor* has gotten such wide usage, a modern reader might mistakenly think that the emphasis on the words *primary health care* is about *care* and expect that the term represents what individual care professionals provide in their clinics when caring for the sick. The Alma-Ata Declaration is anything but a manifesto about the primacy of the clinic. The Alma-Ata Declaration is partly about *care*, but it is mostly about *primary*. It is also first about health—promoting, supporting, and empowering communities to improve health—rather than treating disease. To try to avoid the pitfalls about where to put emphasis in the terminology, throughout the book we refer to the topic of the declaration as "PHC." The most actionable and specific definition of PHC is contained in Article VII of the 1978 declaration.

The Alma-Ata Declaration defines PHC as having seven principles (figure I.1). The first principle notes that PHC evolves from economic and sociocultural and political circumstances so that its research base includes social science and biomedicine. Second, PHC must address the health concerns of a time and place, emphasize creating conditions that prevent disease, and address curative and rehabilitative services. Third, PHC must do things for whole populations at a time, such as community health education, safe water, a safe food supply, sanitation, and so on. Fourth, this population response is bigger than the health sector and must include agriculture, housing, public works, and communications, and all these relevant sectors need to coordinate. Fifth, communities and individuals must take part in planning, organizing, and controlling PHC so that they draw in both the nation's and their own resources in making their places healthier. Sixth, PHC must be inclusive and comprehensive, giving priority to those most in need. Seventh, PHC must include multiple cadres of health workers—physicians, nurses, midwives, community health workers, and traditional practitioners—who work as a team and respond to the expressed needs of their community.

Reading the Alma-Ata principles makes it clear that in 1978, there was a lot of attention on the social determination of disease. For some biomedical specialists, invoking social determinants is the cue to exit the stage. If it cannot be fixed with a drug or surgery, it is anathema to some members of the

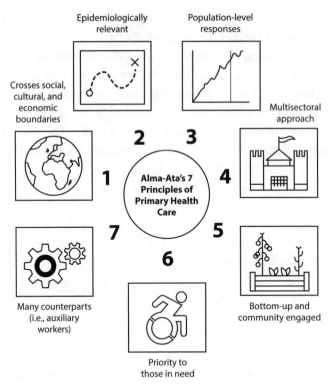

Epidemiologically relevant

Population-level responses

Crosses social, cultural, and economic boundaries

Multisectoral approach

2 3

1 Alma-Ata's 7 Principles of Primary Health Care 4

7 5

6

Many counterparts (i.e., auxiliary workers)

Priority to those in need

Bottom-up and community engaged

Figure I.1. The seven principles of primary health care listed in Article VII of the Alma-Ata Declaration.

medical community. However, for the participants at Alma-Ata, the announcement that disease was socially determined was the opening curtain. The preparatory studies commissioned by the WHO and UNICEF on health progress in countries such as China, Cuba, Jamkhed in India, and Central Java in Indonesia had shown dramatic transformation in social determinants of disease that did not rely on the slow march of economic growth (Djukanovic and Mach 1975; Newell 1975). Participants announced with confidence that coordinated actions by groups of people could address social determinants and recruit community members in cooperation to make their communities healthier. To paraphrase Carl Taylor, the Alma-Ata Declaration did not offer a global solution to all health problems, but it offered a global approach to finding local solutions (Taylor and Taylor-Ide 2002). These local approaches are complementary and foundational to successful implementation of the big vertical approaches that seem to dominate global health

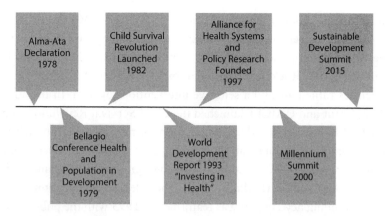

Figure I.2. Timeline of the evolution of primary health care and selective interventions.

today. Attention to PHC bridges the chasm between global paradigms, policies, and politics, and their realization in a place.

Diverging Pathways since 1978

There are parallel and diverging histories of what happened after the Alma-Ata Conference. Like most events of the Cold War, versions vary between Westerners and the Global South. Figure I.2 shows a timeline of key events since the Alma-Ata Conference.

The Western Aid Agency Version of Global Health since Alma-Ata

In the West, the dominant narrative is that economic constraints derailed the PHC agenda (see chapter 1 for details). For those who chose to interpret PHC as a project of constructing networks of health care delivery facilities to offer "primary clinical care," the PHC agenda would put massive demands on limited public sector funds. Many of the poorest countries, especially in Africa, went through the 1980s with badly managed budget deficits that were countered and compounded by structural adjustment policies of the World Bank and the International Monetary Fund (Lawn et al. 2008). The landmark paper by Julia Walsh and Kenneth Warren (1979) outlines a purportedly more economical approach of selective health interventions that emphasized a small set of high-impact packages such as oral rehydration, vaccination, and promotion of breastfeeding. The Ford and Rockefeller Foundations sponsored a conference in Bellagio, Italy, in April 1979, where the Walsh and Warren approach was the centerpiece of discussions attended by Robert McNamara of the World Bank; James Grant, who went on to direct UNICEF; and John Gillian of USAID (Rockefeller Foundation 1979). These leaders of Western aid agencies rallied around a selective interventions agenda. In the autumn of 1982, Grant and UNICEF launched the Child Survival Revolution to promote GOBI-FFF, which stood for growth monitoring, oral rehydration, breast-feeding promotion, immunizations, family planning, female education, and food supplements. UNICEF raised funds from both the World Bank and the Rockefeller Foundation (Packard 2017). The selective interventions era entered a continuing heyday that was reaffirmed in 1993 with the publication of the World Bank's *World Development Report: Investing in Health*. The report introduced economic methods to rationalize investments in selective interventions on the grounds of dollars spent per health outcome gained.

A generation of Western-trained health economists was then put to work buttressing an approach to global health policy-making that emphasized the primacy of discrete, specific, and tangible interventions as the pathway to achieving good health at a low cost. The work of health policy has devolved into rational selection of a portfolio of the most cost-effective interventions to minimize the burden of disease within a given health sector budget. Persisting today, many textbooks and curricula in global health treat the topic of global health as a cavalcade of interventions. Students of global health often build careers around specializing in a disease area or in an intervention area. Advocates press for more priority and funds for their specific disease silo. It is still challenging for public health students and professionals to learn practical skills in population health promotion, community organizing, convening, and building coalitions and partnerships, even though this is what a career in PHC would require.

The Alma-Ata Declaration's version of PHC put the emphasis on community capability to plan and respond to local disease burden. Needing to include the community was the key lesson learned (and apparently forgotten) in the wake of the failure of malaria eradication (Newell 1988). In contrast, the selective interventionists put the emphasis on interventions and belatedly recognized that interventions occur in the context of health systems and with influence from a wide array of social factors. Cries for "greater health system strengthening" emanated from all corners whenever the interventionists ran into bottlenecks from a lack of coordination or community buy-in. The WHO's Alliance for Health Policy and Systems Research was founded in 1997 and has been instrumental in developing a professional society called

Health Systems Global to coordinate scholarship on health systems. Many of the participants in this community still see health systems strength as a means to an end—the end being delivering the list of interventions. Chapter 4 offers details on how the Global Polio Eradication Initiative has realized the necessity of stronger health systems to achieve its single goal. Chapter 5 shows how PHC aligns well with the realization of Sustainable Development Goals (SDGs). Few continue the rallying cry of the Alma-Ata Declaration's vision that communities that had good PHC would be resilient solvers of whatever health issues came their way and that they would initiate solutions to their problems that address root causes far beyond the scope of typical interventions.

The foreign aid to support interventions has not necessarily been bad or harmful. These interventions have saved millions of lives, and it is hard to make the case that the alternative course of history might have been Western investments in PHC and the strength of multisectoral, community-engaged, bottom-up health systems. Western aid agencies have embraced three-to-five-year project cycles and the need to measure activities for external accountability. Distributing health commodities such as bed nets, HIV drugs, vaccines, and family planning supplies is eminently countable, unlike improving multisectoral community engagement. Because of their remit, aid agencies might not be well configured to be the doers or enablers of PHC.

Although Western aid agencies might be forgiven for not taking on a direct role in PHC themselves, their interventionist work plan has constrained the way much of the world thinks and speaks about global health. Westerners make an outsize contribution to international scholarship, writing, speaking, and thinking about global health. Graduate students who come for advanced training in global health in Western institutions receive the Western interventionist paradigm and transmit it back to institutions of higher learning in Africa, Asia, and Latin America. The domination of discourse has kept much more of the spotlight on selective interventions as opposed to PHC.

Ultimately, the design of the Millennium Development Goals (MDGs) cemented the primacy of the Western focus on interventions and achieved a new global consensus around a restrictive definition of development that was measured as outcomes and not as capabilities to achieve outcomes (Pritchett and Kenny 2013). The MDGs included two health goals to lower under-5 mortality and maternal mortality that interlocked well with a mechanistic focus on siloed interventions (UN Millennium Project 2005). At the Millennium Summit in 2000, all 191 UN member nations pledged toward eight

goals including goals to reduce under five mortality by two-thirds and to reduce the maternal mortality ratio by 75%. A group of epidemiologists produced a model called the Lives Saved Tool (LiST), designed to predict how
many children's lives would be saved by investing in each of more than a
dozen interventions (Fox et al. 2011). As the pendulum swung to the extreme
of mechanistic global health policy-making, a preventable child death was no
longer seen as the outcome of social conditions but as the absence of specific
interventions (Black et al. 2003; Jones, Steketee, et al. 2003). It did not matter
who financed them or organized them, or how the interventions were
implemented—success toward MDGs could occur if the interventions
marched forward. Critics noted how the MDG paradigm was self-serving for
the industry of foreign assistance (Easterly 2009; Donini 2012). An NGO
could point out how a low-income country's health statistics were not on
track to reach the MDGs and justify an allotment of foreign aid to parachute
in an intervention whose costs were duly estimated (Bryce et al. 2005).

Views on Global Health from the Global South

Annual health spending in 2015 amounted to $9 trillion, of which $833 billion was spent by low- and middle-income countries (Bishai and Cardona
2017) (figure I.3). Despite their domination of discourse about health spending in low- and middle-income countries, Western donors only contributed
$46 billion, which is less than 6% of spending. In contrast, citizens' out-of-
pocket and tax-based spending represents most health spending in low- and
middle-income countries.

In the wake of the Alma-Ata Conference of 1978, several countries stuck
to, or returned to, the original seven principles of PHC. Countries like Sri
Lanka, Nepal, Vietnam, Bangladesh, Ethiopia, and Cuba are now some of the
leading success stories in achieving good health at a low cost. They embraced
and implemented selective interventions, too. The two approaches need not
be in conflict. Good PHC makes interventions work better and helps sustain
them.

In bringing these success stories to light, this book decidedly focuses on
whole country stories. This is not meant to say that PHC is solely the job of
national ministries of health or that national scale is always desirable and
practical. PHC can involve both the national and subnational levels. However, national-level health policymakers can set up incentives, institutions,
and career pathways that make subnational units much more likely to get
PHC to succeed. The opposite has occurred in many countries not featured

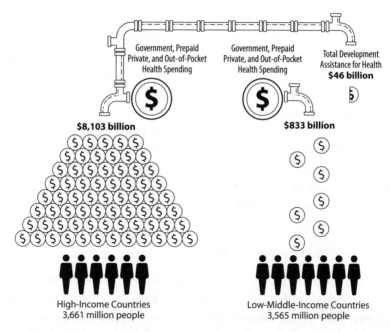

Figure I.3. Aggregate health spending. High-income countries are those with a gross domestic product (GDP) per capita > 12,000 $US, and low-middle-income countries are those with a GDP per capita < 12,000 $US. Source: Bishai 2017

in this book. In most countries, ministries of health divide into administrative units based on the interventions they will carry out. The districts divide themselves as well. It is typical to see divisions for immunizations, TB, HIV, maternal and child health, noncommunicable disease control, laboratories, and the like, with limited ability, incentive, or interest in collaborating and operating as a system. Moreover, many countries experience a "patchwork" array of NGOs, government programs, other externally funded initiatives, and community-led activities that are uncoordinated and create chaos, inefficiency, and subpar outcomes. An emerging best practice (described in chapter 3) to align actors and activities is the creation of crosscutting units of public health practice quality. These units help all the vertical programs attune to how their work can improve the conduct of community-engaged, multisectoral, population-level PHC both at the national and subnational levels.

Inside any community, the pressing suffering of those already sick will force policy concern to get them cures and clinical care. The world will not make progress by reducing our attention to taking care of sick people or reducing our international collaborations for standard interventions in global health. Instead, we need to add back more emphasis on the PHC practices outlined in the 1978 Alma-Ata Declaration and reemphasized in the 2018 Astana Declaration. What can we learn from countries who built their health systems around comprehensive PHC? What do they know about getting people to make it their job to ask if the community's whole health system is working? We must rediscover and recommit to the best practices that have served these countries in making their communities take ownership of their health. For Western donors, PHC has been the ugly stepchild and never the darling of any external donor with a three-year project cycle. However, for countries, community participation in understanding root contributors to ill health and ways to address their priorities using all available resources across all relevant sectors is the best pathway to make sustained progress.

The Continuing Relevance of PHC

There are five factors that ensure the continuing relevance of PHC.

1. *The long-term trend is for less and less reliance on foreign aid for health.* As we saw in figure I.3, foreign assistance is miniscule in comparison to domestic spending for health. Over time, flows of development aid will be decreasing and not increasing. Economic growth is enabling middle-income countries to graduate out of needing aid. The agencies responsible for targeted interventions like GAVI, the Vaccine Alliance, have explicit criteria for countries to graduate off assistance and to develop exit strategies where financing for the interventions is maintained. With the decline of Western spending on global health will come the replacement of Western domination of the global health paradigm by voices from the Global South.

2. *The epidemiological transition to noncommunicable disease makes PHC more relevant.* While it is tempting to think of a selective interventions approach to noncommunicable diseases (NCDs), this approach cannot scale. The risk factors for conditions such as car crash injuries, cancer, heart disease, diabetes, violence, obesity, and so forth do not lend themselves to the distribution of commodities. Approaches to address these risk factors cross sectors and include transportation, food, law enforcement, housing, and social order. Sustaining solutions needs long-term political battles to legislate new regulations and new efforts in enforcement. It requires new ways of cooperating with neighbors to sustain norms of healthier behavior. This is the strength of PHC approaches.

3. *The threat of global pandemics makes PHC essential.* Among the many lessons learned from the recent outbreaks of the Ebola and Zika viruses was the weaknesses of local-level public health operations. These weaknesses in-

cluded not only delayed detection of the outbreaks but a lack of community trust in the public health officials who labored to enact control measures among the susceptible population. In countries that undertake PHC, there is a commitment to build ongoing relationships between public health professionals and the community. Building trust takes time. The investment pays off by improving outbreak detection and speeding up the enactment of control measures.

4. *The upward trend in universal health coverage requires PHC.* As people's incomes grow, the proportion of people covered by health insurance grows. This happens because workers get jobs in the formal sector, where it is easier to offer health insurance. It also occurs because economic growth leads to more ability to demand and pay the taxes or premiums needed for health insurance. Governments will predictably undertake more insurance regulation, and they will offer more governmental health insurance. The growth of health insurance can lead to the inclusion of community concerns in the types of covered services. The interests of insurers become aligned with the methods of PHC in making communities more engaged in population-level health promotion and prevention.

5. *PHC is aligned with SDGs.* In 2015, the UN General Assembly agreed on a new set of seventeen global goals to replace the MDGs. These seventeen goals are inherently more multisectoral, and their achievement requires communities that are committed to social justice and have their own capability to achieve it. These new goals range from a commitment to "no poverty" to a commitment to creating "sustainable communities" to a goal to commit to use "partnerships for the goals." The bottom-up pathways to achieving these goals make PHC more relevant than ever. (See chapter 5 for more.)

Summary

This book is divided into two parts. Part I discusses the legacy of Alma-Ata and offers both a narrative history (chapter 1) and a quantitative examination of global health trends (chapter 2). Practical tools to implement PHC are covered in chapters 3 and 6 using supervisory coaching to help health workers practice public health or engage community members as partners. The relevance of PHC to prevailing priorities in vertical disease control is the topic of chapter 4, and the relevance of PHC to the SDGs is covered in chapter 5.

Part II has assembled country case studies of PHC implementation at the national level since the Alma-Ata Declaration of 1978. Each chapter takes a national perspective to describe how PHC was integrated into the health system. Each country faced slightly different political and cultural constraints, and each took a slightly different path. It turned out that many of the countries that adopted PHC did so in the shadow of civil war. Examples are Bangladesh, Nepal, Sri Lanka, and Vietnam. Obviously, there is no law of history that declares that the victors of a civil war will focus on health and basic needs, but our cases show that this is not exceptional.

The roots of the PHC approach described in 1978 appealed to both Western and Communist bloc countries because of dismay about the slow pace of progress in malaria eradication in the 1950s and 1960s. The PHC approach offered a bit of something for everyone, but comprehensive PHC insisted on a population-level, community-controlled, multisectoral approach as well as evidence-based, basic health care carried out by doctors, nurses, community health workers, and others.

At the Astana Conference of 2018, there was a widespread recognition that ongoing trends will make PHC more relevant than ever. The SDGs, the future scaling down of foreign aid, and the transition to more and more noncommunicable health problems and pandemics requiring multisectoral efforts to address social causes are important reasons to pay attention to success stories in PHC.

This book can help readers get ready for the future by learning lessons from the success stories of countries that have made the most progress in attaining health for all.

REFERENCES

Bishai, D., and C. Cardona. 2017. "Aggregate health spending." *Lancet* 390 (10095): 647.

Black, R. E., S. S. Morris, and J. Bryce. 2003. "Where and why are 10 million children dying every year?" *Lancet* 361 (9376): 2226–2234.

Bryant, J. H. 1969. *Health and the developing world*. Ithaca, NY: Cornell University Press.

Bryce, J., R. E. Black, N. Walker, Z. A. Bhutta, J. E. Lawn, and R. W. Steketee. 2005. "Can the world afford to save the lives of 6 million children each year?" *Lancet* 365 (9478): 2193–2200.

Cueto, M. 2004. "The origins of primary health care and selective primary health care." *Am J Public Health* 94 (11): 1864–1874.

Djukanovic, V., and E. P. Mach. 1975. *Alternative approaches to meeting basic health needs in developing countries*. Geneva: WHO.

Donini, A. 2012. *The golden fleece: Manipulation and independence in humanitarian action*. Sterling, VA: Kumarian Press.

Easterly, W. 2009. "How the Millennium Development Goals are unfair to Africa." *World Dev* 37 (1): 26–35.

Fox, M. J., R. Martorell, N. van den Broek, and N. Walker. 2011. "Assumptions and methods in the Lives Saved Tool (LiST): Introduction." *BMC Public Health* 11 (Suppl. 3): I1.

Jones, G., R. W. Steketee, R. E. Black, Z. A. Bhutta, and S. S. Morris. 2003. "How many child deaths can we prevent this year?" *Lancet* 362 (9377): 65–71.

Lawn, J. E., J. Rohde, S. Rifkin, M. Were, V. K. Paul, and M. Chopra. 2008. "Alma-Ata 30 years on: Revolutionary, relevant, and time to revitalise." *Lancet* 372 (9642): 917–927.

Litsios, S. 2002. "The long and difficult road to Alma-Ata: A personal reflection." *Int J Health Serv* 32 (4): 709–732.

———. 2008. *The third 10 years of WHO*. Geneva: WHO.

Newell, K. 1975. *Health by the people*. Geneva: WHO.

———. 1988. "Selective primary health care: The counter revolution." *Soc Sci Med* 26 (9): 903–906.

Packard, R. 2017. *A history of global health*. Baltimore: Johns Hopkins University Press.

Pritchett, L., and C. Kenny. 2013. "Promoting millennium development ideals: The risks of defining development down." Center for Global Development Working Paper 338.

Rockefeller Foundation. 1979. Health and population in developing countries: A Bellagio conference, April 18–21.

Taylor, C. E., and D. Taylor-Ide. 2002. *A just and lasting change: When communities own their own futures*. Baltimore: Johns Hopkins University Press.

UN Millennium Project. 2005. *Investing in development: A practical plan to achieve the Millennium Development Goals*. New York: United Nations Development Programme.

US Census Bureau. 2013. "Historical estimates of world population." https://www.census.gov/data/tables/time-series/demo/international-programs/historical-est-worldpop.html.

Walsh, J. A., and K. S. Warren. 1979. "Selective primary health care: An interim strategy for disease control in developing countries." *N Engl J Med* 301 (18): 967–974.

Wheelis, M. 2002. "Biological warfare at the 1346 siege of Caffa." *Emerg Infect Dis* 8 (9): 971–975.

World Bank. 1993. *The world development report: Investing in health*. New York: Oxford University Press.

PART ONE

Primary Health Care Foundations

CHAPTER ONE

Primary Health Care

History, Trends, Controversies, and Challenges

HENRY B. PERRY

The people of the world—and the so-called bottom billion in particular—require and have the right to expect a strong and equitable system of primary health care. Primary health care (PHC) in the context of global health, and from the standpoint of the most disadvantaged populations around the world, represents the undisputed long-term core strategy for improving health through health programs (as opposed to overall poverty reduction and broad development). Ironically, PHC has been until recently one of the most neglected topics on the global health agenda. This chapter explores PHC in the context of global health by revisiting and updating the definition of primary care that was enunciated in the 1978 Alma-Ata Declaration and reaffirmed in the 2018 Astana Declaration. The chapter connects PHC to the context of today's global health landscape and evidence base by reflecting on the history of the PHC movement since 1978 and by looking to the near-term future for the global health and development agenda that is geared toward achieving the UN Sustainable Development Goals, attaining universal health coverage (UHC), and ending preventable child and maternal deaths.

The waning of interest in and support for PHC that occurred over the three decades following the 1978 International Conference on Primary Health Care held in Alma-Ata, USSR (now Almaty, Kazakhstan), has recently reversed. The fortieth-anniversary celebration at Astana, Kazakhstan, in 2018 and the Declaration of Astana provided an opportunity to reaffirm support for PHC, to rethink the basic concepts of PHC, and to consider how a stronger and more equitable PHC system can help the world achieve Health for All sooner rather than later (World Health Organization, Ministry of Health of Kazakhstan, and United Nations Children's Fund 2018).

The current renewed interest in PHC can be attributed to several converging trends, the most important of which is a growing awareness of the magnitude of remaining unmet basic health needs throughout the world. Although from a global perspective, enormous gains have been made in disease control and mortality reduction, still more than one billion people have never seen a health care provider (GHWA 2011). Of the seventy-four countries with 97% of the world's maternal and child deaths, only four achieved the 2015 Millennium Development Goals (MDGs) for maternal and child health (Victora et al. 2016), with progress in sub-Saharan Africa for all the health-related MDGs lagging far behind the rest of the world (World Health Organization and United Nations Children's Fund 2012; United Nations 2015). AIDS (acquired immunodeficiency syndrome), tuberculosis, and malaria—all readily preventable or treatable diseases—still claim almost three million lives a year (World Health Organization 2018a, 2018b, 2016). All of these health challenges remain despite vast improvements in the financial resources and technical knowledge with which to combat these tragedies. The number of deaths occurring each year from readily preventable or treatable conditions should be widely considered as among the greatest moral and ethical failures of our current era.

A second reason that interest and support for PHC is now waxing is the recognition that the population coverage of most basic and essential services that fall within the realm of PHC among low-income populations remains below 60% (Victora et al. 2015). (An exception is the coverage of immunizations and vitamin A supplementation, which has benefited from intense and well-coordinated donor funding, policy advocacy, and on-the-ground monitoring.) Basic health-promoting behaviors such as exclusive breastfeeding and handwashing, which we know can be effectively promoted through community-based PHC programs, are still far from the norm.

Third, the decades-long emphasis on specific disease control programs and selective top-down initiatives are increasingly recognized to have forestalled emphasis on strengthening PHC programs and community-based health service delivery.

Julia Walsh and Kenneth Warren titled their highly influential 1979 article "Selective Primary Health Care: An *Interim* Strategy for Disease Control in Developing Countries" (emphasis added). This title shows prescience: for more and more countries, the "*interim*" is over and it is time to get down to the business of building the foundational structures that can help the world achieve and sustain Health for All.

Fourth, the effectiveness of community mobilization, participation, and empowerment in improving population health now has a stronger evidence base for supporting the utilization of basic and essential services and for promoting healthy behaviors. Fifth, the emergence of adult chronic diseases as the major global disease burden of the future makes primary prevention as well as health services for screening and treatment of chronic diseases a top priority. Hence, the need for a functioning PHC system to address this coming burden is obvious since repeated contact with the health system is a prerequisite for chronic disease prevention and control.

Origin of the Term *Primary Health Care* and Organization of Primary Health Care in Developed Countries

The term *primary health care* is generally ascribed to the Dawson Report, which was presented to Parliament in Great Britain in 1920 (Dawson 1920). The report, chaired by Lord Dawson of Penn, was concerned with the "Future Provision of Medical and Allied Services." The report arose from a recognition that the organization of medical care at that time was insufficient and that "it fails to bring the advantages of medical knowledge adequately within reach of the people." Its general principle was that medical services should be "distributed according to the needs of the community." The report also recognized that, while medical care had been previously provided primarily in the home, increasingly, services would need to be provided in facilities with laboratory and radiology services.* It also recognized that preventive and curative medicine "cannot be separated on any sound principle, and any scheme of medical services must be brought together in close co-ordination." Interestingly enough, the report does not actually use the term *primary health care* but does introduce the term *primary health center*.

Early Approaches to Provision of Primary Health Care in Developing Countries

In the early part of the twentieth century, medical services for disadvantaged populations in many low-income countries that were based on modern medical science were pioneered mostly by Christian medical missionaries. These

---

*The original use of the term in 1920 was *primary health care center*, not *primary health care services*, as a way, perhaps, to stress the need for facility-based care in addition to the dominant home-based care that had been the norm up to that time. At present, we seem to need to stress the importance of outreach because the emphasis more recently has been on facility-based care.

services were provided mostly in facilities, particularly hospitals. Mission hospitals accounted for 50% to 80% of hospital beds in many developing countries at that time. Local government health services were poorly developed.

Francophone and other European colonies not under British rule gave emphasis to specific priority diseases (*grandes endémies*), such as sleeping sickness, elephantiasis, and leprosy. Mobile units provided preventive and curative care for these conditions. They also provided curative care to large numbers of people who came to mass gatherings rather than offering services at static facilities. Anglophone countries and colonial health services in Africa and India were beginning to be involved in disease control efforts (e.g., for hookworm, malaria, and yellow fever). In China, early hospitals were mainly established by Christian medical missions, and a national public health system began in the 1920s in response to the emergence of an epidemic of pneumonic plague (United Nations Children's Fund 2008).

Thus, we can see that from the beginning of the twentieth century, both disease-specific (selective) approaches to improving health and more comprehensive facility-based approaches to providing health services were emerging. In developing countries in the early part of the twentieth century, more comprehensive approaches to reaching the entire population beyond facilities had not emerged until the 1930s, with the development of the Ding Xian Project one hundred miles south of Beijing.

The Ding Xian Project was developed by C. C. Chen, an experienced Yale-educated literacy expert who had developed methods for mass education among the rural poor, and Dr. John B. Grant, who was the first professor of public health at the Peking Union Medical College under an arrangement with the Rockefeller Foundation (Taylor-Ide and Taylor 2002). There, in the absence of any formally trained health workers and facilities, "farmer scholars" were trained to administer simple treatments at home using sixteen essential and safe drugs, to give talks and demonstrations on health and hygiene, to maintain clean water supplies, to vaccinate for smallpox, and to record births and deaths. These farmer scholars were the world's first example of what we know today as community health workers (CHWs), and this program served as the prototype for China's national "barefoot doctor" program that emerged in the 1950s. At that time, China had one of the highest death rates in the world (a crude death rate of 25 per 1,000 population and an infant mortality rate of 200 per 1,000 live births) (Sidel 1972). More than one million barefoot doctors received three months of training in traditional Chinese medicine as well as Western medicine (Sidel 1972). They were not formally doctors, though, and their work would be described today as community-based PHC since a range of basic curative and preventive services were being provided outside of health facilities.

In the early 1940s in India, the foundations for PHC in India were laid by the Health Survey and Development Committee, most widely known as the Bhore Committee. The committee was established in 1943 to review the existing health conditions of India and to make recommendations for the future of health services in the country. It was chaired by Sir Joseph Bhore and included some of the international public health luminaries of the day, including Dr. Grant. After working in China in the 1930s, Grant had become the director of the All India Institute of Hygiene and Public Health in Calcutta. The committee met regularly and submitted its report in 1946. The report called for the initial development of primary health centers that would each serve forty thousand people and have for their staff two medical officers, four public health nurses, one nurse, four midwives, four trained *dais* (midwives), two sanitary inspectors, two health assistants, one pharmacist, and fifteen other lower-level workers. The plan called for the later development of "primary health units" with hospitals of seventy-five beds and other services for each ten thousand to twenty thousand people (Community Health 1946). The influence of the Dawson Report from England twenty years earlier is notable.

Iran was an early pioneer in the formal training of CHWs who became early prototypes of its current program of professionalized CHWs, called *behvarzes*. In 1942, Iran initiated the Behdar (meaning "healer") Training Project and in 1972 the West Azerbaijan Project and the Village Behdar Training Scheme to train local people to address the health concerns of the rural poor (Assar and Jaksic 1975; Amini et al. 1983; Ronaghy et al. 1983). These early experiences formed the basis of Iran's current rural national PHC system of thirty thousand behvarzes providing services at seventeen thousand health houses for twenty-three million Iranians (Perry, Zulliger, et al. 2017). The two-year training of the behvarzes is unique in that its focus is on group discussions, role-playing exercises, and working at a model health house set up at each training center (Shadpour 2000). More than 90% of the population has ready access to these health houses, contributing to Iran's strong progress in improvement of its population's health in the 1980s and 1990s (Shadpour 2000). The current program is a compelling example of comprehensive PHC because it not only provides ready access to care but also works with community members and with other sectors to address the social determinants of health (Javanparast et al. 2011).

It was, however, the Chinese barefoot doctor experience that resonated throughout the developing world in the 1960s and 1970s, and provided an inspiration and encouragement to a number of nascent community-oriented programs—particularly in Latin America, where modern health services had not yet reached populations in need. In addition, innovative approaches to addressing health needs in developing countries with few formally trained health professionals and severely constrained financial resources were beginning to accumulate. It was becoming apparent that Western approaches to medical care that had been developed in Europe and the United States were not going to be widely available in many developing countries for a long, long time, and some serious rethinking was needed regarding how to improve the health of people in developing countries.

At the same time, an influential group of international health leaders had become concerned that the work of medical missions in developing countries was also failing to reach many of the world's most vulnerable people because of the missions' focus on hospital care. They began discussions in 1963 and carried out fieldwork that demonstrated that the hospital-based curative services established by medical missions' programs had a limited impact on the health of the populations served by their programs and that at least half of hospital admissions were for preventable conditions. In fact, one report found that the health of people who lived close to a mission hospital was no better than the health of people who lived far away (Arole, Kasaje, and Taylor 1995). Ethical issues were emerging about the lack of attention to people who did not have access to hospitals or who needed preventive and curative services not readily available at these facilities.

Thus, the stage was set at the Christian Medical Commission, established in 1968 in Geneva as a semiautonomous body of the World Council of Churches, to begin to explore a new concept of PHC that was adapted to the needs of developing countries. Among the distinguished people participating in these discussions were Dr. William Foege, Dr. John Bryant, and Dr. Carl Taylor.[†] In fact, it was in this venue that the term *primary health care* began to be used to refer to practical approaches for working with communities in low-income settings to address priority health problems (McGilvray 1981; Litsios 2004).

[†]Foege went on to lead the US Centers for Disease Control and Prevention as well as to serve as advisor to the Bill and Melinda Gates Foundation. Bryant went on to serve as dean of Columbia University's Mailman School of Public Health and to make seminal contributions to the practice of PHC through his leadership at the Aga Khan University's Karachi campus. Taylor's background is discussed in more detail later in this chapter.

This led to high-level discussions between staff at the Christian Medical Commission and staff at the World Health Organization as well as to serious thinking at WHO about how to address the growing gap between the Western approach to medical care with its highly curative, facility-based orientation and the practical possibilities for addressing the health needs of poor people in developing countries. The dialogue was encouraged by Dr. Halfdan Mahler, the executive director of WHO at that time, who had spent ten years in India working with WHO on tuberculosis control and was intimately familiar with medical missions work there (Litsios 2004).

One of the outcomes of this dialogue was an influential volume edited by Kenneth Newell, then director of the Strengthening of Health Services Division at WHO, titled *Health by the People*, which highlighted case studies from around the world based on engaging the community in partnership in addressing health needs (Newell 1975). This volume includes examples from Cuba, China, Iran, and, most importantly, the Comprehensive Rural Health Project in Jamkhed, India. It provided the inspiration for the International Conference on Primary Health Care in 1978, sponsored by WHO and the United Nations Children's Fund, where a concept of PHC that was relevant to developing countries was fully developed and embraced.

Primary Health Care as Defined in the 1978 Alma-Ata Declaration

The 1978 International Conference on Primary Health Care at Alma-Ata, USSR (now Almaty, Kazakhstan), was the largest and most representative global health conference that had been held up to that time, with representatives of 134 governments and 67 international organizations (Cueto 2004). The choice to host the conference in the USSR at the height of the Cold War is a complex and interesting story itself (Litsios 2002). Its landmark three-page declaration has turned out to be one of the pivotal documents for the development of the concepts, principles, and ideals related to PHC that are applicable to all peoples everywhere regardless of the context. The Alma-Ata Declaration expanded the narrow concept of PHC as ambulatory care provided by doctors and nurses in facilities to a much broader definition that resonated with the needs of poor counties. The declaration defined PHC as:

> Essential health care based on practical, scientifically sound and socially
> acceptable methods and technology made universally accessible to individu-
> als and families in the community through their full participation and at a

cost that the community and country can afford to maintain at every stage of their development in the spirit of self-reliance and self-determination. It forms an integral part both of the country's health system, of which it is a central function and main focus, and of the overall social and economic development of the community. It is the first contact of individuals, the family and community with the national health system bringing health care as close as possible to where people live and work, and constitutes the first element of a continuing health care process. (World Health Organization and United Nations Children's Fund 1978)

This definition has broad legitimacy and has consistently been affirmed since as the "gold standard" for PHC, even though its lofty ideals have led some to consider it aspirational and unrealistic. The conference also called for the achievement of Health for All through PHC by the year 2000—still an unrealized goal that will remain with us for most of the twenty-first century.

Walsh and Warren and Selective Primary Health Care

Only one year following the Alma-Ata Conference, Julia Walsh and Kenneth Warren, in their seminal 1979 article "Selective Primary Health Care," promoted selective PHC as an "interim strategy for disease control in developing countries." Although they do not give a formal definition of PHC or of selective PHC in their article, it is apparent that they are referring to the control of priority endemic diseases using cost-effective interventions. They state that the goal of PHC as defined at Alma-Ata is "above reproach, yet its very scope makes it unattainable because of the cost and numbers of trained personnel required" (967). They state (incorrectly, in my view) that basic PHC is oriented to "provide health workers and establish clinics for treating all illnesses within a population," and they argue that selective PHC is "potentially the most cost-effective type of medical intervention" (972). The concept of selective programmatic measures continues to guide much thinking and global action for improving health in developing countries despite having been introduced as an interim approach (Hall and Taylor 2003).

GOBI, Selective Primary Health Care, and the First Child Survival Revolution

In the early 1980s, James P. Grant had become executive director of UNICEF. He was the son of Dr. John B. Grant and had grown up in China as well as in India. He was not a physician but rather had graduated from Harvard Law School and had spent his early career working in international development. Two years after assuming his position, he heard a young pediatrician, Dr. Jon Rohde, then working in Haiti, give a presentation titled "Why the Other Half Dies." Dr. Rohde highlighted the potential of selected interventions, most notably immunizations and oral rehydration solution, to reduce child mortality in poor countries (Bornstein 2007). John Grant hired Rohde as his special assistant and also as the UNICEF representative in India, positions he had held for more than a decade. Under John Grant's dynamic global leadership, with strong technical support from Rohde and many others, UNICEF led the way to what was then referred to as the Child Survival Revolution,[‡] saving millions of lives through this approach (Taylor and Jolly 1988; Bornstein 2007). One of the outcomes of this emphasis was the joint WHO and UNICEF Expanded Programme on Immunization, which had also been fueled by enthusiasm surrounding the eradication of smallpox through immunization in 1978. With the continued recognition of the importance of good nutrition (and the demonstration of the health benefits of exclusive breastfeeding during the first six months of life), the concept of GOBI was established during the mid-1980s: *G* stood for growth monitoring, *O* for oral rehydration for diarrhea, *B* for breastfeeding, and *I* for immunizations.[§]

Selective Primary Health Care and Family Planning

In the 1970s and 1980s, there was focused attention on the perils of rapid population growth and the need to give priority to family planning programs over other programs for health. This led to the "verticalization" of family planning programs. Ministries of health in many countries were forced by external donors to divide their programs into two "wings"—a health wing and a family planning wing—so that comingling of donor family planning funds and their programs could not be "diluted" by funds and programs for other health-related priorities. Part of the underlying donor philosophy was that family planning was a higher priority than other programs since investments in health would only worsen the population explosion by creating more mouths to feed and more population to reproduce.

[‡]This is often referred to now as the *First Child Survival Revolution* in anticipation of another major push to improve child survival.
[§]Two *F*s were added for food supplements and family planning, and then a later *F* was added for female education.

This concept is now known to be shortsighted. Data from the fertility declines in low-income countries in the late twentieth century support a very different concept first enunciated by Taylor and referred to as the child survival hypothesis. It states that women will not have fewer children until they know that the ones they have are going to survive (Taylor, Newman, and Kelly 1976; Connelly 2008). Selective funding by external donors for family planning as well as for GOBI paved the way for addressing subsequent priorities such as HIV/AIDS, malaria, and tuberculosis with highly targeted vertical programs. To global policymakers and donors, the urgency produced by the immediate threat of these three diseases—and particularly HIV/AIDS—outweighed the benefits of long-term investments in comprehensive PHC programming.

The Effect of the Global Economic Recession and National Structural Economic Limitations on the Alma-Ata Movement

The Alma-Ata movement faced a near-fatal setback in the 1980s as a result of the major global recession of that time. Governments of poor countries were unable to meet their debt payments, and the International Monetary Fund along with the World Bank had to step in and provide short-term loans to many countries so they could meet their debt payments. These countries had to agree to structural adjustment policies in order to obtain these loans, as neoliberalism and free-market ideologies (including a reduced role for the state) drove these policies. Among the policies were those that were designed to limit government spending. The end result was reductions in spending on government-funded health care and education (Stubbs et al. 2017). Funds were not available to strengthen and expand PHC services. In this context, selective PHC became the more feasible alternative approach (Packard 2016; Rifkin 2018).

Progress with More Comprehensive Approaches to Community-Focused Primary Health Care during the Past Three Decades

Despite the flourishing of selective PHC since the 1980s and the rapid loss of enthusiasm and funding for comprehensive PHC as envisioned at Alma-Ata, important new approaches have emerged that have gradually gained traction, along with evidence of their effectiveness.

Key Individuals in the Evolution of Primary Health Care

Several important figures played a key role in developing and implementing models of primary health care (PHC). It is important to note the extraordinary influence of Dr. John B. Grant and Mr. James P. Grant, the father-son pair. Many refer to John B. Grant as the father of PHC in its more comprehensive form of preventive and curative services for impoverished populations because of his contributions to the Ding Xian Project in the 1930s, the first PHC project in a developing country using current concepts of PHC. John B. Grant was an important influence in the development of PHC in India through his leadership at the All India Institute of Public Health and his participation on the Bhore Committee.

Dr. John B. Grant's son, Mr. James P. Grant, was a forceful champion of selective PHC for child survival (Jolly 2001; Bornstein 2007). The school of public health at BRAC University in Bangladesh (oriented to community-based PHC), established in 2004, is named after him. Dr. John B. Grant's grandson and son of Mr. James P. Grant, also named John Grant, served as the first director of the United States Agency for International Development's (USAID) Child Survival and Health Grants Program for US-based nongovernmental organizations (NGOs) in the mid-1980s. This program was an influential force in the development of community-based PHC.

Dr. Halfdan Mahler, the Danish physician who served an extraordinary three terms as director general of the World Health Organization (WHO) from, 1973–1988, is widely considered to have been WHO's most effective director general. Mahler was the champion of the Alma-Ata concept of PHC, with its emphasis on the integration of services, equity, and community participation. The philosophical, as well as the practical programmatic, differences between the selective approach championed by James Grant and the more comprehensive primary approach championed by Halfdan Mahler were apparent and a source of ongoing tension.

Dr. Carl Taylor, who founded the Department of International Health at the Johns Hopkins School of Public Health in 1968, has been called the "acknowledged leader of PHC over the second half of the twentieth century" (Rohde 2002, n.p.). Taylor was a close friend of John B. Grant, Halfdan Mahler, and James P. Grant. He was also, at Mahler's request, a leader of the 1978 Alma-Ata Conference and one of the authors of the Alma-Ata Declaration. Carl Taylor fully understood and appreciated the tension between comprehensive and selective primary care. Taylor would describe long train rides in China with James Grant where they would debate into the wee hours of the morning the pros and cons of comprehensive and selective approaches. Taylor took great pains to remind James Grant, having known James Grant's father quite well, that his father would have come down strongly on the side favoring the comprehensive approach (Taylor 2010).

Carl Taylor was a foundational figure in PHC, having started his career as a medical missionary in north India in the late 1940s and soon thereafter teaching at the Harvard School of Public Health while developing pioneering field studies in PHC in north India in the 1950s. In the 1960s, he founded the Department of International Health at Johns Hopkins and left a lasting imprint on the academic discipline we now call international health and, increasingly, global health.

Key Individuals in the Evolution of Primary Health Care, continued

In the 1960s and 1970s, Carl Taylor led one of the first PHC operations research projects of the twentieth century: the Narangwal Project. The Narangwal Project and Taylor's mentorship together influenced a generation of leaders of PHC—most notably Drs. Rajanikant and Mabelle Arole, Dr. Miriam Were of Kenya, and Drs. Rani and Abhay Bang. Others inspired and influenced by Taylor's vision of PHC include Dr. Nils Daulaire (who led major global health initiatives at USAID, the Global Health Council, and the US Department of Health and Human Services), Dr. Rudolph Knippenberg (who served for many years as chief health advisor at the United Nations Children's Fund [UNICEF]), and Dr. Mary Taylor (formerly senior program officer at the Gates Foundation and influential advisor for global health programs).

Dr. Jon Rohde, mentioned previously, is another foundational figure in the global PHC movement, positioned as he was to serve as global advisor for health and nutrition to James Grant and also as UNICEF representative of India from 1982 to 1995. It was his oral presentation and paper that inspired James Grant to pursue the selective approach to child survival, and he has championed child survival through broader approaches to PHC as well over the past half-century. He is the author of many articles and books on topics related to child survival and health for all.

Drs. Rajanikant and Mabelle Arole were a husband-wife team who learned about the Narangwal Project as students at Johns Hopkins, where they were mentored by Taylor. Following their studies at Hopkins, they went off to an isolated area of central India and established a pioneering comprehensive PHC program that was featured in Kenneth Newell's book *Health by the People* (1975) and was the most influential force for the vision of PHC embodied in the Alma-Ata Declaration. They established one of the first CHW programs in India and led the way with practical approaches to community and women's empowerment and to addressing the social determinants of health. Their program, the Jamkhed Comprehensive Rural Health Project, was a prototype for and remains one of the best full expressions of PHC as defined at Alma-Ata. Jamkhed is a model of what PHC should be for impoverished populations in the twenty-first century, with activities that qualify for the working redefinition of PHC established for this chapter, including surgical care and inpatient beds at their health center (Arole and Arole 1994; Arole 2002; Perry and Rohde 2019). Carl Taylor continued to visit Jamkhed periodically and took great pride in the work established there and in the influence the program had nationally and internationally. Rajanikant Arole achieved national prominence in health affairs in India and served as the NGO representative of the National Rural Mission upon its establishment in 2005. The National Rural Mission set the policies for the creation of accredited social health activists, which now number one million throughout India. Mabelle Arole later became a regional advisor for UNICEF for South Asia and promoted the Jamkhed model throughout the region.

Drs. Abhay and Rani Bang are a husband-wife team who, like the Aroles, came to Johns Hopkins to study and were influenced by Carl Taylor and the Narangwal Project. They established a pioneering PHC program in

Gadchiroli, in central India as well. Their program, the Society for Education, Action and Research in Community Health (SEARCH), has been a leading field site for community-based research on health and on the development and testing of community-based approaches to improve maternal and child health, most notably through community case management of childhood pneumonia and home-based neonatal care (Bang et al. 1990; Bang et al. Reddy 2005; SEARCH 2013).

Dr. David Sanders has served as an intellectual architect of the current global PHC movement. He started out as a physician working in Zimbabwe with the relief organization Oxfam and as a faculty member at the University of Zimbabwe, where he helped establish Zimbabwe's national community health worker program in the 1980s. He moved to South Africa in 1992, working initially with the African National Congress on health policy development and in 1993 as professor and founding director of the newly established Public Health Program (which has since become the School of Public Health) at the University of Western Cape. He has had a long association with the People's Health Movement, serving as a member of its Global Steering Council. He was a frequent voice at national and international health meetings, pleading for a stronger commitment to the principles of comprehensive PHC as defined at Alma-Ata. He was also a prominent spokesperson for, as well as an activist engaged in, the wider political struggle for improving health and health care for disadvantaged populations and for addressing the broader social determinants of health and the political framework required to achieve that. He is the coauthor of one of the classic books in global health, *Questioning the Solution: The Politics of Primary Health Care and Child Survival* (1997).

Community-Oriented Primary Health Care

Community-oriented primary health care (COPC) emerged in the 1950s in South Africa as an approach to engage PHC centers and their staffs in proactively addressing the health needs of the community rather than simply attending to patients who come to the facility for care. Through COPC, the community plays a key role in prioritizing health problems and making management decisions, and it encourages medical practitioners to engage with community health problems. It links medical practice with public health.

COPC is defined as a "continuous process by which primary care is provided to a defined community on the basis of its assessed health needs through the planned integration of public health practice with the delivery of primary care services" (Mullan and Epstein 2002, 1750). COPC has served as the model for the community health center movement in the United States. These community health centers (now called federally qualified health centers) are governed by a local board of directors and provide health care to underserved populations. The community has control over decisions of the

Key Organizations in the Evolution of Primary Health Care

The Jamkhed Comprehensive Rural Health Care Project was founded in 1970 by the physician team Rajanikant and Mabelle Arole. It has focused its work on a comprehensive approach to primary health care (PHC), including multisectoral actions, women's and community empowerment, and community-based services provided by community health workers (CHWs). It has served as one of the world's foremost training sites in PHC, with more than forty-two thousand people at all levels from throughout India and more than three thousand people from one hundred countries around the world coming to Jamkhed for short courses during which villagers do much of the teaching (Jamkhed Comprehensive Rural Health Project 2013; Perry and Rohde 2018).

The Society for Education, Action and Research in Community Health (SEARCH) was founded by physicians Abhay and Rani Bang in 1983. It is one of the world's foremost field research sites on community-based PHC. Its rigorous small-scale studies of community-based management of childhood pneumonia and home-based neonatal care have changed the global landscape of PHC (SEARCH 2013). In addition, their program is the world's foremost example of the census-based, impact-oriented (CBIO) approach, which is the most promising means for productively engaging the natural and potentially productive tension between vertical and comprehensive approaches to PHC (Perry et al. 1999).

BRAC (established in 1972 as the Bangladesh Rural Advancement Committee) exemplifies the principles of PHC defined at Alma-Ata (see also chapter 7). Operating almost exclusively outside of health facilities at the grassroots level through a multidisciplinary approach with women's savings and action groups (called voluntary organizations) as the key agents of change, BRAC works in all fields of development, including health, and has become one of the world's leaders in community-based PHC. I had the special privilege of nominating BRAC for the $1 million annual Gates Award in Global Health, which they won in 2003.

BRAC is now the largest NGO in the world, having learned how to successfully take its programs to scale while at the same time creating mechanisms by which these programs can be largely self-sustained with locally generated income. BRAC is now a global force for poverty alleviation, with programs in eleven countries in Africa and Asia. Its programs reach 130 million people: 120 million in Bangladesh and 10 million in other countries. Its CHW program in Bangladesh has 130,000 Shasthya Shebikas, making it one of the largest CHW programs in the world. BRAC has been a global leader in both selective and comprehensive approaches to PHC, making it an interesting case study from the standpoint of examining the tensions between them. Shasthya Shebikas provide comprehensive, community-based services while linking effectively to vertical disease control programs for immunizations, family planning, nutrition, tuberculosis, and many others (Chowdhury et al. 1997; Perry 2000; Standing and Chowdhury 2008). It now has an exemplary PHC program for mothers and children in the urban slums developed by way of a grant from the Gates Foundation—the Manoshi Project, which also embodies CBIO principles. Of BRAC's $1 billion budget, 85% is generated internally through commercial activities owned and operated by BRAC (Chowdhury and Perry 2010).

The People's Health Movement is a global network bringing together grassroots health activists, civil society organizations, and academic institutions from around the world, particularly from low- and middle-income countries. It has a presence in seventy countries. Its framework for action is its People's Charter for Health, which endorses the Alma-Ata Declaration and affirms health as a social, economic, and political issue but above all as a fundamental human right. In 2005, when I attended the People's Health Assembly in Cuenca, Ecuador, Dr. Halfdan Mahler symbolically passed the "Olympic flame" of the spirit of Alma-Ata to the People's Health Movement—in part an expression of his frustration that WHO had not done more to nurture this flame. The People's Health Movement has provided an alternative world health report from time to time (in 2006, 2008, 2011, and 2018) called Global Health Watch, which has been influential in highlighting in particular the social and political dimensions underlying the health problems of disadvantaged people in low- and middle-income countries.

The United States Agency for International Development's (USAID) Child Survival and Health Grants Program (CSHGP) and the CORE Group have together provided a leadership role in forging community-based programming for maternal and child health and for advancing the child survival agenda. The CSHGP, initiated in 1986 following Congress's historic earmark for child survival funding, supported US-based nongovernmental organizations (NGOs) to implement child survival projects. As mentioned previously, it was initially headed by John B. Grant's grandson and James Grant's son, John Grant.

Until its termination in 2018, the program provided funding and technical support to US-based NGOs (called private voluntary organizations, or PVOs, by USAID).

Although the amount of money provided annually by the CSHGP was modest and actually declined in real terms over time (it remained constant in US dollars at around $20 million per year), the nature of the program proved catalytic for virtually all of America's leading NGOs working in global maternal and child health. The process of requiring baseline and household coverage surveys of key child survival indicators, preparation of a detailed implementation plan (based on the results of the baseline household survey), and midterm and final evaluations (based also on follow-up household surveys) led by independent consultants provided NGOs with a new approach to the professionalization of their programming. These evaluations, together with the technical support for interventions available through USAID, led to a transformation of programming for many NGOs, and this approach spread to local NGOs throughout the world who collaborated on these child survival projects.

The project evaluations accumulated by USAID through this program over the past three decades constitute the most extensive library of child survival programming in the world. After decades of experience with these programs, NGOs learned the value of sharing experiences, knowledge, and ideas about how to best improve child survival programming. This was possible in part by attending annual conferences for grant recipients. One individual described the program this way: "What began in this simple spirit of openness quickly gained momentum as participants realized significant savings in time, thought and resources—all made possible by collaborating." The group realized that this "community of practice" model was also fertile ground for the creation of new knowledge and ideas as well (CORE Group 2013). This association of NGOs became a formal legal entity in 2000 and called itself the CORE Group (from Collaboration and Resources for Community Health). It committed itself to "technical excellence in integrated, community-based global health programming" (CORE Group 2019, n.p.). The CORE Group is now a global force for community-based PHC through its technical resources that are used widely around the world by programs implementing community-based interventions for maternal and child health. It has created opportunities for networking among program managers and continues the facilitation of sharing relevant programming experiences in community-based PHC. The CORE Group Polio Project, in operation since 1999, has played an instrument role in stopping poliovirus transmission in hard-to-reach and resistant populations such as Uttar Pradesh, India; Angola; Ethiopia; and now South Sudan and Nigeria by pioneering community-based PHC programs that reach every household (Losey et al. 2019). The lessons learned from this experience hold great promise for strengthening health programs in underserved areas around the world (Perry et al. 2019).

National Actors That Have Influenced Primary Health Care

Other chapters in this book cover national case studies of countries that pursued PHC strategies to great results since 1978. Nepal (chapter 9) has been a global leader in the development of community-based PHC

services through its cadres of CHWs, most notably female community health volunteers. Progress despite Nepal's difficult terrain and political instability is noteworthy (BASICS II, the MOST Project, and USAID 2004; Gottlieb 2007; Henry B. Perry 2016; Perry, Zulliger, et al. 2017).

Bangladesh (chapter 7) also developed strong community-based PHC programs that have made possible high population coverage of immunizations, oral rehydration therapy for treatment of diarrhea, and family planning services, among other interventions (Perry 2000; El Arifeen et al. 2013). Bangladesh has also been a global leader in addressing the social determinants of health—most notably by improving the educational status of women.

Rwanda, Eritrea, and Ethiopia are beginning to stand out. Ethiopia's progress is particularly notable (chapter 8) for its massive expansion of PHC services beginning in 2003 with the training of one full-time, government paid health extension worker for every twenty-five hundred people and one voluntary CHW for every five households. Ethiopia has seen rapid progress in reducing child and maternal mortality as well as controlling HIV/AIDs, tuberculosis, and malaria, and in reducing undernutrition in children, making it one of the few countries in the world to achieve the Millennium Development Goals for Health by the year 2015 (Admasu, Balcha, and Getahun 2016; Admasu, Balcha, and Ghebreyesus 2016; Assefa et al. 2018; Assefa et al. 2019). The Federal Ministry of Health of Ethiopia is now hosting the newly emerging International Institute for Primary Health Care for training delegations from throughout Africa and beyond in strengthening of PHC services and the experience of Ethiopia in this effort (International Institute for Primary Health Care-Ethiopia 2018)

Although they are not covered extensively in this book, Brazil and Thailand are also notable. Brazil is emerging as a global model for PHC for low-income countries. As a low-income country itself fifty years ago, Brazil gradually built a PHC program that has been effective in making services available to its population and in achieving equity and proactive preventive services through home visits to every household by CHWs who work as members of family health teams based at health centers (Rice-Marquez, Baker, and Fischer 1998; Jurberg and Humphreys 2010; Kleinert and Horton 2011). Brazil has had one of the most rapid declines in under-5 child mortality in the world and has achieved one of the most equitable distributions of health service coverage and health status among low- and middle-income countries. Its CHW program is now the model for South Africa's new CHW program, and this influence will likely spread throughout southern Africa. As an example of its commit- ment to equity and PHC, Brazil's government was one of the first to ensure free universal access to treatment for HIV/AIDS with antiretroviral medication.

Thailand ranks first among low-income countries (those with a gross national income of less than US$5,000 per person) in terms of progress in reducing its mortality among children younger than 5 years of age (Rohde et al. 2008). It achieved all of the Millennium Development Goals in the early 2000s. This extraordinary success was achieved during a time of rapid economic development, so expanded funding for health services was available. All interventions were fully integrated into a PHC network and were implemented through district health systems, with ten to twelve health centers in a health district each serving five thousand people. Nurses and public health workers are the backbone of the rural health system and provide community-based services, including home visits, with a strong emphasis on health promotion and prevention (Patcharanarumol et al. 2011).

organization's board of directors, as community members are required to constitute a majority of the board. The COPC movement guided the development of the Tanzanian Essential Health Interventions Project (1997–2004), which has influenced the development of PHC in the country ever since (Tollman, Doherty, and Mulligan 2006).

The Emergence of Community-Based Primary Health Care and Community Health Workers

Beginning with the previously mentioned case studies in the WHO book *Health by the People*, there has been a gradually accelerating accumulation of evidence and experience demonstrating that services provided in the community outside of health facilities, either alone or in coordination with facility-based care, can be effective in improving health. Perhaps the most important pioneering field research study of this type was the Narangwal Project (1967–1973) in rural north India. The Narangwal Project was a four-cell experimental design that tested various combinations of program interventions for improving maternal and child health using community-based workers and engaging in a collaborative partnership with the community (Kielmann et al. 1983; Taylor et al. 1983). This was one of the first (in a group of only ten) projects constituting the world's evidence at that time, reported by Davidson Gwatkin, Janet Wilcox, and Joe Wray in 1980, showing that child mortality and nutrition can be improved through PHC interventions if they have a strong outreach component that reaches a high proportion of the target population.

The Narangwal Project either directly or indirectly spawned other seminal field projects and research activities that have demonstrated the power of community-based PHC. Notable scions include the Jamkhed Comprehensive Rural Health Project, established in 1970, and the SEARCH Project in Gadchiroli, established in 1985. The Jamkhed Project was one of the archetypes for the Alma-Ata Conference described in WHO's *Health by the People*, published in 1975. Jamkhed used community participatory approaches, including illiterate village health workers, to make dramatic health gains in a short period of time, including a decline in the infant mortality rate from 176 deaths per 1,000 live births to 20 deaths per 1,000 live births (Arole and Arole 1994; Perry and Rohde 2019). SEARCH carried out some of the first studies demonstrating the effectiveness of using illiterate CHWs to diagnose and treat childhood pneumonia and provide home-based neonatal care (Bang et al. 1990; Bang et al. 1999; Bang, Bang, and Reddy 2005).

Community-based work in Haiti at the Hospital Albert Schweitzer (Berggren, Ewbank, and Berggren 1981) and in Bolivia through the Andean Rural Health Project, now Curamericas Global (Perry et al. 1998; H. B. Perry, Shanklin, and Schroeder 2003), in the 1970s and 1980s led to the emergence of the census-based, impact-oriented approach to PHC (Perry et al. 1999), which attempts to find a "middle way" to respond to both the broad health needs within a population and the epidemiological priorities in a way that can achieve measurable results (Mosley 1988). The CBIO approach gave prominence to the process of mapping and identifying homes and inhabitants in a defined program area, home visitation, surveillance and registration of vital events, and provision of health education and health services in the home or nearby—approaches that are now widespread, including application on a national level in Ethiopia, a country of one hundred million people.

CBIO provided a foundation for the emergence of the Care Group model, an approach to community-based PHC in which a low-level health promoter meets every two to four weeks with groups of women volunteers who then share an educational message with ten or so households for which they are responsible. This approach, utilized in more than thirty child survival projects around the world, has shown marked expansion of coverage of key child survival interventions, reductions in under-5 mortality, and improvements in child undernutrition (Edward et al. 2007; Perry et al. 2010; Davis et al. 2013).

Similar to the Care Group model are widespread women's groups practicing participatory learning and action (PLA). PLA groups have now been tested in a series of randomized-controlled trials. A meta-analysis of these studies demonstrates substantial reductions in maternal and neonatal mortality (Prost et al. 2013). Community-based approaches have a firm evidence base as part of effective health programming in resource-constrained settings (Rohde and Wyon 2002; Rosato et al. 2008; Black et al. 2017). Community-based approaches also have the added benefit of strengthening community accountability and making programs more responsive to community needs.

Over the past three decades, there has been extensive experience in implementing community-based child survival projects led by nongovernmental organizations (NGOs) working in collaboration with ministries of health but working alongside them rather than through them. This has produced a rich experience of community-based approaches that have produced dramatic improvements in coverage of key child survival interventions. Unfortunately, even though these projects often undergo rigorous evaluations, only a few of these have been published in the peer-reviewed literature (Perry et al. 1998; Perry, Shanklin, and Schroeder 2003; Edward et al. 2007; Davis et al. 2013; Ricca et al. 2013).

In 2004, WHO produced an extensive review of the importance of family and community practices for improving child health (Hill, Kirkwood, and Edmond 2004). An updated review of the effectiveness of community-based approaches for improving maternal, neonatal, and child health has been produced as well (Freeman et al. 2012; Perry, Rassekh, Gupta, Wilhelm, et al. 2017; Jennings et al. 2017; Sacks et al. 2017; Freeman et al. 2017; Schleiff et al. 2017; Perry, Sacks, et al. 2017; Perry, Rassekh, Gupta, and Freeman 2017; Black et al. 2017).

The Alma-Ata Declaration called for services to be provided "as close as possible to where people live and work," and for services to be provided by health teams composed of "physicians, nurses, midwives, auxiliaries and community workers as applicable, as well as traditional practitioners as needed." This gave impetus for the development of national-level CHW programs in a number of countries across Africa and South Asia. Unfortunately, for multiple reasons including poor selection of CHW candidates, inadequate training and supervision, and a decline in public sector funding during the 1980s, many of these programs failed, leading to a loss of enthusiasm thereafter.

However, with the growing scientific evidence of the capacity of CHWs to reduce under-5 mortality through interventions such as home-based neonatal care (Lassi, Haider, and Bhutta 2010) and community case management of pneumonia, diarrhea, and malaria (Young et al. 2012), and with the growing realization that countries such as Brazil, Bangladesh, Nepal, and Ethiopia are making strong progress in reducing child mortality through the development of strong CHW programs, there has been justifiably renewed interest in CHWs and in scaling up national CHW programs. A high-level push is now underway for deploying one million CHWs in rural Africa, one for every 650 rural inhabitants (Singh and Sachs 2013).

The Growing Recognition That Facility-Based Care Alone Will Not Accelerate Progress in Achieving Health Gains

One important theme to emerge during the first decade of the twenty-first century has been the limitation of health facilities by themselves to improve the health of impoverished populations where resources are scarce. The Integrated Management of Childhood Illness was a major effort of WHO and UNICEF in the late 1990s and early 2000s to develop a scientific basis for health workers at peripheral facilities to diagnose and treat childhood illness (World Health Organization 2013). This was an attempt to integrate several vertical child health programs sponsored by external donors, most notably the control of acute childhood respiratory diseases and diarrheal diseases. IMCI attempted to bring in nutritional counseling as well as recognition and treatment of childhood undernutrition, although it was obvious to those who worked in field settings that facility-based programs were not going to be effective without a strong community-based component since in the great majority of settings the utilization of services at facilities would never achieve high levels of population coverage of key child survival interventions. It has been widely known and demonstrated since the 1960s that the rate of utilization of health facilities decreases exponentially with one's distance from the facility (King 1966). Nevertheless, the underlying philosophy at WHO seemed to be that if the quality of facility-based services for treatment of childhood illness could be improved, then families would seek out care for their sick children at these facilities, thereby reducing under-5 mortality rates.

This hypothesis was put to a rigorous test in a twelve-country study of IMCI led and funded by WHO and UNICEF in the late 1990s and early 2000s. As this effort was moving forward, the NGO child survival community (and in particular NGOs supported by the United States Agency for International Development's Child Survival and Health Grants Program) had experienced success with community-based approaches in child survival programming, resulting in what today is referred to as C-IMCI, or community-based IMCI (Winch et al. 2002).

The findings from a $10 million evaluation of the IMCI Program in twenty-one countries were finally published in 2005 and demonstrated no impact on under-5 mortality, though the quality of care provided at facilities did improve, and the cost per illness treated was lowered (Bryce and Victora 2005; Bryce et al. 2005). The community-based component of IMCI was never well implemented during the twelve-country study, and enormous obstacles were encountered in the training of health care providers and supplying them with the needed medicines.

This and the broader lack of evidence for the effectiveness of strengthening facility-based care in improving population health further reinforced the importance of community-based approaches in improving population health. As further research on these issues has progressed, the unwillingness of parents to take sick children to health facilities has become increasingly apparent. One recent randomized trial has demonstrated that outcomes are better when sick children meeting the criteria for referral are treated by CHWs in the community (Bari et al. 2011). The explanation for this is twofold: (1) the additional time lost in obtaining care at a facility leads to a lower chance of success if the child's condition is worsening rapidly, even with high-quality care, and (2) the (presumed) improved quality of care obtained at a facility does not provide that much additional benefit over the quality of care provided by a properly trained and supported CHW. The most current available evidence now indicates that the expansion of community-based platforms for delivery of interventions that have been demonstrated to be effective outside of health facilities provided by community-level workers would save 2.3 million lives of mothers and their offspring per year globally compared to 0.8 million lives by expanding the coverage of services that can be provided in health centers and 0.9 million lives by expanding the coverage of services in hospitals (Black et al. 2016; Black et al. 2017).

The Selective versus Comprehensive Primary Health Care Debate

The debates of the past three decades between those who favor selective vertical approaches to PHC and those who favor comprehensive horizontal approaches have been bitter, with those who give priority to impact and cost-effectiveness favoring the former and those who give priority to community participation and responding to the interests and needs of communities favoring the latter (Hall and Taylor 2003; Cueto 2004; Magnussen, Ehiri, and Jolly 2004). But, of course, both approaches are essential, though unfortunately most donor and high-level technical support has gone to selective vertical approaches.

In an address in 2009, Dr. Margaret Chan, director general of WHO, stated: "I think we can now let a long-standing and divisive debate die down. This is the debate that pits single-disease initiatives against the agenda for strengthening health systems. . . . As I have stated since taking office, the two approaches are not mutually exclusive. They are not in conflict. They do not represent a set of either-or options. It is the opposite. They can and should be mutually reinforcing. We need both" (Chan 2009).

Trying to find ways of building on the best of both approaches (e.g., through "diagonal" approaches) has been an important theme in the literature over this time (Mosley 1988; Taylor and Jolly 1988; Sepulveda et al. 2006; Taylor 2010). As discussed in detail in chapter 4, which looks at the particular case of polio control, there is deep complementarity between vertical and horizontal approaches, and both have to be pursued. The donor-led *interim* emphasis on selective interventions instead of comprehensive PHC (Walsh and Warren 1979) is increasingly giving way to the compelling logic for simultaneously pursuing both vertical and horizontal programs to achieve the synergy.

The Movement for Universal Health Coverage: Implications for Primary Health Care

UHC is a growing global movement called for initially by the World Health Assembly in 2005. As defined by World Health Assembly Resolution 58.33 (2005): "Universal coverage is defined as access to key promotive, preven-

M. Chan, "Why the world needs global health initiatives." High-Level Dialogue on Maximizing Positive Synergies between Health Systems and Global Health Initiatives, Venice, Italy, June 22, 2009.

tive, curative and rehabilitative health interventions for all at an affordable cost, thereby achieving equity in access. The principle of financial-risk protection ensures that the cost of care does not put people at risk of financial catastrophe. A related objective of health-financing policy is equity in financing: households contribute to the health system on the basis of ability to pay. Universal coverage is consistent with WHO's concepts of health for all and primary health care" (World Health Assembly 2005). The connection of the concept of UHC to PHC with the Alma-Ata Declaration and the goal of Health for All is obvious from the aforementioned quotation, which comprises the first words of the World Health Assembly resolution. The previous full definition expresses a concept of comprehensive coverage because the interventions are "promotive" and "preventive" as well as curative.

This movement is, in principle, "a fairer, more efficient financing that pools risk and encourages prepayment to share health-care costs equitably across the population" (Latko et al. 2011, 2162). As Frenk and de Ferranti (2012) observe: "Universal health coverage sits at the intersection of social and economic policy. Introduction of reforms that promote universal coverage is not only the right thing to do on ethical grounds; it is also the smart thing to do to achieve economic prosperity. The paradox of health care is that it is one of the most powerful ways of fighting poverty, yet can itself become an impoverishing factor for families when societies do not ensure effective coverage with financial protection for all" (863–864).

UHC has been called the "third global health transition," following the demographic transition (when low mortality and fertility rates replace high mortality and fertility rates) and the epidemiologic transition (when the burden of noncommunicable diseases and conditions grows as the burdens of infectious diseases and maternal/neonatal conditions diminish) (Rodin and de Ferranti 2012).

The movement for UHC is deeply embedded in Article 25 of the Universal Declaration of Human Rights, which proclaims that everyone has the right to a standard of living adequate for health, including medical care, and the right to security in the event of sickness or disability (United Nations General Assembly 1948). It is also deeply embedded in WHO's constitution, which states that "the enjoyment of the highest attainable standard of health is one of the fundamental rights of every human being without distinction of race, religion, political belief, economic or social condition" (World Health Organization 1948).

The movement for UHC has the potential to provide more funds for PHC services; improve the fairness of funding a collective public good; reduce the potential for unjust economic setbacks as a result of expenditures for health care, particularly among the very poor; and, most importantly, expand access to primary health care. For the foreseeable future, it is impossible to envision how UHC can, in fact, be meaningfully achieved without a full-fledged expansion of CHW programs in low-income settings, where it will take more than a generation (if not two or three) to overcome the existing shortages of health care professionals, their concentration in more urban settings, and the great distances that people living in rural areas often have to traverse to reach a health facility.

In practice, many of the subsequent speeches, symposia, and studies on UHC have subtly altered the emphasis of the movement, reducing the definition to coverage with financing for curative and individually delivered services of health care. The original and full definition of coverage, which includes population-level, multisectoral, community-based health promotion and prevention, is very much aligned with the comprehensive PHC approaches described throughout this book.

Current Controversies and Challenges Facing Primary Health Care

As is readily apparent from the history presented previously, the quest to achieve Health for All through PHC has faced an abundance of controversies and challenges. Many of these persist presently, and new ones are emerging. What follows is a selective set of the most pressing questions.

To What Extent Can a Core Package of Primary Health Care Functions and Activities Be Identified?

The concept of UHC implies a need to define the package of promotive, preventive, curative, palliative, and rehabilitative services to include. How might one go about defining such a core package? The most logical ways to approach a problem like this were pioneered by Dr. John Wyon in north India in the 1960s (Wyon and Gordon 1971), Carl Taylor in north India in the 1970s (Kielmann et al. 1983; Taylor et al. 1983), Rajanikant and Mabelle Arole in central India in the 1970s (Arole and Arole 1994), Drs. Warren and Gretchen Berggren in Haiti in the 1970s (Berggren, Ewbank, and Berggren 1981), Abhay and Rani Bang in central India in the 1980s (Bang et al. 1990), and Dr. Henry Perry in Bolivia in the 1980s (Perry et al. 1999). This approach is now called the CBIO approach (Perry and Davis 2015). It involves the development of a partnership between a health program and a population, using local surveillance carried out by routine home visits to define epidemiological priorities (the most frequent, serious, readily preventable or treatable conditions in the population) and to help the communities in the population identify what their health priorities are. Unsurprisingly, almost always in low-income settings, the community's health priorities revolve around improving curative care services. Then, with the available resources (financial, infrastructure, and human), a plan is developed with the community that addresses program priorities, which are a combination of epidemiological and community-defined priorities. Thus, the actual content of the services would vary from place to place and over time, depending on the local situation.

But even within this framework, is there still an essential set of services that should comprise the core of PHC. Table 1.1 is an attempt to define this core starting point of a community's deliberation on priorities. Strategies for working with communities to define local priorities based on locally available resources and local health needs, and strategies for working in partnership with communities to make these services universally accessible (through shared financing, community mobilization, and utilization of CHWs and participatory women's groups) are still poorly developed in most low-income settings. Further development of these strategies and assessing their effectiveness in typical field settings represents one of the great frontiers in PHC for the twenty-first century.

The Neglected Demand-Side Solutions to Strengthening Primary Health Care

The lack of a consumer orientation to the provision of health services in low-income countries, especially those services provided by ministries of health, has often led to a lack of compassionate care and, not surprisingly, marked dissatisfaction in and distrust of health systems, particularly among the poorest inhabitants of low-income countries. In large health care organizations, and particularly those operated by ministries of health, there has been too often a lack of local accountability, leading to absent staff, frequent staff turnovers, lack of supplies and equipment, and so on.

The concept of community participation in PHC is strongly emphasized in the Alma-Ata Declaration, with its call for the following:

> The people have the right and duty to participate individually and collectively in the planning and implementation of their health care.

Table 1.1. A proposed set of core primary health care services for disadvantaged communities in low-income countries

---

Core Preventive Primary Health Care Services

Immunizations promoted by WHO
Micronutrient supplementation
Antenatal care
Detection of hypertension in adults
Screening for HIV, tuberculosis, and syphilis
Distribution of insecticide-treated bed nets in malaria-endemic areas and intermittent preventive treatment of malaria in pregnant women and children
Promotion of good dental health

Core Promotive Primary Health Care Services

Promotion of good nutrition (exclusive breastfeeding during the first six months of life, appropriate complementary feeding after six months of age, and so forth)
Promotion of handwashing, access to clean water and sanitation
Promotion of healthy household behaviors for good maternal and child health, in addition to promotion of good nutrition (promotion of importance of birth spacing, household cleanliness, and warning signs of pregnancy and serious childhood illness, for which care should be sought)
Promotion of smoking cessation, weight reduction for those who are obese, and physical activity for those who are sedentary

Core "Curative"* Primary Health Care Services

Diagnosis and treatment of common ailments and conditions (e.g., eye and skin infections, acute respiratory infection, and diarrhea) and pain management
Management of serious childhood illness
Management of serious mental illness
Initial management of obstetrical complications (removal of retained placenta, management of preeclampsia, and initial management of eclampsia, obstructed labor, postpartum hemorrhage, and puerperal sepsis)
Provision of first-line family planning services (oral birth control pills, condoms, injectable contraceptives, contraceptive implants)
Recognition of and referral of life-threatening conditions to a higher-level facility
Continued treatment and management of conditions of patients referred down from a higher-level facility for ongoing follow-up care

Core Rehabilitative Services

Physical therapy for those recovering from injury
Assistance to those in the community with long-term disabilities (e.g., blindness, deafness, limb loss, mental retardation, and congenital deformities) and to their families

---

*Putting *curative* in quotation marks serves to highlight the fact that not all conditions will be curable—whether it is HIV infection, hypertension, some forms of mental illness, and so forth.

Primary health care is essential health care . . . made universally accessible to individuals and families in the community through their full participation at a cost that the community and country can afford to maintain at every stage of their development in the spirit of self-reliance and self-determination.

Primary health care . . . requires and promotes maximum community and individual self-reliance and participation in the planning, organization, operation and control of primary health care . . . and to this end develops through appropriate education the ability of communities to participate.

Primary health care . . . relies . . . on health workers . . . suitably trained socially and technically to work as a health team and to respond to the expressed health needs of the community. (World Health Organization and United Nations Children's Fund 1978)

Community-oriented PHC is a pillar of PHC, and this involves working in partnership with communities to help them improve their health.

Roles of More- and Less-Qualified Personnel

The 1978 Alma-Ata Declaration calls for the inclusion of the full spectrum of PHC providers, from mothers in the home to CHWs, auxiliary workers, nurses, and physicians. In resource-constrained settings, and even in resource-rich settings such as the United States, the team approach to provision of health services leads to the best-quality services and to the most cost-efficient use of available resources. (Even in the United States, inequities in health status and in the utilization of health services has led to a recent and rapid growth in the use of CHWs [Perry, Zulliger, and Rogers 2014]). The global experience now is vast in the suitability and advisability of delegating to lesser-trained staff many tasks and responsibilities that were once the sole purview of physicians or graduate nurses. WHO recently convened a task force to recommend which tasks for maternal, neonatal, and child health could be safely and appropriately delegated to lower-level staff, including CHWs (Dawson et al. 2014). Although not without controversy still, the weight of the evidence continues to strongly support the full engagement of carefully selected lower-level workers to carry out many well-defined tasks and responsibilities as long as these persons are carefully trained and well supervised.

Remuneration and Other Incentives for Frontline Workers

The remuneration of frontline health workers is a current source of controversy, particularly with respect to whether it is appropriate for health programs to engage CHWs on a voluntary, nonsalaried basis. Although the amounts of money paid to frontline workers are modest, the vast numbers of these workers mean that the implications of these policies are substantial, especially when the funding comes from a central government source. On the one hand, there is the charge that engaging CHWs without remuneration is unjust exploitation, while, on the other hand, there is the reality that communities have people who are eager to serve their neighbors on a voluntary basis. If funding scarcity were not a problem, then payment would, of course, be desirable. However, there are examples of CHW programs that made initial commitments to pay their workers but then could not maintain that commitment, leading to a crumbling of the program. This happened in Nepal in the early 1980s, and later these workers, who had become inactive, were recruited back as female community health volunteers. If the creation of an expectation for a salary is established and then the program cannot sustain that expectation over time, the program is worse off than if it had originally started with volunteer CHWs who had no expectation of a salary.

In NGO child survival programs, there are many examples of volunteer CHWs who receive no formal salary but who receive some kind of "incentives"—special recognition from the community, release from certain community responsibilities, special privileges in accessing health services, and so forth. The most balanced approach to this issue is to not expect from volunteers more than a modest amount of work (e.g., no more than four to five hours per week) and, if ongoing financial remuneration is to be provided, to be confident that this support can be maintained on a sustainable basis.

In 2019, WHO released guidelines to countries for CHW programs that include, among other things, recommendations regarding remuneration of CHWs. WHO has proposed that CHWs be remunerated "with a financial package commensurate to the job demands, complexity, number of hours, training, and roles that they undertake" (Cometto et al. 2018; World Health Organization 2018c). Another important recommendation related to remuneration is that CHWs should *not* be paid exclusively or predominantly according to performance-based incentives because current evidence indicates that such a policy leads CHWs to focus on those aspects of the work related to remuneration and to neglect other important activities that are not tied to remuneration.

Impact of Global Trends on the Evolution of Primary Health Care for the Disadvantaged in Low-Income Countries

Anticipating the specific influences of global forces and trends on PHC is, of course, impossible, but we can be sure of a few things. For example, more and more of the disadvantaged in low-income countries will be living in urban slums, and technological advances will bring new diagnostic and laboratory tests within the reach of low-cost PHC programs. Innovations like mHealth will make it easier for people to receive useful health-related messages, for people to communicate with their health care provider, and for different members of the health team to communicate among themselves, with great potential for improving the quality of care. As the population ages, chronic, noncommunicable diseases will increasingly dominate the burden of disease. AIDS will have become a chronic disease, and PHC will be increasingly focused on care of the elderly. Socioeconomic development will lead to higher living standards and higher educational levels, and this will increase the demand for and consumption of PHC services. Continuing improvements in the educational level of women and their level of empowerment will also produce an increase in the demand for and the consumption of PHC services.

Toward a Rebirth and Revisioning of Primary Health Care

In recent scholarship related to PHC, there is a persistent theme: The concept of PHC as articulated at Alma-Ata is valid and needs to be maintained. But at the same time, there is a broadly held view that we are now at a time for a renewal and revitalization of PHC and perhaps even a redefinition of PHC for the twenty-first century, leading to a full-fledged fulfilment of the ideas that emerged at Alma-Ata.

In recognition of the twenty-fifth anniversary of the Alma-Ata conference, which took place in 2003, the Pan American Health Organization convened a series of events and dialogues culminating in a 2007 position paper on renewing PHC in the Americas. Their report states that there is "a growing recognition that PHC is an approach to strengthen society's ability to reduce inequities in health; and a growing consensus that PHC represents a powerful approach to addressing the causes of poor health and inequality" (Pan American Health Organization 2007, 2). In celebration of the thirtieth anniversary of the Alma-Ata Declaration, *The Lancet* published a series of papers titled "Alma-Ata: Rebirth and Revision." The lead editorial by *The Lancet* team stated that "the Alma-Ata Declaration revolutionized the world's interpretation of health. Its message was that inadequate and unequal health care was unacceptable: economically, socially, and politically" ("A Renaissance in Primary Health Care," 2008, 33).

Dr. Margaret Chan, then director general of WHO, in her lead editorial to the series, remarked: "With an emphasis on local ownership, primary health care honoured the resilience and ingenuity of the human spirit and made space for solutions created by communities, owned by them, and sustained by them" (Chan 2008). One of the articles in the series expressed the same idea this way: "The very idea of health for all energised workers and fueled new efforts in many countries to improve service coverage, especially for previously underserved communities. The inherent focus on equity, the necessity of reaching the unreached and involving them not only in the benefits of health care, but more importantly, in the decisions and actions that collectively make health, was at once novel and revolutionary. Thus, the precepts of social justice became an integral part of health planning" (Lawn et al. 2008, 919).

The 2018 Astana Conference marked the latest rededication to the principles of PHC. During Astana's closing plenary, Dr. Carissa Etienne, director of PAHO and regional director for the Americas of WHO, drew a standing ovation with her resounding injunction: "Ladies and gentlemen, primary health care must form a central part of the strategy for transforming health systems to achieve universal access to health and universal health coverage" (Pan American Health Organization 2018). In his address to the World Health Assembly in 2019, Dr. Tedros Adhanom Gebreyesus, director general of WHO, affirmed the centrality of PHC for achieving Health for All (Tedros 2019):

> The Declaration of Astana, endorsed by all 194 Member States last year, was a vital affirmation that there will be no UHC without PHC. Primary health care is where the battle for human health is won and lost. Strong primary health care is the front line in defending the right to health, including sexual and reproductive rights. It's through strong primary health care that countries can prevent, detect and treat noncommunicable diseases. It's through strong primary health care that outbreaks can be detected and stopped before they become epidemics. And it's through strong primary health care that we can protect children and fight the global surge in vaccine-preventable diseases like measles. . . . Of course, strong primary health care depends on having a strong workforce, working in teams. Doctors, nurses, midwives, lab technicians, community health workers—they all have a role to play."

At that same meeting, the World Health Assembly passed a historic, first-ever resolution on CHWs (World Health Assembly 2019). This resolution recognizes the essential role the CHWs play in delivering PHC and calls for further development of CHW programs, better integration of these programs into health systems, and stronger support for CHW programs from health systems. Of particular note is that this resolution also calls for strong efforts at monitoring and evaluating CHW programs "in order to ensure a strong evidence base for their promotion" (World Health Assembly 2019).

Now is the time to convert this rhetoric into a genuine renaissance in PHC to better serve the disadvantaged in low-income settings. PHC is the means for achieving the highest attainable standard of Health for All people, and now, as the world celebrates the fortieth anniversary of the Alma-Ata Declaration, is the time for a renewed focus on the principles outlined at Alma-Ata. Health for all—the elimination of disparities in access to health services and in health status—was not achieved by the year 2000 and may not be achieved by the year 2100, but it will eventually be achieved. This a common quest that all humanity shares.

REFERENCES (SEE PAGE 341 FOR FULL CITATIONS FOR BOXED TEXT)

Amini, F., M. Barzgar, A. Khosroshahi, and G. Leyliabadi. 1983. *An Iranian experiment in primary health care: The West Azerbaijan project*, edited by M. King. Oxford: Oxford University Press.

Arole, M., and R. Arole. 1994. *Jamkhed—a comprehensive rural health project.* London: Macmillan Press.

Arole, M., D. Kasaje, and D. Taylor. 1995. "The Christian Medical Commission's role in the worldwide primary health care movement." In *Partnerships for social development: A casebook*, edited by Independent Task Force on Community Action for Social Development. Franklin, WV: Future Generations.

Assar, M., and Z Jaksic. 1975. "A health services development project in Iran." In *Health by the people*, edited by K. W. Newell, 112–127. Geneva: World Health Organization.

Bang, A. T., R. A. Bang, S. B. Baitule, M. H. Reddy, and M. D. Deshmukh. 1999. "Effect of home-based neonatal care and management of sepsis on neonatal mortality: Field trial in rural India." *Lancet* 354 (9194): 1955–1961.

Bang, A. T., R. A. Bang, and H. M. Reddy. 2005. "Home-based neonatal care: Summary and applications of the field trial in rural Gadchiroli, India (1993 to 2003)." *J Perinatol* 25 (Suppl. 1): S108–22.

Bang, A. T., R. A. Bang, O. Tale, P. Sontakke, J. Solanki, R. Wargantiwar, and P. Kelzarkar. 1990. "Reduction in pneumonia mortality and total childhood mortality by means of community-based intervention trial in Gadchiroli, India." *Lancet* 336 (8709): 201–206.

Bari, A., S. Sadruddin, A. Khan, Iu Khan, A. Khan, I. A. Lehri, W. B. Macleod, M. P. Fox, D. M. Thea, and S. A. Qazi. 2011. "Community case management of severe pneumonia with oral amoxicillin in children aged 2–59 months in Haripur district, Pakistan: A cluster randomised trial." *Lancet* 378 (9805): 1796–803.

Berggren, W. L., D. C. Ewbank, and G. G. Berggren. 1981. "Reduction of mortality in rural Haiti through a primary-health-care program." *N Engl J Med* 304 (22): 1324–1330.

Black, R. E., C. Levin, N. Walker, D. Chou, L. Liu, M. Temmerman, and DCP RMNCH Authors Group. 2016. "Reproductive, maternal, newborn and child health: Key messages from *Disease Control Priorities 3rd edition*." *Lancet* 388 (10061): 2811–2824.

Black, R. E., C. E. Taylor, S. Arole, A. Bang, Z. A. Bhutta, A. M. R. Chowdhury, B. R. Kirkwood, N. Kureshy, C. F. Lanata, J. F. Phillips, M. Taylor, C. G. Victora, Z. Zhu, and H. B. Perry. 2017. "Comprehensive review of the evidence regarding the effectiveness of community-based primary health care in improving maternal, neonatal and child health: 8. Summary and recommendations of the Expert Panel." *J Glob Health* 7 (1): 010908.

Bornstein, D. 2007. *How to change the world: Social entrepreneurs and the power of new ideas*, 247–61. Oxford: Oxford University Press.

Bryce, J., and C. G. Victora. 2005. "Ten methodological lessons from the multi-country evaluation of integrated management of childhood illness." *Health Policy Plan* 20 (Suppl 1): i94–i105.

Bryce, J., C. G. Victora, J. P. Habicht, R. E. Black, and R. W. Scherpbier. 2005. "Programmatic pathways to child survival: Results of a multi-country evaluation of integrated management of childhood illness." *Health Policy Plan* 20 (Suppl 1): i5–i17.

Chan, M. 2008. "Return to Alma-Ata." *Lancet* 372 (9642): 865–866.

Chan, M. 2009. "Why the world needs global health initiatives." High-Level Dialogue on Maximizing Positive Synergies between Health Systems and Global Health Initiative. Venice, Italy, June 22.

Cometto, G., N. Ford, J. Pfaffman-Zambruni, E. A. Akl, U. Lehmann, B. McPake, M. Ballard, M. Kok, M. Najafizada, A. Olaniran, O. Ajuebor, H. B. Perry, K. Scott, B. Albers, A. Shlonsky, and D. Taylor. 2018. "Health policy and system support to optimise community health worker programmes: An abridged WHO guideline." *Lancet Glob Health* 6 (12): e1397–e1404.

Community Health. 1946. "Health Survey and Development Committee (Bhore Committee)." Accessed June 24, 2019. http://www.communityhealth.in/~commun26/wiki/index.php?title=Health_Survey_and_Development_Committee.

Connelly, M. 2008. *Fatal misconceptions: The struggle to control world population*. Cambridge, MA: Belknap Press.

Cueto, M. 2004. "The origins of primary health care and selective primary health care." *Am J Public Health* 94 (11): 1864–1874.

Davis, T. D., C. Wetzel, E. Hernandez Avilan, C. de Mondoza Lopes, R. P. Chase, P. J. Winch, and H. B. Perry. 2013. "Reducing child global undernutrition at scale in Sofala Province, Mozambique, using Care Group volunteers to communication health messages to mothers." *Glob Health Sci Pract* 1 (1): 35–51.

Dawson, A. J., J. Buchan, C. Duffield, C. S. Homer, and K. Wijewardena. 2014. "Task shifting and sharing in maternal and reproductive health in low-income countries: A narrative synthesis of current evidence." *Health Policy Plann* 29 (3): 396–408.

Dawson, B. E. 1920. *Interim report on the future provision of Medical and Allied Services 1920 (Lord Dawson of Penn)*. London: His Majesty's Stationary Office. http://www.sochealth.co.uk/healthcare-generally/history-of-healthcare/interim

-report-on-the-future-provision-of-medical-and-allied-services-1920-lord-dawson -of-penn/.

Edward, A., P. Ernst, C. Taylor, S. Becker, E. Mazive, and H. Perry. 2007. "Examining the evidence of under-five mortality reduction in a community-based programme in Gaza, Mozambique." *Trans R Soc Trop Med Hyg* 101 (8): 814–822.

Freeman, P., H. B. Perry, S. K. Gupta, and B. Rassekh. 2012. "Accelerating progress in achieving the millennium development goal for children through community-based approaches." *Glob Public Health* 7 (4): 400–419.

Freeman, P. A., M. Schleiff, E. Sacks, B. M. Rassekh, S. Gupta, and H. B. Perry. 2017. "Comprehensive review of the evidence regarding the effectiveness of community-based primary health care in improving maternal, neonatal and child health: 4. Child health findings." *J Glob Health* 7 (1): 010904.

Frenk, J., and D. de Ferranti. 2012. "Universal health coverage: Good health, good economics." *Lancet* 380 (9845): 862–864.

Gwatkin, D. R., J. R. Wilcox, and J. D. Wray. 1980. *Can health and nutrition interventions make a difference?* Washington, DC: Overseas Development Council.

Hall, J. J., and R. Taylor. 2003. "Health for all beyond 2000: The demise of the Alma-Ata Declaration and primary health care in developing countries." *Med J Aust* 178 (1): 17–20.

Hill, Z., B. Kirkwood, and K. M. Edmond. 2004. *Family and community practices that promote child survival, growth and development: A review of the evidence.* Geneva, Switzerland: World Health Organization.

Jennings, M. C., S. Pradhan, M. Schleiff, E. Sacks, P. A. Freeman, S. Gupta, B. M. Rassekh, and H. B. Perry. 2017. "Comprehensive review of the evidence regarding the effectiveness of community-based primary health care in improving maternal, neonatal and child health: 2. Maternal health findings." *J Glob Health* 7 (1): 010902.

Jolly, Richard, ed. 2001. *Jim Grant: UNICEF visionary.* Florence, Italy: UNICEF Office of Research-Innocenti.

Kielmann, Arnfried A., Carl E. Taylor, C. DeSweemer, R. L. Parker, D. Chernichovsky, William A. Reinke, Inder S. Uberoi, D. N. Kakar, N. Masih, and R. S. S. Sarma. 1983. *Volume 1. Child and maternal health services in rural India: The Narangwal experiment. Integrated nutrition and health care.* 2 vols. Baltimore: Published for the World Bank [by] Johns Hopkins University Press.

King, Maurice Henry. 1966. *Medical care in developing countries: A primer on medicine of poverty and a symposium from Makerere,* edited by M. King. London: Oxford University Press.

Lassi, Z. S., B. A. Haider, and Z. A. Bhutta. 2010. "Community-based intervention packages for reducing maternal and neonatal morbidity and mortality and improving neonatal outcomes." *Cochrane Database Syst Rev* 11: CD007754.

Latko, B., J. G. Temporao, J. Frenk, T. G. Evans, L. C. Chen, A. Pablos-Mendez, G. Lagomarsino, and D. de Ferranti. 2011. "The growing movement for universal health coverage." *Lancet* 377 (9784): 2161–2163.

Lawn, J. E., J. Rohde, S. Rifkin, M. Were, V. K. Paul, and M. Chopra. 2008. "Alma-Ata 30 years on: Revolutionary, relevant, and time to revitalise." *Lancet* 372 (9642): 917–927.

Litsios, S. 2002. "The long and difficult road to Alma-Ata: A personal reflection." *Int J Health Serv* 32 (4): 709–732.

————. 2004. "The Christian Medical Commission and the development of the World Health Organization's primary health care approach." *Am J Public Health* 94 (11): 1884–1893.

Magnussen, L., J. Ehiri, and P. Jolly. 2004. "Comprehensive versus selective primary health care: Lessons for global health policy." *Health Aff (Millwood)* 23 (3): 167–176.

McGilvray, J. 1981. *The quest for health and wholeness.* Tubingen, Germany: German Institute for Medical Missions.

Mosley, W. H. 1988. "Is there a middle way? Categorical programs for PHC." *Soc Sci Med* 26 (9): 907–908.

Mullan, F., and L. Epstein. 2002. "Community-oriented primary care: New relevance in a changing world." *Am J Public Health* 92 (11): 1748–1755.

Newell, Kenneth W., ed. 1975. *Health by the people.* Geneva, Switzerland: World Health Organization.

Packard, R. M. 2016. *A history of global health: Interventions into the lives of other people.* Baltimore: Johns Hopkins University Press.

Pan American Health Organization. 2007. *Renewing primary health care in the Americas: A position paper of the Pan American Health Organization/World Health Organization (PAHO/WHO).* Washington, DC: Pan American Health Organization/World Health Organization.

————. 2018. "PAHO director Dr. Carissa Etienne's closing remarks at Global Conference on Primary Health Care—Astana, Kazakhstan, October 2018." Accessed June 24, 2019. https://www.paho.org/hq/index.php?option=com_content&view=article&id=14760:dr-carissa-etienne-director-paho-closing-remarks-at-global-conference-on-primary-health-care&Itemid=2270&lang=en.

Perry, H., and T. Davis. 2015. "The effectiveness of the census-based, impact-oriented (CBIO) approach in addressing global health goals." In *Aid Effectiveness in Global Health*, edited by E. Beracochea, 261–278. New York: Springer.

Perry, H., N. Robison, D. Chavez, O. Taja, C. Hilari, D. Shanklin, and J. Wyon. 1998. "The census-based, impact-oriented approach: Its effectiveness in promoting child health in Bolivia." *Health Policy Plann* 13 (2): 140–151.

————. 1999. "Attaining health for all through community partnerships: Principles of the census-based, impact-oriented (CBIO) approach to primary health care developed in Bolivia, South America." *Soc Sci Med* 48 (8): 1053–1067.h

Perry, H., O. Sivan, G. Bowman, L. Casazza, A. Edward, K. Hansen, and M. Morrow. 2010. "Averting childhood deaths in resource-constrained settings through engagement with the community: An example from Cambodia." In *Essentials of Community Health*, edited by J. Gofin and R. Gofin, 169–174. Sudbury, MA: Jones and Bartlett.

Perry, H., R. Zulliger, K. Scott, D. Javadi, J. Gergen, K. Shelley, L. Crigler, I. Aitken, S. H. Arwal, N. Afdhila, N. Worku, J. Rohde, Z. Chowdhury, and R. Strodel. 2017. "Case studies of large-scale community health worker programs: Examples from Afghanistan, Bangladesh, Brazil, Ethiopia, India, Indonesia, Iran, Nepal, Niger, Pakistan, Rwanda, Zambia, and Zimbabwe." Accessed June 24, 2019. https://www.mcsprogram.org/resource/case-studies-large-scale-community-health-worker-programs-2/?_sfm_resource_topic=community-health.

Perry, H. B., B. M. Rassekh, S. Gupta, and P. A. Freeman. 2017. "Comprehensive review of the evidence regarding the effectiveness of community-based primary health care in improving maternal, neonatal and child health: 7. Shared character-istics of projects with evidence of long-term mortality impact." *J Glob Health* 7 (1): 010907.

Perry, H. B., B. M. Rassekh, S. Gupta, J. Wilhelm, and P. A. Freeman. 2017. "Compre-hensive review of the evidence regarding the effectiveness of community-based primary health care in improving maternal, neonatal and child health: 1. Rationale, methods and database description." *J Glob Health* 7 (1): 010901.

Perry, H. B., and J. Rohde. 2019. "The Jamkhed Comprehensive Rural Health Project and the Alma-Ata vision of primary health care." *Am J Public Health* 109 (1): 699–704.

Perry, H. B., E. Sacks, M. Schleiff, R. Kumapley, S. Gupta, B. M. Rassekh, and P. A. Freeman. 2017. "Comprehensive review of the evidence regarding the effectiveness of community-based primary health care in improving maternal, neonatal and child health: 6. Strategies used by effective projects." *J Glob Health* 7 (1): 010906.

Perry, H. B., D. S. Shanklin, and D. G. Schroeder. 2003. "Impact of a community-based comprehensive primary healthcare programme on infant and child mortality in Bolivia." *J Health Popul Nutr* 21 (4): 383–395.

Perry, H. B., R. Zulliger, and M. M. Rogers. 2014. "Community health workers in low-, middle-, and high-income countries: An overview of their history, recent evolution, and current effectiveness." *Annu Rev Public Health* 35:399–421.

Prost, A., T. Colbourn, N. Seward, K. Azad, A. Coomarasamy, A. Copas, T. A. Houweling, E. Fottrell, A. Kuddus, S. Lewycka, C. MacArthur, D. Manandhar, J. Morrison, C. Mwansambo, N. Nair, B. Nambiar, D. Osrin, C. Pagel, T. Phiri, A. M. Pulkki-Brannstrom, M. Rosato, J. Skordis-Worrall, N. Saville, N. S. More, B. Shrestha, P. Tripathy, A. Wilson, and A. Costello. 2013. "Women's groups practising participatory learning and action to improve maternal and newborn health in low-resource settings: A systematic review and meta-analysis." *Lancet* 381 (9879): 1736–1746.

"A renaissance in primary health care." 2008. *Lancet* 372 (9642): 863.

Ricca, J., N. Kureshy, K. Leban, D. Prosnitz, and L. Ryan. 2013. "Community-based intervention packages facilitated by NGOs demonstrate plausible evidence for child mortality impact." *Health Policy Plan* 29 (2): 204–216.

Rifkin, S. B. 2018. "Health for all and primary health care, 1978–2018: A historical perspective on policies and programs over 40 years." Oxford Research Encyclope-dia of Global Public Health. Oxford University Press. Accessed June 18, 2019. https://doi.org/10.1093/acrefore/9780190632366.013.55.

Rodin, J., and D. de Ferranti. 2012. "Universal health coverage: The third global health transition?" *Lancet* 380 (9845): 861–862.

Rohde, Jon E., and John Wyon, eds. 2002. *Community-based health care: Lessons from Bangladesh to Boston.* Boston: Management Sciences for Health (in collaboration with the Harvard School of Public Health).

Ronaghy, H. A., J. Mehrabanpour, B. Zeighami, E. Zeighami, S. Mansouri, M. Ayato-lahi, and N. Rasulnia. 1983. "The middle level auxiliary health worker school: The Behdar Project." *J Trop Pediatr* 29 (5): 260–264.

Rosato, M., G. Laverack, L. H. Grabman, P. Tripathy, N. Nair, C. Mwansambo, K. Azad, J. Morrison, Z. Bhutta, H. Perry, S. Rifkin, and A. Costello. 2008. "Community participation: Lessons for maternal, newborn, and child health." *Lancet* 372 (9642): 962–971.

Sacks, E., P. A. Freeman, K. Sakyi, M. C. Jennings, B. M. Rassekh, S. Gupta, and H. B. Perry. 2017. "Comprehensive review of the evidence regarding the effectiveness of community-based primary health care in improving maternal, neonatal and child health: 3. Neonatal health findings." *J Glob Health* 7 (1): 010903.

Schleiff, M., R. Kumapley, P. A. Freeman, S. Gupta, B. M. Rassekh, and H. B. Perry. 2017. "Comprehensive review of the evidence regarding the effectiveness of community-based primary health care in improving maternal, neonatal and child health: 5. Equity effects for neonates and children." *J Glob Health* 7 (1): 010905.

Sepulveda, J., F. Bustreo, R. Tapia, J. Rivera, R. Lozano, G. Olaiz, V. Partida, L. Garcia-Garcia, and J. L. Valdespino. 2006. "Improvement of child survival in Mexico: The diagonal approach." *Lancet* 368 (9551): 2017–2027.

Shadpour, K. 2000. "Primary health care networks in the Islamic Republic of Iran." *East Mediterr Health J* 6 (4): 822–825.

Sidel, V. W. 1972. "The barefoot doctors of the People's Republic of China." *N Engl J Med* 286 (24): 1292–1300.

Singh, P., and J. D. Sachs. 2013. "1 million community health workers in sub-Saharan Africa by 2015." *Lancet* 382 (9889): 363–365.

Stubbs, T., A. Kentikelenis, D. Stuckler, M. McKee, and L. King. 2017. "The impact of IMF conditionality on government health expenditure: A cross-national analysis of 16 West African nations." *Soc Sci Med* 174 (February): 220–227.

Taylor, C., and R. Jolly. 1988. "The straw men of primary health care." *Soc Sci Med* 26 (9): 971–977.

Taylor, C. E. 2010. "What would Jim Grant say now?" *Lancet* 375 (9722): 1236–1237.

Taylor, C. E., J. S. Newman, and N. U. Kelly. 1976. "The child survival hypothesis." *Popul Stud (Camb)* 30 (2): 263–278.

Taylor, C. E., R. S. S. Sarma, Robert L. Parker, William A. Reinke, and R. Faruqee. 1983. *Volume 2. Child and maternal health services in rural India: The Narangwal Experiment. Integrated family planning and health care*. Baltimore: Johns Hopkins University Press.

Taylor-Ide, Daniel, and Carl E. Taylor. 2002. "Ding Xian: The first example of community-based development." In *Just and lasting change: When communities own their futures*, 93–101. Baltimore: Johns Hopkins University Press.

Tollman, S., J. Doherty, and J. Mulligan. 2006. "General primary care." In *Disease control priorities in developing countries*, edited by D. T. Jamison, J. G. Breman, A. R. Measham, G. Alleyne, M. Claeson, D. B. Evans, P. Jha, A. Mills, and P. Musgrove, 1193–1209. New York: World Bank and Oxford University Press.

United Nations. 2015. *The Millennium Development Goals report 2015*. Accessed June 24, 2019. http://www.un.org/millenniumgoals/2015_MDG_Report/pdf /MDG%202015%20rev%20(July%201).pdf.

United Nations Children's Fund. 2008. *The state of the world's children 2008: Maternal and newborn health*. New York: United Nations Children's Fund.

United Nations General Assembly. 1948. "Universal declaration of human rights." United Nations. Accessed June 24, 2019. http://www.ohchr.org/EN/UDHR/Documents /UDHR_Translations/eng.pdf.

Victora, C. G., J. H. Requejo, A. J. Barros, P. Berman, Z. Bhutta, T. Boerma, M. Chopra, A. de Francisco, B. Daelmans, E. Hazel, J. Lawn, B. Maliqi, H. Newby, and J.

Bryce. 2016. "Countdown to 2015: A decade of tracking progress for maternal, newborn, and child survival." *Lancet* 387 (10032): 2049–2059.

Walsh, J. A., and K. S. Warren. 1979. "Selective primary health care: An interim strategy for disease control in developing countries." *N Engl J Med* 301 (18): 967–974.

Winch, P. J., K. Leban, L. Casazza, L. Walker, and K. Pearcy. 2002. "An implementation framework for household and community integrated management of childhood illness." *Health Policy Plan* 17 (4): 345–353.

World Health Organization. 1948. *Constitution of the World Health Organization.* Accessed September 6, 2019. http://www.who.int/governance/eb/who_constitution _en.pdf.

———. 2013. "Integrated Management of Childhood Illness (IMCI)." Accessed June 24, 2019. http://www.who.int/maternal_child_adolescent/topics/child/imci/en/.

———. 2016. "10 facts on malaria." Accessed June 24, 2019. http://www.who.int /features/factfiles/malaria/en/.

———. 2018a. "HIV/AIDS." Global Health Observatory (GHO) data. Accessed June 24, 2019. http://www.who.int/gho/hiv/en/.

———. 2018b. "How many TB cases and deaths are there? Situation in 2017." Global Health Observatory (GHO) data. Accessed June 24, 2019. http://www.who.int/gho /tb/epidemic/cases_deaths/en/.

———. 2018c. *WHO guideline on health policy and system support to optimize community health worker programmes.* Accessed June 24, 2019. https://apps.who.int /iris/bitstream/handle/10665/275474/9789241550369-eng.pdf?ua=1.

World Health Organization, Ministry of Health of Kazakhstan, and United Nations Children's Fund. 2018. "Global Conference on Primary Health Care: 25–26 October 2018—Astana, Kazakhstan." Accessed June 24, 2019. http://www.who.int /primary-health/conference-phc/.

World Health Organization and United Nations Children's Fund. 1978. "Declaration of Alma-Ata: International Conference on Primary Health Care." Accessed June 24, 2019. http://www.who.int/publications/almaata_declaration_en.pdf.

———. 2012. *Building a future for women and children: The 2012 report.* Accessed September 6, 2019. http://www.countdown2015mnch.org/documents/2012Report /2012-complete-no-profiles.pdf.

———. 2018. "Declaration of Astana." Accessed June 24, 2019. https://www.who.int /docs/default-source/primary-health/declaration/gcphc-declaration.pdf.

World Health Assembly. 2005. *Sustainable health financing, universal coverage and social health insurance: World Health Assembly Resolution 58.33 (2005).* World Health Organization (Geneva). Accessed September 6, 2019. http://www.who.int /health_financing/documents/cov-wharesolution5833/en/.

———. 2019. "Community health workers delivering primary health care: Opportunities and challenges." World Health Organization. Accessed June 24, 2019. http://apps .who.int/gb/ebwha/pdf_files/WHA72/A72_R3-en.pdf.

Wyon, J. B., and J. E. Gordon. 1971. *The Khanna Study: Population problems in the rural Punjab.* Cambridge, MA: Harvard University Press.

Young, M., C. Wolfheim, D. R. Marsh, and D. Hammamy. 2012. "World Health Organization / United Nations Children's Fund joint statement on integrated community case management: An equity-focused strategy to improve access to essential treatment services for children." *Am J Trop Med Hyg* 87 (Suppl. 5): 6–10.

CHAPTER TWO

Identifying Countries with Exceptionally Rapid Gains in Life Expectancy

A Quantitative Approach

CAROLINA CARDONA AND DAVID BISHAI

There have been countless efforts to compare national progress in health and development. The method used in the comparison depends on the question being asked. Simple questions like, "Which country has the highest life expectancy at birth (LEB)?" or "Which country has the highest gross domestic product (GDP) per capita?" are easily answered by a simple ranking. However, seeing the top performers in any given year or decade offers very little insight into how countries got that way. Achieving better health and prosperity can take decades. Observing high performers this year can be very misleading to anybody willing to believe that the policies of this year's high performers are best practices to emulate. If the goal of cross-country comparison is to find "best" practices and policies, one has to do better than setting up a simple ranking.

There have been very influential exercises to derive best practices in national health policies that were based on quantitative rankings of dubious provenance. For example, in 1985, the Rockefeller Foundation convened a Bellagio Conference to focus on four "success story" countries and states: China, Costa Rica, Sri Lanka, and Kerala state in India (Balabanova et al. 2013). The empirical evidence for China, Sri Lanka, and Kerala being "success stories" lay in a study by John Caldwell, who ranked countries in order of per capita gross national product (GNP) and by infant mortality rate to find countries whose infant mortality rates were twenty-five places or higher than their GNP rank (Caldwell 1986). With this metric, Caldwell identified Kerala, Sri Lanka, and China as the top three high-performing countries. Their 1982 rank of infant mortality rate was seventy-five, sixty-two, and forty-six points higher than their 1982 rank of GNP per capita. The Caldwell metric would have placed Burma, Jamaica, India, Zaire, Tanzania, and Kenya next in order of success stories and then tenth would have been Costa Rica. However, it suited both Caldwell and the 1985 Rockefeller agenda to catapult Costa Rica to global stardom. Despite a degree of arbitrariness, the Caldwell study was a partial step forward for methodology because it insisted that a ranking of health performance needed to be done with respect to national resources (e.g., GNP per capita) that might potentially be available to achieve better health. Caldwell's analysis was rudimentary, and subsequent efforts attempted to control for more social determinants of health in addition to national income and have used multivariate methods. For example, the World Health Report (2000) ranked national health systems by regressing life expectancy on health spending, controlling for national schooling attainments and GDP, to identify countries whose health was better than would be predicted by the regression (World Health Organization 2000). Randall Kuhn followed up the Caldwell analysis in 2010 and found continued success of China, and added focus on Vietnam, Cuba, and Costa Rica (Kuhn 2010). In *Good Health at Low Cost 25 Years On*, also supported by Rockefeller Foundation, the authors chose "success stories" almost entirely based on subjectivity. They purposively chose to focus on Bangladesh, Kyrgyzstan, and Tamil Nadu as success stories without undertaking an empirical quantitative demonstration that these countries were progressing faster than others (Balabanova et al. 2013). Success story countries have been interrogated for lessons in how countries can achieve better than expected results in population health given their limited resources in order to find routes that could be followed by other limited populations (Halstead, Walsh, and Warren 1985; Caldwell 1986; Balabanova, McKee, and Mills, 2011).

Whether success story countries are chosen subjectively or based on objective data analysis, there is always a presumed counterfactual that "success" means performing *better than expected* and the performance that is expected is based in part on economic resources. A rigorous demonstration that resources (and how they were used) mattered for health had been released in 1975 by S. H. Preston. The Preston Curve emphasized a strong empirical connection between current resources and current health indicators. The Preston Curve graphically demonstrates that improvements in the economies of the poorest countries are typically accompanied by improvements in population health (Preston 1975). The curve shows that higher income is associated with a much higher life expectancy. Furthermore, the association begins to weaken for countries at much higher levels of national income, above around $10,000 per person. Economists see the Preston Curve as an input–output relationship in which countries can input economic resources and receive an output of better population health. From this viewpoint, countries that are obtaining higher than average health outputs from a given input would seem to be investors worth imitating.

From an economic perspective, a success story would be a country for whom a small amount of inputs from the national economy are able to generate a larger than average increase in health or life expectancy. A quantitative implementation of this idea would need to control for a country's starting position in both its health status and its economic status, and look for countries with the steepest slope. Importantly, an analysis would have to attend to timing. Money spent on creating population health can sometimes save lives instantly in situations where there is an ongoing infectious epidemic that must be halted. However, money spent on health more typically saves lives over decades in situations where investments gradually build a population's herd immunity by vaccinating many cohorts of children, or where cleaner air, cleaner water, and safer food is produced through generations of regulatory improvements. So a search for success needs to look for connections between economic resources in the past and subsequent health gains. Finally, a successful country may have achieved success in previous decades under previous policies that have not been maintained. A search for "best practices" would be wise to avoid declaring any policies worthy of emulation unless they were in place during the decades of superior performance. The list of best-performing countries changes across decades, and the list is different based on whether a country is starting with a high or low life expectancy (Cardona and Bishai 2018).

The chapters in the current volume of national success stories are about countries that were chosen purposively and selectively. They were chosen not only because have they achieved improvements in health but also because they had pursued a comprehensive, multisectoral primary health care (PHC) strategy. This book is much more about the nuts and bolts of comprehensive PHC implementation than it is a book that aims to prove that comprehensive PHC will hasten health gains. The widespread acclaim for the Astana Declaration by more than 114 countries is manifest evidence of interest in PHC already. The goal of most chapters in this volume is to inform implementation.

Nevertheless, out of curiosity, it would be nice to know whether countries embracing comprehensive PHC have performed well in measures that attempt to rank success in transforming national resources into better health. Building on past attempts to judge success, we use multivariate methods to control for each country's starting position on the Preston Curve in terms of both starting GDP per capita and starting LEB. Our measure of success will be a dynamic one based on the slope of the Preston Curve—ΔLEB per Δ(GDP per capita). This slope measure reflects how much health a country can get from each new dollar added to the economy. We are mindful that GDP is badly flawed as an indicator of the distribution of economic gains, but, frankly, to achieve a large increase in LEB from an increase in GDP signifies that a country is distributing gains from its economy so they benefit vulnerable people. Better measures of GDP distribution are available, but they do not extend to as many countries, and they do not cover as many decades. Life expectancy also leaves out data on nonfatal disabilities, but it does summarize age-specific mortality rates across all age groups, with somewhat higher weights given for the earlier age groups. Again, data availability leaves no better alternative for a health measure. We are concerned that in many cases, LEB has not actually been measured but has been statistically imputed based on GDP per capita. In our analysis, we flag suspicious cases like these.

One of the practical things that emerges from this project is that the ΔLEB per Δ(GDP per capita) metric for any given country is not always heading in the same direction in any given year. If a country has a recession, Δ(GDP per capita) will be negative. If a country has a massive epidemic, ΔLEB will be negative. If both events occur, ΔLEB divided by Δ(GDP per capita) will be positive—but positive for the wrong reasons. Having a very positive slope of ΔLEB/Δ(GDP per capita) because life expectancy falls dramatically during small economic recessions is not a signal of success, and we have to exclude countries that show a negative ΔLEB and Δ(GDP per capita).

To quantitatively search for success stories, we confined our search to time periods when the input–output relationship holds—where both life expectancy and GDP per capita are simultaneously growing. Along the way, we categorize the various possible trajectories that countries can take along their sojourn through the space of progress in life expectancy and GDP per capita. Once countries are classified by their progress in life expectancy and GDP per capita, we identify the exemplary countries with celebratory progress in both their economy and health. We stipulate that the only cases worth emulating are countries in which there is simultaneous health growth and economic growth. No national planner wants to know how to achieve a situation where health is growing but the economy is failing, nor the reverse, where the economy grows and health fails. Planners should want to achieve both health and prosperity.

After undertaking a detailed analysis of these health and wealth growth spells in the cross-country database for the past fifty years, we were able to find a list of best-performing countries that changes over time. Our list of exemplary countries achieving good health at low cost or "punching above their weight" is ever changing.

Methodology

This section describes the methods used in our search for superior performance in transforming economic growth into subsequent improvements in population health. In order to compare countries to peers who were at a similar phase in the epidemiological transition, countries were divided into four strata based on their population health: $LEB < 51$, $51 \leq LEB < 61$, $61 \leq LEB < 71$, and $LEB \geq 71$. Over time, each country was reclassified into a new stratum whenever its life expectancy crossed one of the aforementioned thresholds. Between 1960 and 2009, most countries left a lower stratum to join a higher one. Many countries crossed two or three life expectancy strata, contributing country-years of observation in multiple strata.

Data

Data were obtained for a set of 189 countries on LEB and GDP per capita over a fifty-year period, 1960–2009, from publicly available databases.

Country data for GDP per capita adjusted by purchasing power parities (PPPs) (in international dollars, fixed 2011 prices) were obtained from the Gapminder compilation (Gapminder 2018b). GDP data for 1990 to 2009 came from the World Bank World Development Indicators (World Bank 2018), and prior to 1990 most GDP data came from the Maddison Project (Maddison Project 2013). For a detailed explanation by country, please refer to Gapminder Documentation 001 (GD001) (Gapminder 2018a).

Data on LEB were also obtained from Gapminder (Gapminder 2016). Data from 1990 to 2009 were retrieved from the Global Burden of Disease Study 2015, from the Institute for Health Metrics and Evaluation, University of Washington–Seattle (Gapminder 2016). Data prior to 1990 used Gapminder Historic Life Expectancy Data, whose main sources are the Human Mortality Database (Human Mortality Database 2013) and World Population Prospects—the 2010 revision (United Nations Population Division 2011). See Gapminder Documentation 004 (GD004) (Gapminder 2014) for a detailed explanation of sources by country and year.

Criteria for Typology

Countries were classified into five typologies according to the three-year moving average (MA) of the ten-year gains in the log of LEB and to the three-year MA of the ten-year gains in the log of GDP per capita. We used the log transformation to rein in outliers who had anomalously large GDP per capita growth. Gains were defined as the difference between the current observation and the observation ten years ago for every ith country, $i = 1, \ldots,$ 189, in t years, $t = 1960, 1961, \ldots, 2009$. For example, three-year gains of LEB_i were defined as the difference between $\text{LEB}_{i,t}$ and $\text{LEB}_{i,t-10}$. We identified five typologies as follows:

1. Preston behavior:
    a. Three-year MA of the ten-year gains in the log of $\text{LEB}_{i,t} \geq 0$, and
    b. Three-year MA of the ten-year gains in the log of $\text{GDP}_{i,t} \geq 0$;
2. Health growth and economic recession:
    a. Three-year MA of the ten-year gains in the log of $\text{LEB}_{i,t} \geq 0$, and
    b. Three-year MA of the ten-year gains in the log of $\text{GDP}_{i,t} < 0$;
3. Health decline and economic growth:
    a. Three-year MA of the ten-year gains in the log of $\text{LEB}_{i,t} < 0$, and
    b. Three-year MA of the ten-year gains in the log of $\text{GDP}_{i,t} \geq 0$;
4. Health decline and economic recession:
    a. Three-year MA of the ten-year gains in the log of $\text{LEB}_{i,t} < 0$, and
    b. Three-year MA of the ten-year gains in the log of $\text{GDP}_{i,t} < 0$;
5. Suspiciously linear:
    a. Three-year MA of the ten-year gains in the log of $\text{LEB}_{i,t} \leq 1.01 *$ three-year MA of the ten-year gains in the log of $\text{LEB}_{i,t-1}$, and
    b. Three-year MA of the ten-year gains in the log of $\text{LEB}_{i,t} \geq .99 *$ three-year MA of the ten-year gains in the log of $\text{LEB}_{i,t-1}$, and
    c. Three-year MA of the ten-year gains in the log of $\text{LEB}_{i,t} \neq 0$.

To check robustness, we also tried different intervals to define LEB and GDP gains besides ten-year gains. We checked gains across one, five, and ten years. Our robustness test showed that the choice of interval did not have a big impact. In a comparison of the results using five-year versus ten-year gains, our 9,450 country-years of observation were, respectively, distributed as follows: 66.0% versus 65.8% had Preston behavior, 16.3% versus 15.3% had LEB growth and economic recession, 4.8% versus 3.5% had epidemic and economic growth, 3.8% versus 3.9% had epidemic and economic recession, and 9.1% versus 11.5% had suspiciously linear data. For this study,

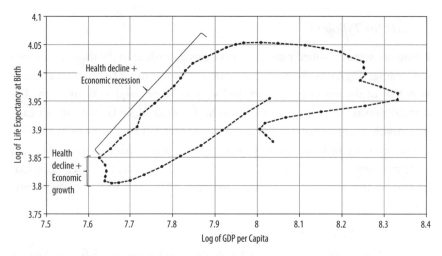

Figure 2.1. Trajectory in life expectancy and gross domestic product (GDP) per capita for a typical country, Zambia.

we considered ten-year gains to define the typology of the countries and committed to an analysis in which enduring longer-term gains in population health was the basis.

Figure 2.1 maps the trajectory of a typical country on the Preston axes of Log of Life Expectancy at Birth and Log of Gross Domestic Product per Capita, illustrating that typical countries do not have classic Preston behavior all the time. This country was slowly climbing the canonical Preston Curve from 1962 to 1967 and climbing again from 2000 to 2009. From 1980 to 1999, the country had declining health. Its economy also declined from 1968 to 1995. From 1960 to 1962, it had health improvements while also having economic declines. In determining whether this country qualifies as a success story, we only examined its performance during the times that it had positive health gains *and* economic gains. Over the fifty years of analysis, most countries went back and forth between typologies. Countries simply do not have constant economic growth nor constant improvements in their life expectancy across years. Epidemics and economic recessions happen almost everywhere, leading most countries to contribute country-years of observation across multiple typologies. Figure 2.2 shows the typology of various trajectories in the LEB-GDP plane for the same country, using the decadal gains in the log of LEB and the log of GDP per capita. Quadrant I groups country-years of observations with a Preston behavior—both the three-year MA of the decadal gains in the log of LEB and GDP per capita are positive—while quadrants II, III, and IV group country-years with positive decadal gains in

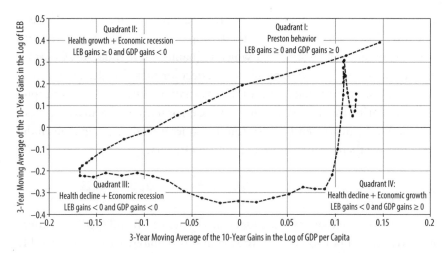

Figure 2.2. Typology of various trajectories in the progress of life expectancy at birth (LEB) and gross domestic product (GDP) per capita plane for a typical country, Zambia.

the log of LEB and an economic recession, country-years with an epidemic and an economic recession, and country-years with an epidemic and economic growth, respectively.

Definition of Good Performance

Our metric for good performance is based on the slope of the relationship between the three-year MA of the log of LEB and the three-year MA of the log of GDP per capita. The analysis was performed separately for each country, for decades 1960 to 1969, 1970 to 1979, 1980 to 1989, 1990 to 1999, 2000 to 2009, and by LEB stratum to confine comparisons of countries with similar LEB starting points in a given decade. The analysis was very much like a repeated tournament where each country could enter its slope for contention in each of five decades. In each decade, there were four competitive divisions in which the country could contest based on the four strata of LEB (LEB < 51, LEB between 51 and 61, LEB between 61 and 71, and LEB ≥ 71). Only country intervals showing Preston behavior were included. In the analysis, the slope of the Preston Curve was measured separately for each country and each decade as β_1 in an ordinary least squares regression model of each country's performance.

$$\text{MA of } (\log \text{ of LEB}_{i,t}) = \beta_0 + \beta_1 * \text{MA of } (\log \text{ of GDP}_{i,t}) + \varepsilon_i$$

Subscript t indicates that each country could potentially compete for distinction in each separate decade and its slope results would be entered into comparison in the LEB strata for which it qualified in that decade. Constant term β_0 serves as a country-specific fixed effect for each decade, and β_1 is our coefficient of interest that captures the association between GDP per capita and LEB during the decade. Finally, ε_i is the error term. In the analysis, countries had to be in a given LEB stratum for at least three years in a given decade to have their results registered in that category.

Results

Most countries had positive decadal gains in their LEB and GDP per capita; however, the proportion of countries with this typology varies considerably across life expectancy levels. Figure 2.3 shows the distribution of country-years across typologies by LEB stratum. The results show that as LEB increases, there is a greater proportion of countries with canonical Preston behavior. Among countries from the lowest LEB stratum (LEB < 51), 50.7% had a Preston behavior, and this proportion rose to 77.3% among countries from the highest LEB stratum (LEB ≥ 71). The reason for this is straightforward: benefiting from Preston behavior is a necessary condition to ascend into a high LEB stratum, whereas having repeated epidemics and economic recessions (and not Preston behavior) is compatible with long spells of having LEB < 51.

Between the 1960s and the 1990s, the proportion of countries with Preston behavior decreased across decades within each LEB stratum and started to increase again in the 2000s. In the 1960s, the proportion of country-years with Preston behavior in the lowest and highest LEB stratum was 67.2% and 93.5%, respectively. This proportion decreased to 9.3% and 64.3% in the 1990s for countries in the lowest and highest LEB stratum, respectively.

Figure 2.3 also shows that the proportion of countries with positive increases in their decadal gains in LEB during an economic recession was higher among countries from the lowest LEB stratum (LEB < 51) and among countries from the second stratum (51 ≤ LEB < 61).

Over the 9,450 country-years analyzed (189 countries observed over five decades), 6,218 country-years—more than half of those examined—exhibited positive decadal gains in their life expectancy and economic growth. These countries were ranked by decade and LEB stratum based on their ability to increase their rate of change of LEB given an increase in their GDP per capita. Figure 2.4 displays the top five countries in each decade with the great-

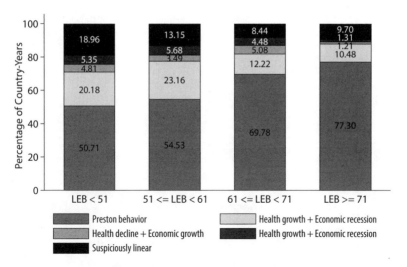

Figure 2.3. Typology distribution of country-years by life expectancy at birth (LEB) stratum based on the three-year moving average of the ten-year gains of the log LEB and the log of gross domestic product per capita. There were 9,450 observations of country-years.

est rate of change—the list only includes countries with a Preston behavior. One might have expected to find the list of the top five countries to be consistent across decades by LEB stratum. However, the majority of top performers changed across decade and LEB stratum. There were some exceptions in the bottom three strata, where countries made the list more than twice, but no country made the list more than twice in the highest LEB stratum.

Countries with outstanding progress in the bottom three strata were Mali and Nepal—they achieved high LEB growth during periods of minimal economic growth. Mali was in the lowest LEB stratum (LEB < 51) from the 1960s to the mid-1990s. In this stratum, it ranked third during the 1970s and 1980s, and first during the 1990s. Mali's greatest decadal gains in LEB and GDP per capita occurred in the 1980s. It was able to increase LEB by an average of 8.13 (SD 0.15) years per decade while having an average GDP increase of 117 (SD 112) (international) dollars. Mali transitioned to the second LEB stratum (51 ≤ LEB < 61) in the mid-1990s and remained there in the 2000s. The country ranked second in the 1990s and fifth in the 2000s, with an average increase of 0.218 (SE 0.047) and 0.534 (SE 0.052) in its LEB given a one (international) dollar increase in its GDP per capita (P < 0.01). Nepal made the top five list four times between the 1960s and the 2000s. It ranked fifth in the 1960s (LEB < 51), second in the 1980s (51 ≤ LEB < 61), and second

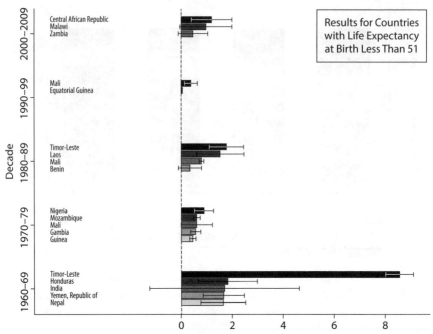

Coefficient on Gross Domestic Product (GDP) per Capita in Regression of
Life Expectancy on GDP per Capita

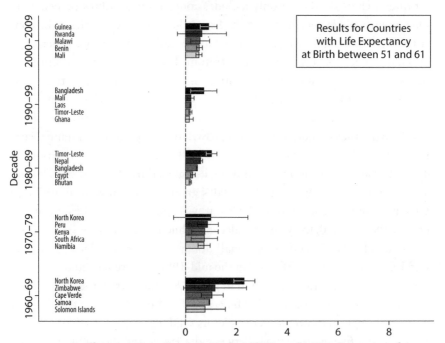

Coefficient on Gross Domestic Product (GDP) per Capita in Regression of
Life Expectancy on GDP per Capita

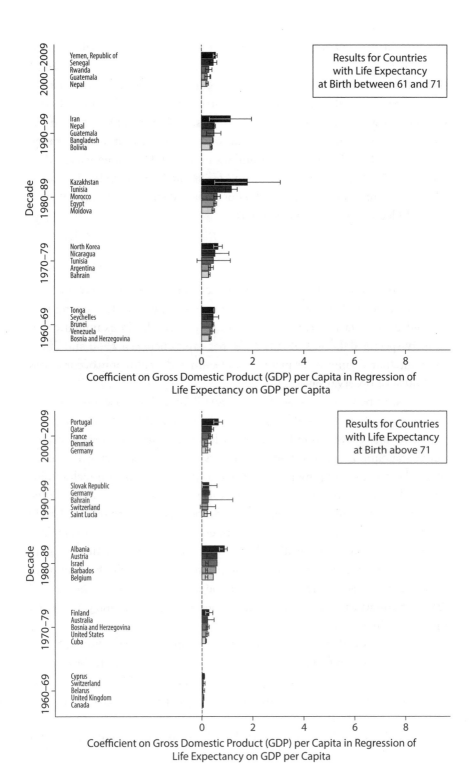

Figure 2.4. Top five economies with a Preston behavior, by strata and decade.

and fifth in the 1990s and 2000s ($61 \leq LEB < 71$). For Nepal, the greatest rate of change was 1.648 (SE 0.350) in the 1960s, when it had a $LEB < 51$ ($P<0.01$). Other countries featured in the current volume achieved distinction: Cuba was ranked fifth among countries with $LEB \geq 71$ in the 1970s. Bangladesh was ranked highly in the 1980s, and even ranked first in the 1990s among countries with a LEB between 51 and 61, and third among countries with a LEB between 51 and 61 in the 1980s. Ghana was ranked fifth in the 1990s. Stalwarts from *Good Health at Low Cost* (1985) such as China, Sri Lanka, and Costa Rica did not achieve distinction, and Kerala was not included because it is not a country.

Conclusion

We show that contrary to assumptions, the canonical Preston Curve relationship where both LEB and GDP per capita are simultaneously growing fails to hold up in a large proportion of country-years. In an examination of country-specific data on LEB and GDP per capita between 1960 and 2009, we found that simultaneous increases in health and wealth only occur in less than 60% of observations.

The list of best-performing countries is still limited because it is often the case that a country looks like it is deriving a high health output from minimal economic growth simply because it has had a prolonged spell of economic stagnation, and health improvements are simply occurring as a result of secular trends set up by past introductions of public health technology. Thus, what often appear to be "top-performing" countries in climbing the Preston Curve frequently appear successful because of stagnant and barely positive economic growth. The project of empirically identifying exemplary countries achieving good health at low cost or "punching above their weight" needs to reexamine foundational assumptions about (1) whether countries are actually engaged in transforming economic growth into better health and (2) what counts as a valid comparison group for a given country at a given time depending on its starting LEB.

Our analysis settled these questions by excluding countries whose ten-year trajectories were typified by worsening economies and worsening health. We also compared countries in similar ten-year brackets of LEB and in the same calendar decade. Very few countries remain top performers across many decades. Consistently exceptional performers were Mali, Nepal, and Bangladesh. The details of Nepal's and Bangladesh's configurations of their health systems around comprehensive PHC are covered elsewhere in the current volume. Cuba and Ghana also achieve distinction and are covered, too.

REFERENCES

Balabanova, Dina, Martin McKee, and Anne Mills. 2011. *Good health at low cost 25 years on: What makes a successful health system?* Oxford: Oxford University Press.

Balabanova, Dina, Anne Mills, Lesong Conteh, Baktygul Akkazieva, Hailom Banteyerga, Umakant Dash, Lucy Gilson, Andrew Harmer, Ainura Ibraimova, and Ziaul Islam. 2013. "Good health at low cost 25 years on: Lessons for the future of health systems strengthening." *Lancet* 381 (9883): 2118–2133.

Caldwell, John. 1986. "Routes to low mortality in poor countries." *Popul Dev Rev* 12 (2): 171–220.

Cardona, C., and D. Bishai. 2018. "The slowing pace of life expectancy gains since 1950." *BMC Public Health* 18 (1): 151.

Gapminder. 2014. Gapminder documentation 004: New life expectancy data. http://www.gapminder.org/data/documentation/gd004/.

Gapminder. 2016. "Life expectancy at birth (years)." Version 2016 10 12.

Gapminder. 2018. Gapminder Documentation 001: GDP per capita, constant PPP dollars. Available at https://www.gapminder.org/data/documentation/gd001/.

Halstead S. B., Walsh J. A., Warren K. S., Rockefeller Foundation. *Good health at low cost: Proceedings of a conference held at the Bellagio Conference Center, Bellagio, Italy, April 29–May 3, 1985.* New York, NY: Rockefeller Foundation, 1985.

Human Mortality Database. 2013. Life expectancy at birth. Berkeley: University of California.

Kuhn, Randall. 2010. "Routes to low mortality in poor countries revisited." *Popul Dev Rev* 36 (4): 655–692.

Maddison Project. 2013. Maddison historical statistics. University of Groningen. https://www.clio-infra.eu/Indicators/GDPperCapita.html.

Max Planck Institute for Demographic Research. http://www.mortality.org or www.humanmortality.de.

Preston, S. H. 1975. "The changing relation between mortality and level of economic development." *Popul Stud* 29 (2): 231–248.

United Nations Population Division. 2011. "Life expectancy at birth, both sexes." In *World population prospects: The 2010 revision—Life expectancy at birth, both sexes.* United Nations Population Division.

World Health Organization. 2000. *World Health Report.* Geneva: World Health Organization.

World Bank. 2018. World development indicators: GDP per capita, PPP (constant 2011 international $). https://data.worldbank.org/indicator/NY.GDP.PCAP.PP.KD.

Strategies to Improve Comprehensive Primary Health Care Performance in a District

CLAUDIA PEREIRA, DAVID BISHAI, AND MELISSA SHERRY

For policymakers who want to start improving comprehensive primary health care (PHC), it is often daunting to know where to begin. PHC connects many sectors and involves many different players, so it defies a desire to work from planned blueprints. Unlike a campaign to distribute oral rehydration solution, bed nets, or media messages, there is no pipeline from inputs to outputs to outcomes. Contrasting with commodity coverage campaigns, there is no coverage metric for PHC that counts the numbers of people receiving comprehensive multisectoral population-level PHC.

However, there are ways to benchmark and measure PHC performance. Implementation of PHC becomes the introduction of routine policies and procedures that regularly use these measurements to keep improving PHC and public health operations. This can be done via self-assessments and external assessments (Pan American Health Organization 2001; Alwan, Shideed, and Siddiqi 2016). There can be a disconnect between measures of national performance and performance at the provincial and district levels (Bellagio District Public Health Workshop Participants 2017). Because PHC performance happens close to the people, attention to what is happening outside of the central level is crucial.

In this chapter, we describe an approach that marries total quality improvement approaches, supportive supervision, and benchmark measures of essential public health functions (EPHFs) to improve PHC performance. The tools for this approach were worked out in pilot studies conducted in Botswana, Mozambique, and Angola, and can be applied in a variety of settings.

Advantages of a Public Health Functions Approach to Primary Health Care

PHC has been misunderstood by many. Both the Alma-Ata and Astana Declarations list so many aspirations that PHC might seem amorphous and difficult to pin down. Many confuse the term *primary care* used by many North Americans to describe generalists' clinical services with the *primary health care* term referring to the systematic community transformation described in the Alma-Ata Declaration that is the focus of this book. The 1979 introduction of the term *selective primary health care*, which was supposed to be an interim strategy to engage external donor support for top down vertical programs, has made the landscape even more confused (Walsh and Warren 1979; Newell 1988).

To a first approximation the following equation can serve:

PHC = Primary Care + (Population-Level, Multisectoral, Community-Controlled Public Health)

In other words, comprehensive PHC is the public health system. It surrounds, subsumes, and complements the conduct of primary care and does the community work necessary for health promotion. Despite the conceptual expansiveness of comprehensive PHC, its budgetary profile is tiny. Population-level public health activities are carried out by small cadres of public health practitioners with budgets that are between 1% and 5% as large as the clinical workforce. The basic fact is that sick people seeking clinical services are far more willing to spend money and to create political priority for the cure of their suffering and pain. Healthy people who have not yet become sick are not vocal about their condition—they seldom pay much money to stay healthy, and they are almost never a political force advocating for public spending. When doctors, nurses, pharmacists, and hospital staff worry about the bottom line of their financial support, they will turn toward curing sick people because that pays the bills—preventing sickness for whole populations does not. Cure crowds out prevention in every health system on earth (Bishai et al. 2014). In this chapter, we address the "crowd-out" syndrome and attend to the goal of making measures that can drive systems to achieve comprehensive PHC.

Measurement of comprehensive PHC is the foundation of a system where staff are assigned permanent roles in fostering the execution and improvement of comprehensive PHC. What gets measured gets managed, so developing a workable agenda for PHC measurement is the key to implementation

(Bitton et al. 2017; Veillard et al. 2017). Unsurprisingly, the primary care–clinical services dimension has benefited from much more progress in measurement. The numbers and proportions of children receiving vaccines, mothers receiving attended deliveries, and HIV patients getting antiretrovirals are eminently measurement friendly. But if implementation of the PHC agenda settles for measuring just the easily measurable part of PHC, then implementation will succumb to the predictable and universal syndrome in which clinical, curative operations crowd out the population-level preventive operations.

We describe efforts from a variety of countries to use a checklist of things that need to happen when comprehensive PHC is being implemented effectively. With a checklist and a system for improving performance measures, PHC can be effectively scaled up and intensified.

We do not offer a "universal blueprint" but propose a set of feasible steps that can engage each participant in the health system in finding their own role in improving PHC. Unlike a battle plan where vast armies of people and supplies must coordinate movement and activity in time and space, the implementation of PHC is bottom up and crowd sourced. The key is to unlock and energize a community's preexisting public health assets by systematically making them aware of how their contributions fit into the work of making a population and a place get healthier.

Necessary Preconditions

What makes the steps we propose feasible is that the required new elements are catalysts, not the main ingredients. Comprehensive PHC is multisectoral, but the sectors only need to be coordinated, not created. PHC engages civil society, but it does not have to develop the fundamental institutions of a government. There are preconditions that must prevail to enable PHC, but they are not prohibitive. The major and sometimes most limiting precondition is a desire to improve comprehensive PHC that is shared by leadership and spreads through the ranks. The commitment to building horizontal strength in community-based, multisectoral, population-level prevention is a spark that needs to be carefully tended. Powerful forces will always reward a focus on high-tech, curative specialty services. These services are accompanied by opportunities to allocate large budgets and manage large numbers of workers. Yet in every generation emerge leaders who realize the imperative to work upstream to stop the social and environmental conditions that fill the clinics with preventable sickness and suffering. Enlightened leaders are all

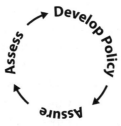

Figure 3.1. Public health core functions.

around, but they are not everywhere. Their commitment to build comprehensive PHC is a necessary precondition.

The second precondition to sustain PHC is a cadre of workers who have job titles placing them squarely in the realm of public health. Some countries call them *district health officers*, but they can also be public health operatives serving in a hospital, an accountable care organization, a health insurance pool, or even in a large private corporation. Public health spilled out of the exclusive provenance of government-run health departments long ago, and this chapter is relevant to both public health officers and professionals whose public health practice is outside government units.

Envisioning Improved Comprehensive Primary Health Care Performance in a District

What would it be like to be in a place with top-notch comprehensive PHC? What would one see happening? What would people be doing, knowing, and thinking? Describing the ideal in broad terms is a pathway to deriving a set of specifics.

A place with comprehensive PHC would be a place characterized foremost by widespread awareness of what the leading upstream health threats were. Citizens, politicians, and public health technocrats would all share a coherent mental model of what imperiled the people's health. The understanding would include but also go far beyond familiarity with relative magnitudes of disease incidence, prevalence, and burden. They would share consensus about the local distribution of social risk factors, including reduced livelihoods, stigma, and exclusion. There would be shared understanding of social and biological geography, locating physical risks in the air, water, food supply, and roadways. This knowledge would be common knowledge. Clergy would know, school principals would know, business leaders would know, and local politicians would know, and they would all talk through their options to address these problems together. The many and varied community members would transform their awareness to actions that they are responsible for. Through regular check-ins, they would hold one another accountable for working together. Part of what they would need to do would require resources from outside. Since this is an ideal version of PHC, there would be safe, accessible, high-quality primary medical care that has an outreach service and stays responsive to community oversight.

From those general features, we can identify the three specific linked processes: assessment, policy development, and assurance. In comprehensive PHC, these core functions of an aware health system are executed collaboratively across multiple segments and sectors of the community (Centers for Disease Control and Prevention 2018). Table 3.2 offers one possible list of EPHFs, but each setting may establish its own list. Many different parties participate in these core functions, but a strong PHC system will assign a district health officer or public health director to steward the process. This leader will have a core set of professional staff with skills in surveillance, basic epidemiology, health promotion, community relations, and health policy. However, the public health staff will *not* bear the burden of executing and assuring that public health policies are carried out. Public health professionals convene and engage members of the community to work together.

Assessment, policy development, and assurance (figure 3.1 on page 71) are well aligned with the seven principles of PHC listed in the Alma-Ata Declaration, as shown in table 3.1. However, the Alma-Ata–inspired execution of the public health cycle puts members of the community at the center of policy development and includes them in executing assurance strategies. The public health professionals in this paradigm ally their technical skills in epidemiological surveillance with convening operations to listen and form consensus among the multiple partners in a community who will execute health promotion across multiple sectors.

Ongoing Supportive Supervision for Primary Health Care

This section lays out a model of an ongoing program of supportive supervision staffed by a public health practice quality support unit. The basic process of PHC strengthening consists of regularly helping the staff of regional and district public health departments assess and improve the quality of their performance. Measurement plays an essential role and is not done for measurement's sake, nor is measurement done in order to give the chief executive a dashboard that they will use to steer the system or report to funding

Table 3.1. Alignment of assessment, policy development, and assurance with the seven elements of primary health care listed in the Alma-Ata Declaration

Phases of the Public Health Cycle	Elements of Primary Health Care Mentioned in Article VII of the Alma-Ata Declaration
Assess	Epidemiologically relevant, community-based strategy Sociocultural, political, and economic background (country-context)
Policy Development	Multisectoral approach and development Bottom-up, community-engaged planning, organization, promotion, and control
Assure	Integrated systems giving priority to those in need Includes multiple counterparts (auxiliary workers) Population-level responses

agencies. Measurement is done so the professional staff of the public health department can see and improve their professional practice. Practice report cards are meant to be shared with all the staff so that a performance improvement plan can be jointly developed by the workers who will carry out the plan. These improvement plans often incorporate customized programs in professional training designed to address perceived gaps.

Naturally, an important part of the strategy should be developing partnerships with local schools of public health, nongovernmental organizations (NGOs), and selected online resources for professional training. Implementation will also require in-house resources in coaching and mentoring. In any public health agency, there will be some staff with experience and skills that can serve to develop the capacity of coworkers if the system provides for this. In federalized health systems, there is a hierarchy of national, provincial, and local levels so that coaches for local workers can be maintained at the provincial level and coaches for the provincial level at the national level, and so forth. Performance improvement coaches (PICs) would use regular participatory measurements of public health practice quality. They would develop practice improvement plans during on-site visits, and they would follow up progress on the plans. The measurements used for practice improvement would necessarily span the entire assessment, policy development, and assurance cycle. Staffing ratios would be about one provincial coach to about twenty municipalities or districts. With this ratio, a coach would have time to make one daylong visit to each site per quarter and maintain weekly or biweekly telephone contact.

The initial visit of the PIC to a district should provide district public health staff with the necessary training on how to use a performance measurement tool to derive a report card and then to coach them in developing a feasible performance improvement plan. The use of the measurement tool and the drafting of an improvement plan is typically done as a team exercise that would be scheduled over one or several days.

Once the performance measurement results are shared, the team will have a clear picture of how they are faring across several dimensions of public health practice and comprehensive PHC. Instead of making a plan that simultaneously addresses all of them, the PIC should ask the team to focus on only two or three high-priority areas. The best way to begin this process is by walking the team through the performance assessment results, focusing on areas that are weak, and discussing strengths and weaknesses. This is the improvement planning phase, which is a key step in achieving quality and improving performance.

The plan should focus on the dimensions of practice that the team participants believe they could improve the most and the areas that they would find most important to address in order to impact the health of the district or municipality. It is important that the participants discuss how they are choosing the particular priorities and why they believe their chosen areas are important since the decisions should not just be based on low scores but on thoughtfully confronting the results from the tool with the current public health reality of the district. Once a decision has been made about which functions to work on, the team should spend time listing the top barriers to improving performance on those functions. This discussion should be guided by asking why they feel that each public health function is not currently being performed at an optimal level. It is important to always emphasize and recognize that funding, resources, and time are a constant problem in any health system, so other types of barriers should be considered because the goal is to gain an in-depth understanding of all the reasons why practices were not being performed at an optimal level at the time of the assessment. At this point, participants should keep in mind that barriers may overlap, and they may include cultural, community, environmental, health system factors or infrastructure-type barriers. The next step is to narrow down the identified barriers to those that are most significant or the most difficult to overcome. Staff should also be able to think through which area has barriers that are the most complicated or insurmountable and which has barriers that are more amenable to change. A ranking system of the easiest and most difficult barriers could be used.

Measuring Comprehensive Primary Health Care and Public Health

Public health practice measurement efforts go back to the early twentieth century (Winslow 1925). In 1925, the American Public Health Association developed an appraisal form and later an evaluation schedule to help public health departments document their performance (Derose et al. 2002). The Centers for Disease Control and Prevention (CDC) developed a list of "ten public health practices" in 1989 (Dyal 1995), which later evolved into the list of "ten essential services" (Derose et al. 2002) that has been used to benchmark practice in the United States. To avoid confusion about the word "services," this list of ten things that public health agencies do is usually called the "ten essential public health functions" (EPHFs). In the United States, the CDC has developed a widely modified package of measurement instruments for EPHFs called the National Public Health Performance Standards Program that are used in many local and state health departments. The measurements of performance are the foundation of performance improvement (Corso et al. 2000; Upshaw 2000). The ten canonical EPHFs are shown in table 3.2.

In the late 1990s, the World Health Organization (WHO) developed a task force to examine the concept of EPHFs. A group of 145 public health experts from all of the world's regions were queried using the Delphi method to determine priorities and make recommendations for member countries. The consensus was that country health ministries and regional offices need to work to define national-level lists of what is deemed essential and that the list should vary from country to country (Bettcher et al. 1998). WHO has encouraged its regional offices to develop context-specific measurements of EPHFs, and these have been carried out in regional offices for all of the Americas (Bettcher

et al. 1998), resulting in the landmark study, *Public Health in the Americas*, spearheaded by Pan American Health Organization (PAHO) regional director George Alleyne (PAHO 2001). Several WHO regional offices have developed measurement tools to assist ministries in assessing performance (Martin-Moreno et al. 2016; World Health Organization Regional Office for the Eastern Mediterranean 2017). The CDC has worked with the International Association of National Public Health Institutes to develop exercises, such as the Staged Development Tool, that help national-level public health officials assess their public health functions and form policies to prioritize improved performance (Barzilay et al. 2018).

In a parallel and somewhat confusing development, the Primary Health Care Performance Indicator (PHCPI) project has produced a suite of PHC vital signs profiles to gather core indicators of what it calls "PHC." However, in practice, the PHC measures are about the clinical primary medical care system and have little overlap with EPHFs. The conceptual framework for PHCPI is designed explicitly to move inputs into service delivery to produce service outputs and clinical outcomes (Veillard et al. 2017). The PHC vital signs profile has indices to measure access to clinical services, quality of clinical services, and social equity in access to clinical services. Most countries that have used it so far have not attempted to use the index of performance of population health. Perhaps in the future, the well-developed EPHF toolkits developed by the CDC and WHO will find a way to help PHCPI users develop assessments of a more comprehensive concept of PHC.

There has been substantial effort to engineer the content of PHC performance measurement tools; however, in practice the procedures for developing that content are equally important. Inclusion, participation, and transparency matter. This lesson was learned the hard way in the Canadian province of Ontario, where the provincial Ministry of Health developed and published a set of Ontario Public Health Standards (OPHS) designed to bring accountability to the practice of local boards of health (Schwartz et al. 2014). The OPHS included fourteen indicators and drew data from existing sources in the local system. Managers and chief medical officers of the public health units referred that the indicators that were chosen were "not indicative of the effectiveness of our services," "lacking relevance to us," "number counting," and being "beyond our control." They also said that the accountability system related more to a bureaucratic compliance with the OPHS than generating learning to improve performance and the health of the local population. Approaches that define standards independently from the providers who will use those standards are likely to fail, as their understanding of what drives performance often does not take into account important nuances of daily work (Forster and Walraven 2012).

The Use of EPHFs in Karnataka, India

Karnataka, a state in India, experienced considerable growth in the 1990s. Despite economic improvements, in the early 2000s the need to tackle disparities in health outcomes across several indicators was clear. In order to improve health outcomes, the approach of targeting EPHFs was taken by considering a broader perspective on public health, in which the participation of public health actors would play a key role.

The State Government of Karnataka created an independent task force to address the health sector through such a perspective and to allocate resources by setting up systems for public accountability. The system performance was to be examined against a list of core public health functions. With the support of the World Bank, a project was launched using this considerably novel approach. It was expected that by addressing the system through a wider lens, all aspects of public health would be assessed and addressed, and improvements would be observed in the outcomes that were considered most important, such as maternal and child health and infectious diseases.

Results-based EPHF indicators were developed and assessed over the following fifteen years. This approach required training and a change of culture to achieve results and sustain the changes in the long term. In practical terms, health was addressed at the local level through district health officers in a continuous process of working closely with those who executed public health toward assessment and policy development considering EPHFs. DHOs achieved consensus on the EPHF to prioritize and made recommendations for action.

Many improvements were observed, including an increase in the number of deliveries taking place in a health facility (from 65% to 94%). Among poor women, the percentage rose from 35% to 77%. In addition, health personnel were training in the areas of organizational development and quality assurance, which are crucial for the continuous process of assessment and reassessment required by EPHFs. Positive results were observed in all EPHFs, including health promotion in the areas of food safety and communicable and noncommunicable diseases, and linking people to health services, with a successful cervical cancer screening program and the implementation of regulations and public laws (World Bank 2003, 2018).

Based on all these reflections about existing assets and strengths, and the number of barriers and level of difficulty of the barriers to be overcome, the team should finally be able to choose a small number of public health functions that they would like to focus on.

There are a few different ways a team could go about focusing on a chosen function, but one would be to consider the top challenges and the root causes of those challenges as well as the resources available and the types of barriers faced. The participants should have a clear understanding of the most significant challenges to improving their performance.

The next phase would be to brainstorm ideas on ways to overcome challenges given the resources. It is crucial to open space to creatively consider the strengths that do exist in the community. Staff should think about partners they could work with to overcome those challenges. Such partners could be influential people in the community, NGOs working in health or development, other government workers (across sectors), or government-affiliated contractors. The idea is to focus on anyone who could be of help and how they could be engaged in the process of improving public health practice. In this step, it is important to consider ways to reach out or cooperate with other stakeholders, even those who may fall outside the government or health sector. There is an opportunity to share the workload of strengthening public health practice with different organizations. Reaching out to them to brainstorm ways to work together, one might consider sharing data, technology systems, or expertise on a given topic, or partnering for health promotion. Steps to engage partners may be as simple as setting up a preliminary meeting to discuss competencies or could be more advanced—for example, putting on a workshop in the district to emphasize the importance of the work needing to be done and inviting multiple potential partners. While the officer(s) should list ideas as to how to engage the partners, the team should also encourage discussion on ways to engage others working in the community and examine which partners may be most likely to help improve public health practice.

The next step is to consider the solutions for overcoming barriers based on their potential *impact* to improve performance and to consider the *feasibility* of the solutions given. For each solution the team has laid out, now they must consider how difficult it would be to carry out. They also have to determine how much impact a solution could have on the system if it were carried out successfully. It is important to focus on one solution at a time, thinking about how feasible and impactful each solution may be simultaneously. For feasibility, the element to consider is the timeline (how soon they could realistically carry out that solution), resources required to carry out the solution (few versus many), and the social or political environment necessary to achieve their solutions. For impact, it would be necessary for staff to consider whether the solution would lead to major changes or minor changes in the achievement of the community's public health goals.

After looking at solutions to improve EPHFs, choosing one that seems most feasible, actionable, and with the highest impact on EPHF strengthening is necessary. The team needs to list steps as to how they should go about carrying out that specific solution. For this step to work, they should break this process down into basic, simple, and clear steps such as "arrange meeting with the local NGO working in the area" or "form team to develop assessment of the availability of technology in the district" all the way through the point where the overall progress should be reevaluated at three or six months. A realistic timeline for the steps listed (improvement plan) should be written down, and dates for completion should be agreed upon among team participants considering a three-month time frame.

A Network of Supportive Performance Improvement Coaches

In this model, after improvement plans have been established, follow-up is an essential step in successfully achieving improvement, as it fosters accountability and continuity of the strategy. Additionally, it is necessary that the PIC maintains constant contact with the local offices, whether it is by making weekly phone calls to follow up on progress or by making use of other communication technologies, such as WhatsApp or SMS to, encourage the continuity of the performance improvement plan. Furthermore, one visit to each district should take place monthly or bimonthly to thoroughly discuss progress and difficulties, and to motivate district health officers and staff.

The network of comprehensive PHC performance improvement would not bring excessive costs. Very frequently, the staff who do the work of PHC are typically already on the payroll, but they are pulled toward clinical services management and deprioritize the more high-yield work of addressing root causes of disease. More importantly, the communitarian approach to convening and identifying community strengths and assets brings new resources to work on health promotion that are not typically a part of clinical health care budgets.

To form an idea of what it might cost, consider a country like Angola, with 173 municipalities. A PHC improvement network would require eight PICs.

They would be responsible for the supportive supervision of about twenty municipalities each, and there would be one coordinator overseeing the work of all coaches. PICs should live in the same, or adjacent, province where the municipality is located to facilitate travel. Considering wages, transportation, per diem, material, and 346 visits to municipalities per year (two per municipality), the estimated costs would be US$700,000. This investment would offer better performance for the many individual disease programs operating in Angola, such as yellow fellow, malaria, tuberculosis, HIV, and Ebola. (For an example, see chapter 4 on PHC's impact on polio control.)

Improving Comprehensive Primary Health Care and Public Health Everywhere

In 2016, the Sixty-Ninth World Health Assembly adopted a resolution for member states to strengthen the EPHF to support achievement of universal health coverage and the Sustainable Development Goals (World Health Organization Executive Board 2016). The mandate recognized the importance of the public health functions as cost-effective, comprehensive, sustainable, and a means to improve health and reduce the burden of the disease while also noting the importance of public health strengthening in achieving the SDGs (World Health Organization Executive Board 2016). Further, it called on the World Health Organization to develop technical guidance on the application of EPHFs; facilitate international cooperation to build necessary institutional, administrative, and scientific capacity to support the EPHF; to take the lead in promoting cooperation and coordination for health systems strengthening in the area of EPHF; and to report to the World Health Assembly on the implementation of this and its contribution to the achievement of 2030 SDG targets (World Health Organization Executive Board 2016).

The World Health Assembly resolution echoes developments in high-income countries as well. In the United States, Public Health 3.0 calls for strengthening public health practice via a focus on the EPHF and a renewed focus on the power of public health to convene sectors and communities to address the social determinants of health (DeSalvo et al. 2016). Public Health 3.0 highlights the role of public health leadership in multisectoral partnerships, emphasizing a need for public health to take on the role of "chief health strategist" in communities in order to bring together community members, public health, and other sectors to address health challenges through locally adapted

Health in All Policies (HiAP) approaches (DeSalvo et al. 2016). In order to achieve this vision of Public Health 3.0, the public health workforce needs to be resourced and trained on how to carry out the EPHFs, which includes how to act as a community convener and mobilizer. A stronger public health workforce that can convene communities and lead change across sectors for health will have significant implications for achievement of the HiAP, One Health, universal health coverage, and, ultimately, the SDG agendas. (See chapter 5.)

Making comprehensive PHC the foundation of health systems that can make progress toward achievement of the SDGs begins with recognition that public health functions are distinct from clinical services and their professional staff needs to realize their full potential and importance in this distinct role. Public health departments require their own resources, leadership, and frameworks for performance measurement in order to avoid being crowded out by clinical service provision. Further, public health departments

Table 3.2. The ten essential public health functions map

Assess	1. *Monitor* health status to identify and solve community health problems. 2. *Diagnose and investigate* health problems and health hazards in the community.
Policy Development	3. *Inform, educate,* and empower people about health issues. 4. *Mobilize* community partnerships and action to identify and solve health problems. 5. *Develop policies and plans* that support individual and community health efforts.
Assure	6. *Enforce* laws and regulations that support individual and community health efforts. 7. *Link* people to needed personal health services and assure the provision of health care when otherwise unavailable. 8. *Assure* competent public and personal health care workforce. 9. *Evaluate* effectiveness, accessibility, and quality of personal and population-based health services. 10. *Research* for new insights and innovative solutions to health problems.

Note: Divided into three continuous operations in a cycle: *assess* health and health threats, *policy development* among the broad community in policy solutions, *assure* that solutions are carried out across multiple sectors.

need a clear mandate that outlines their core functions and allows them to measure their performance, analyze strengths and weaknesses, and act to ensure all functions are carried out, with mentorship and information available on how to continuously improve. An important strategy paper for the United Kingdom suggested ring-fencing public health budgets in the National Health Service so that all citizens would have equal access to high-quality public health operations.

The opportunity to achieve the SDGs through a public health framework is especially appealing because it does not require a new workforce or a new framework. In fact, public health officers are already in place in districts across the world, and the EPHFs framework already provides a structure through which the SDGs can be achieved (see chapter 5). Strengthening public health practice will require retraining and reorientation of the existing public health workforce in order to turn public health workers into community "chief health strategists" capable of using data to convene and mobilize communities and stakeholders for multisector action. The future public health workforce must be trained and motivated to effectively carry out each of the EPHFs in partnership with communities and other sectors. Workers will need resources devoted to strengthening their capacity to practice community-engaged public health and will need ongoing technical assistance and leadership from the World Health Organization with its regional offices and country health ministries to ensure that there is leadership and guidance for district public health officers to become experts in carrying out the EPHF.

REFERENCES (SEE PAGE 341 FOR FULL CITATIONS
FOR BOXED TEXT)

Alwan, Ala, Olla Shideed, and Sameen Siddiqi. 2016. "Essential public health functions: The experience of the Eastern Mediterranean Region." *East Mediterr Health J* 22 (9): 694–700.

Bellagio District Public Health Workshop Participants. 2017. *Public health performance strengthening at districts: Rationale and blueprint for action.* https://www.who.int /alliance-hpsr/bellagiowhitepaper.pdf.

Bishai, D., L. Paina, Q. Li, D. H. Peters, and A. A. Hyder. 2014. "Advancing the application of systems thinking in health: Why cure crowds out prevention." *Health Res Policy Syst* 12 (1):28.

Bitton, A., H. L. Ratcliffe, J. H. Veillard, D. H. Kress, S. Barkley, M. Kimball, F. Secci, E. Wong, L. Basu, C. Taylor, J. Bayona, H. Wang, G. Lagomarsino, and L. R. Hirschhorn. 2017. "Primary health care as a foundation for strengthening health systems in low- and middle-income countries." *J Gen Intern Med* 32 (5): 566–571.

Centers for Disease Control and Prevention. 2018. "The public health system and the 10 essential public health services." Accessed December 27, 2018. https://www.cdc .gov/publichealthgateway/publichealthservices/essentialhealthservices.html.

DeSalvo, Karen B., Patrick W. O'Carroll, Denise Koo, John M. Auerbach, and Judith A. Monroe. 2016. "Public health 3.0: Time for an upgrade." *Am J Public Health* 106 (4): 621–626.

Newell, Kenneth W. 1988. "Selective primary health care: The counter revolution." *Soc Sci Med* 26 (9): 903–906.

Pan American Health Organization. 2001. *Public health in the Americas*. Washington, DC: Pan American Health Organization.

Veillard, J., K. Cowling, A. Bitton, H. Ratcliffe, M. Kimball, S. Barkley, L. Mercereau, E. Wong, C. Taylor, L. R. Hirschhorn, and H. Wang. 2017. "Better measurement for performance improvement in low- and middle-income countries: The Primary Health Care Performance Initiative (PHCPI) experience of conceptual framework development and indicator selection." *Milbank Q* 95 (4): 836–883.

Walsh, J. A., and K. S. Warren. 1979. "Selective primary health care: An interim strategy for disease control in developing countries." *N Engl J Med* 301 (18): 967–974.

World Health Organization Executive Board. 2016. "Strengthening essential public health functions in support of the achievement of universal health coverage." 138th Session Executive Board, World Health Organization.

CHAPTER FOUR

Why Well-Supported Health Systems Are Necessary for Vertical Programs to Succeed

Lessons from Polio Eradication

SVEA CLOSSER

The Global Polio Eradication Initiative (GPEI) is the most far-reaching co-ordinated health project in history. In the thirty years of its existence, the GPEI has repeatedly reached into more than one hundred countries to deliver more than twenty billion doses of oral polio vaccine in special campaigns.* It does this in pursuit of an extremely narrow and very clearly defined goal: total eradication of poliovirus.

Because the GPEI is an eradication program, aiming to reduce incidence of polio to zero in every country in the world, it is global in scope and vertical in design, focusing on a single disease. Polio eradication's magic bullet is a standardized methodology that includes both the delivery of polio vaccine to every child in the world, usually through mass door-to-door campaigns, and intense communication and social mobilization aimed at getting parents to enthusiastically accept the vaccination of their children.

On paper, the methods and goals of the GPEI have always been broader than just the eradication of polio. The seeds of the modern eradication program were planted in an elimination effort in the Americas in the early 1980s, shortly after the Alma-Ata Conference.† In 1984, Brazilian epidemiologist Ciro de Quadros persuaded the Pan American Health Organization and

---

*This number, obtained from the WHO's database of polio eradication campaigns, is so large because many children are vaccinated multiple times. In parts of Pakistan and northern India, for example, one child can easily receive twenty to thirty doses of oral polio vaccine by the time they are 5 years old.

†In this chapter, I use *elimination* to mean the regional reduction to zero of transmission, and *eradication* to mean complete reduction to zero transmission globally of an infectious disease.

United Nations Children's Fund (UNICEF) to support polio elimination. His argument was that polio could be a "banner disease" for immunizations in general (de Quadros 1997, 185; de Quadros 2009). The resulting American project of polio elimination was a collaboration between PAHO, UNICEF, the Rotary Foundation, and the United States Agency for International Development, and was the first major international partnership of United Nations, bilateral, and private agencies in the health sector. All of these agencies said that they supported mass polio immunization campaigns as a way to increase immunization rates in general—as a way of furthering primary health care (PHC) (Hampton 2009).[‡] Rotary's official literature explained that its contribution to the program was named "PolioPlus," "in recognition that control of polio is only one sector of the battle to improve child health, and that PolioPlus should support and complement the goals of the Expanded Programme on Immunization (EPI) of the World Health Organization. Furthermore, it is recognized that EPI itself is part of a broader primary health care strategy to improve child health" (Rotary Foundation 1985, 187).

When polio eradication became a global goal in 1988, it continued to include broader health goals in its language. Routine immunization was, and remains, the first of the "four pillars" of polio eradication. Current policy documents also state commitment to broader health systems issues. The Polio Eradication Endgame and Strategic Plan 2013–2018 includes strengthening of immunization systems as a core objective (Global Polio Eradication Initiative 2013).

Yet in practice, despite these stated commitments, polio eradicators and those championing routine immunization or PHC have sometimes been at odds. In the 1990s, for example, polio eradication got off to a very slow start globally, largely because many in WHO were still skeptical of eradication as a strategy and of polio eradication in particular (Needham and Canning 2003).

Conversely, polio eradication officials have sometimes seen support for broader health goals, even the relatively narrow goal of promoting more routine immunization, as a distraction from the single-minded focus needed to eradicate a disease. In the early 2000s, for example, many (though certainly not all) polio eradication officials were wary of GAVI, the then fledgling initiative aiming to increase rates of routine immunization. They viewed GAVI

[‡]UNICEF's vision of "selective Primary Health Care," which included routine immunization, was more a basket of vertical programs than PHC as conceptualized at Alma-Ata (Cueto 2004).

as a potential threat, a competitor for attention and funding (Global Technical Consultative Group for Poliomyelitis Eradication 2000; Closser et al. 2014).

What the history and current trajectory of polio eradication reveals, however, is that conceptualizing eradication programs in opposition to broader health goals is unhelpful. Strong basic health systems are necessary for the success of vertical programs—even a program like polio eradication, built on vaccination campaigns.

In fact, the Alma-Ata Declaration's definition of PHC provides a helpful guide to the key elements of health systems that facilitate disease eradication. PHC, the Declaration says, "includes at least: education concerning prevailing health problems and the methods of preventing and controlling them; promotion of food supply and proper nutrition; an adequate supply of safe water and basic sanitation; maternal and child health care, including family planning; immunization against the major infectious diseases; prevention and control of locally endemic diseases; appropriate treatment of common diseases and injuries; and provision of essential drugs" (World Health Organization 1978, 2). This list of functions forms a useful, straightforward definition of a strong health system—a clear delineation of what needs to be in place for vertical initiatives to work in ways that benefit both communities and the health systems that serve them.

There is more to the definition of PHC in the Alma-Ata Declaration, and the full scope of PHC as outlined in the document is relevant to successful eradication programs. Community control of and engagement in health systems facilitates trust and goodwill; in contrast, people who feel that their health system is completely unresponsive to their needs are likely to distrust vertical programs. In this chapter, I illustrate the symbiotic shared ecology of eradication goals with comprehensive PHC.

Solid Health Systems Facilitate Quick Elimination of Polio

The elimination of polio proved possible—and often even relatively straightforward—in countries with solid basic health systems. The last case of wild polio in the Americas was in Peru in 1991, seven years after the elimination effort began. This was achieved with a relatively modest effort: just one to three campaigns per year in polio-endemic countries were enough to secure elimination across the hemisphere.

This relatively quick success was possible in the Americas because the polio vaccine provided during campaigns supplemented other population-level institutions in public health. Compared to sub-Saharan Africa and South Asia, the Americas had high rates of routine immunization, as well as good sanitation systems that interrupted fecal-oral transmission of poliovirus (Pan American Health Organization 1995).

Polio was next eliminated in WHO's Western Pacific region in 1997. With a few exceptions in very targeted areas, polio elimination across the region was achieved with just one or two vaccination campaigns per year (Aylward 1997; World Health Organization 2002). As in the Americas, the elimination effort in the Western Pacific was built on high routine immunization rates: although there were areas with low coverage, almost 90% of children across the region got three doses of polio vaccine through routine immunization (World Health Organization 2002).

In these regions of the world with relatively solid health systems, the elimination of polio was not easy—it required enormous efforts in organization and logistics. But, it was doable: With a few vaccination campaigns per year boosting levels of population immunity against poliovirus, the disease disappeared.

Twenty years after polio was eliminated in the Americas and the Western Pacific, it persists in three countries in the world: Afghanistan, Pakistan, and Nigeria.[§] In all of these places, the eradication effort dwarfs what was done in the Americas and the Western Pacific in scope and intensity: many areas in these three countries have seen as many as eleven campaigns per year for the past fifteen years. And yet polio persists.

Part of the reason for polio's continuing transmission in these countries is that their climates and cities provide excellent poliovirus habitat. Poliovirus thrives in hot environments with high population density and poor sanitation—South Asia is a nearly ideal ecological niche.

Yet, India, probably an ideal habitat for polio, managed to eliminate the disease in 2010, through a very intensive program of repeated campaigns. Also, the hot, densely populated state of Punjab in Pakistan rarely sees polio. In both India and the Punjab, high numbers of repeated campaigns were supported by health systems that are in general a bit stronger, according to the definition laid out previously, than those in areas with continuing polio transmission.

[§]In addition to the countries listed here, which have never eliminated polio, there are also outbreaks in some other countries, such as the Democratic Republic of the Congo, that previously achieved elimination.

Armed conflict has had a long-term, serious impact on health services in both Pakistan and Afghanistan. Unlike in other parts of South Asia (see chapters 9 and 11, this volume), health services have been allowed to suffer in the context of war. In Afghanistan's long series of wars, health facilities were neglected or destroyed, and aid for health systems has been woefully inadequate, in part because sanctions limited health aid (Bhutta 2002). In Pakistan, leaders—both military and civilian—have poured resources into national defense, at the expense of sectors like education and health (Suleri 2013). Health indicators in Pakistan are particularly poor in areas bordering Afghanistan, where people often live far from government services—and where polio transmission persists.

In Nigeria, polio transmission occurs in the north, where health services are poor. Rates of routine immunization, for example, are well below 50% across the region (Gunnala et al. 2016). In the south, where health systems are much stronger, polio cases are extremely rare.

If Nigeria, Pakistan, and Afghanistan had stronger health systems with good rates of routine immunization, intensive campaigns would have succeeded in eliminating polio as they had in so many prior situations. But because their health systems often do not provide basic services, especially to the poor and marginalized, polio retains its grip. Vaccine hesitancy is extremely difficult to overcome when the health systems fail to earn the trust of the community.

In fact, wherever basic health services falter, polio transmission often follows. Syria is a clear case in point. The country, which long had solid health systems with routine immunization rates above 90%, had not seen a case of polio since 1995. In 2012, with war, routine immunization rates dropped below 70%. An outbreak of polio ensued in 2013, followed by a second outbreak in 2017.[¶]

The Polio Program Often Supports Strong Health Systems

In 2012, I worked along with a team of other researchers on a project aimed at assessing the impact of polio eradication on routine immunization and

¶The first outbreak was wild polio, while the second was vaccine-derived polio. While wild polio and vaccine-derived polio differ in their sources (vaccine-derived polio, as the name implies, arises when the vaccine virus mutates to virulence), they both are controlled the same way—through achieving high levels of population immunity through vaccination (Kew et al. 2005).

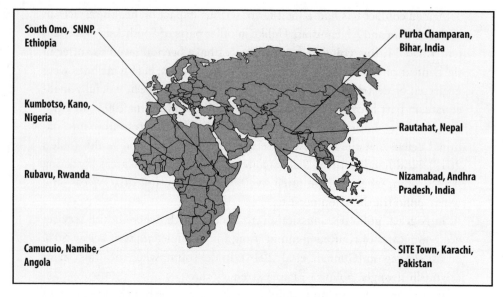

Figure 4.1. Case studies of the relationship between polio eradication and health systems. SNNP = Southern Nations, Nationalities, and Peoples.

PHC (Closser et al. 2014). We went to eight study sites in sub-Saharan Africa and South Asia (figure 4.1), learning about the relationship between polio eradication and other health services by spending time working with and interviewing the staff implementing these programs. We interviewed national and district-level officials, ground-level staff, and parents of children targeted during campaigns. We also carried out participant observation in polio campaigns and primary care activities at community-level health posts.**

We found that in places where health systems are relatively strong, providing services like routine immunization, curative care, and sanitation to large segments of the population, vertical programs such as polio eradication can be beneficial: They often provide additional attention and resources that can help improve coverage of a variety of health interventions.

We saw one example of how this can work in the Indian state of Andhra Pradesh, where the health system is relatively strong, and where polio was eliminated in the early 2000s. To ensure that poliovirus is not reintroduced, there are still a couple door-to-door campaigns per year in Andhra Pradesh. These highly organized and targeted campaigns take extra measures to en-

---

**Our methods are more fully described in an article (Closser et al. 2012), and the full qualitative research protocol is available at http://sites.middlebury.edu/polio_eradication _impacts_study/qualitative-research-guide/.

sure that high-risk populations, such as nomads and people living in urban slums, get vaccinated against polio.

The outreach to high-risk populations that happens during polio campaigns in Andhra Pradesh benefits other health services. In our study, we watched workers checking on the routine immunization status of hard-to-reach children they visited during polio campaigns. This gave planners new information about vaccination coverage in high-risk children.

Our study found another example of the positive benefits of the polio program in Rubavu, a district in Rwanda with relatively strong PHC. There, high-level officials used polio campaigns as an opportunity to visit local health centers. They participated in social mobilization activities and provided feedback to staff. Local health staff told us that these visits were valuable, because they provided officials with a better perspective of the current, on-the-ground challenges faced by health centers, often difficult to convey through reports alone.

Other studies, too, found that a few polio campaigns a year in relatively strong health systems had beneficial effects (Aylward 1997). In the Americas, for example, social mobilization around polio campaigns, which included both communication materials and strong community involvement, were used to educate people about a range of health issues. Later, these social mobilization efforts were used as models for other health programs (Pan American Health Organization 1995).

Using a vertical program to support general health systems, as in these examples, is sometimes called the "diagonal" model of health systems strengthening (Frenk 2006). Such an approach can be effective. However, our study found that the positive impacts of polio eradication were most pronounced in areas with relatively strong health systems. Where health systems were weak, neglected, or damaged by war, the impacts of polio eradication activities on broader health services were complicated.

In Weak Health Systems, a Heavy Emphasis on Polio Can Distort Priorities

In areas with relatively solid routine immunization, polio was generally eliminated in the 1990s with just a few campaigns per year. It was also possible to eliminate polio in some parts of the world with low routine immunization coverage—for example, in much of sub-Saharan Africa—because low population density and climactic factors made the chain of polio transmission relatively easy to break. But in struggling health systems with weak immunization and sanitation programs, particularly in areas of high population density, the GPEI is forced to do much more in its efforts to eliminate poliovirus. In place of two or three door-to-door campaigns, nine or ten campaigns per year are common in polio-endemic areas with weak health systems. This means vastly more time and resources must be expended by health staff in pursuit of polio elimination.

Because this greatly increased effort comes in the context of poor health services generally, it often leads to distorted allocations of effort and money, with polio receiving a wildly disproportionate share of attention and funding in comparison to its disease burden. We saw examples of this in the polio-endemic and recently polio-endemic areas in our study.

Polio campaigns are resource intensive and staff intensive: They require an extensive workforce to carry out planning and supervision, social mobilization, vaccination, and monitoring. Some of this work is done by WHO and UNICEF staff, but given the scale of campaigns, they almost always involve much larger numbers of government health staff.

One of our study sites in India was Purba Champaran, a district in Bihar that had some of India's last polio cases. At the time of our study, just one year after the last case, Bihar was carrying out an intensive schedule of polio campaigns. These labor-intensive campaigns pulled on a range of frontline workers, including auxiliary nurse-midwives (ANMs), female community health workers (ASHAs), and Anganwadi workers (frontline nutrition staff). The majority of workers in these cadres devoted a full seventy-seven days to polio campaigns in 2010.

In addition to polio eradication, frontline health staff in Purba Champaran were tasked with a series of campaign-centered vertical programs. Health officials and workers carried out back-to-back campaigns for polio, measles, and vitamin A. When asked about their responsibilities, ANMs and ASHAs listed vertical programs that they were involved in—a list that bore little resemblance to the ideals of PHC outlined at Alma-Ata.

Even though in practice health workers in Purba Champaran were tasked with a collection of vertical programs, workers and officials were still frustrated by what they viewed as a disproportionate focus on polio compared to other health issues. "Polio, polio," one frustrated immunization official said at a meeting. "When is anyone ever going to pay attention to anything else?"

In the two polio-endemic field sites in our study—Karachi, Pakistan, and Kano, Nigeria—health staff also complained about the mismatch between the focus on polio and on other health priorities. A high-level official in Pakistan commented, "For policy makers, politicians, and bureaucrats, if we talk about immunization they understand it as 'polio,' and not the other way around." Respondents in Kano also said that attention to polio eradication superseded the attention given to all other health issues.

Dissatisfaction with Distorted Priorities Can Hinder Polio Eradication

Dissatisfaction with the focus on polio, in comparison with other health issues, made many workers frustrated and unmotivated in their polio vaccination campaign work. This demotivation did not arise immediately, in the first few years of campaigns. And it was rare in places with just a few polio campaigns per year. Rather, it grew over time with year after year of intensive campaign work. When workers spent a third of their time on polio campaigns for twenty years running, as they have in parts of South Asia and Nigeria, their frustration with their polio campaign work was in many cases serious and deep.

The GPEI is aware of this issue, usually calling it "campaign fatigue." But the issue went beyond fatigue for some workers—they felt frustration and anger. Their primary complaint was the very low per diem given to polio campaign workers, which many experienced as disrespect (Closser et al. 2017). But many also mentioned that, although they felt eradicating polio was a worthy goal, the disproportionate focus on polio reflected disregard for the most pressing health needs of their communities. For example, a low-level official in Karachi, Pakistan, said: "The people have their own priorities, first is water and living in difficult situations, groceries and sanitation. They don't have their basic needs. And the polio campaign has gone on for more than 10 years." Workers repeatedly voiced these frustrations in all of our case studies with more than a few campaigns per year (table 4.1).[††]

Supervisors across these areas said they had trouble getting workers to do good work on polio campaigns. "Polio, polio, polio," said a district-level official in Purba Champaran, India. "Workers, motivators, vaccinators, we have threatened them a lot, from the government side. Now they have closed their ears."

In addition to demotivating workers, repeated campaigns in the context of poor health services contributed to polio vaccine refusals (Closser, Jooma, et al. 2016; Closser, Rosenthal, et al. 2016). Especially when poor and mar-

---

[††]Workers in Nepal, although they only worked on four campaigns in 2011, had just experienced several years running with eleven campaigns per year.

Table 4.1. Polio campaigns, worker motivation, and polio vaccine refusals

Case Study District	Number of Polio Campaigns in 2011	Were Many Workers Frustrated with Repeated Campaigns?	Were There Current Reports of Polio Vaccine Refusals?
Rubavu (Rwanda)	1	No	No
South Omo (Ethiopia)	2	No	No
Nizamabad, Andhra Pradesh (India)	2	No	No
Rautahat (Nepal)	4	Yes	No
Camucuio, Namibe (Angola)	4	No	Yes
Kumbotso, Kano (Nigeria)	8	Yes	Yes
Purba Champaran, Bihar (India)	9 to 10	Yes	No
SITE Town, Karachi (Pakistan)	11	Yes	Yes

Source: Closser, Rosenthal, et al. 2016.

ginalized populations had reasons to distrust the government, it seemed suspicious to them that the same health system that neglected their most severe health needs came to their doorstep with polio vaccine. A national-level official in Nigeria summarized the issue clearly: "The first question [parents] will ask is, 'Why is it that when my child is ill, I go to the health facility, am not able to see the doctor, my child is not treated well by the health personnel, and I buy the medicine, but now workers come to my house to drop off the OPV [oral polio vaccine] to my child who is healthy.' So this is a disconnect."

A frontline health worker in Kano, Nigeria, said: "People raise so many suspicious questions about polio. Some of the non-compliant people often remark that if you go to hospitals, you buy every drug. Then why is it that polio vaccine is given house to house free of charge?"

Another worker in Kano noted: "If boreholes and other essential amenities should be provided to these communities, the polio vaccine would be more acceptable."

Similar sentiments were common in Karachi, Pakistan. A worker there said: "We get asked, Why do we repeatedly go for the polio campaigns? Why are we worried about polio? The people say, 'We have so many other problems.'"

In Camucuio, Angola, where health services had been disrupted or destroyed by civil war, workers also said that refusals were fueled by this dynamic. One worker explained parental refusals this way: "All the time it is polio, polio; so they have this taboo."

Comprehensive Primary Health Care Is the Bedrock of Successful Vertical Programs

Solid health systems providing services including routine immunization, then, are the bedrock on which successful elimination programs are built. Additionally, in these areas vertical programs are likely to support health systems. In areas with relatively strong health systems, polio campaigns provided additional boosts of funding and high-level attention, leading both to the elimination of polio and to broader health system benefits.

When these basic health systems are damaged by war or neglect, even the most well-resourced and intense vertical programs may not be able to eliminate disease. In these areas, vertical programs can exacerbate existing problems (Cavalli et al. 2010). Repeated polio campaigns in the context of poor health services fed a negative feedback loop of worker demotivation and parental vaccine refusal—making the elimination of polio even more difficult. India was able to overcome these challenges, in part by shoring up support for routine immunization and sanitation in polio-endemic areas (Closser et al. 2014). Whether these problems can be surmounted in Nigeria, Pakistan, and Afghanistan remains to be seen.

PHC and vertical programs should not be conceptualized as opposing models of service delivery. Strong basic health services are, in fact, essential for the success of vertical programs. When single-disease programs build on the base of solid public health services, disease elimination is often possible, and vertical programs are likely to have positive health system benefits. In contrast, when vertical agendas are pushed in areas with weak health systems, they are much more likely to fail.

Carl Taylor, the champion of PHC who prepared many documents for the Alma-Ata Conference, made this argument in 1978 in reference to vertical family planning programs. Integrating health services, he argued, led both to administrative efficiencies and greater community acceptance. "By using the rapport created by health care activities that are constantly in demand," he wrote, "acceptance can be enhanced of . . . activities toward which there tends to be ambivalence" (Taylor 1978, 63). The full scope of comprehensive PHC supports and nourishes vertical programs (table 4.2). Without this support, eradication initiatives are likely to flounder.

Smallpox eradication was achieved through a vertical program that required little health system support (Brilliant 1985; Henderson 2009; Foege 2011). However, no other extant disease, with the possible exception of guinea worm, has the epidemiological characteristics to be eradicated that way. The ease of case detection in smallpox, coupled with a highly effective vaccine, made targeted ring vaccination a viable option and required far less mass vaccination. Smallpox eradication is often rightly heralded as a great public health success and a potential model for other programs (Levine 2007). However, the smallpox model of vertical programs, insofar as it existed independent of the broad provision of basic health services, is not a useful model for elimination or eradication programs in the modern world.

Measles, likely to be the next target for eradication, is a case in point. Measles is epidemiologically much more difficult than polio to eradicate. A measles eradication program is likely to face serious problems of parental refusal if measles campaigns are pushed too hard or for too long in areas with generally weak health systems (Omer, Orenstein, and Koplan 2013). This is especially true since measles vaccine, in contrast to oral polio vaccine, requires an injection.

Funding for global health has long neglected basic health system and public health improvements in favor of vertical programs, in part because health security arguments are so compelling to wealthy governments (Rushton 2011; Packard 2016). Funding for polio eradication from major donors such as the United States government, Rotary, and the Bill and Melinda Gates Foundation grew from enthusiasm over the possibility of eradication—and from the fact that many older Americans, including Rotarians, had some personal experience with polio. A similar enthusiasm for funding broad-based public health infrastructure has not existed in these organizations (Storeng 2014). Yet these basic public health services are an essential component of successful vertical programs.

A number of ways forward are possible. The suggestion of a recent Bellagio Conference on public health performance strengthening is one worth exploring: "If a credible plan for public health performance improvement is put forward, one might consider a 'levy' on foreign direct assistance for health (i.e., vertical health programs) and it would be justifiable in the sense that

Table 4.2. Comprehensive primary health care, as conceptualized at Alma-Ata, supports vertical programs

Element of Comprehensive Primary Health Care (from Alma-Ata Declaration Article VII)	How It Helps Vertical Programs
Addresses the main health problems in the community, providing promotive, preventive, curative, and rehabilitative services accordingly.	Vertical programs focusing on a niche issue in an environment where a community's main health issues are not addressed are likely be greeted with distrust and frustration by that community (Greenough 1995; Durbach 2000; Renne 2006; Factor et al. 2013; Closser, Jooma, et al. 2016; Closser, Rosenthal, et al. 2016).
Includes at least: education concerning prevailing health problems and the methods of preventing and controlling them; promotion of food supply and proper nutrition; an adequate supply of safe water and basic sanitation; maternal and child health care, including family planning; immunization against the major infectious diseases; prevention and control of locally endemic diseases; appropriate treatment of common diseases and injuries; and provision of essential drugs.	Proper nutrition, basic sanitation, routine immunization, and control of locally endemic diseases provide a solid foundation that vertical programs need to thrive: • Good nutrition lessens the impact of infectious disease (Caulfield et al. 2004; Black et al. 2008). • Safe water and basic sanitation not only interrupt fecal-oral disease transmission but also reduce rates of diarrhea that make children prone to common infectious diseases (Bartram and Cairncross 2010). • Routine immunization provides population immunity to key diseases. • Control of locally endemic diseases through a PHC approach means putting systems in place to improve health and manage disease (this volume provides many examples of how this can be done). Disease elimination is much easier when these systems exist. • Controlling the diseases that affect local communities most builds trust in the health system (Closser, Rosenthal, et al. 2016). In settings where these systems are functioning, eliminating some infectious diseases is possible (Dowdle and Hopkins 1997).
Involves, in addition to the health sector, all related sectors and aspects of national and community development, in particular agriculture, animal husbandry, food, industry, education, housing, public works, communications, and other sectors, and demands the coordinated efforts of all those sectors.	Intersectoral collaboration is an important—and often challenging—aspect of most vertical programs. Eliminating malaria, for example, requires extensive collaboration across sectors to achieve vector control, communications, and surveillance (Feachem et al. 2009). This remains an understudied and poorly understood aspect of PHC (Lewin et al. 2008) but one with clear importance to single-disease initiatives.

Continued

Table 4.2. continued

Element of Comprehensive Primary Health Care (from Alma-Ata Declaration Article VII)	How It Helps Vertical Programs
Requires and promotes maximum community and individual self-reliance and participation in the planning, organization, operation, and control of primary health care, making fullest use of local, national, and other available resources, and to this end develops through appropriate education the ability of communities to participate.	Community participation in a health system builds trust in that system (Gilson 2003; Perry et al. 2014). As the example of polio illustrates, eliminating diseases in areas where communities do not trust the health system can be extremely difficult (Jegede 2007; Abimbola et al. 2013).
Relies, at local and referral levels, on health workers, including physicians, nurses, midwives, auxiliaries, and community workers, as applicable, as well as traditional practitioners as needed, suitably trained socially and technically to work as a health team and to respond to the expressed health needs of the community.	Most vertical programs rely on local health workers as their foot soldiers. When ground-level workers are technically skilled, know their communities well, and are trained to be responsive to local needs, they are able to skillfully navigate the communities they serve (Ballard et al. 2018). A robust health workforce is essential to the success of many vertical programs (Brugha et al. 2010). Effective health workers are also trusted by their communities (Gilson et al. 2005)—and trust in local health workers has proven to be a key issue in securing disease elimination.

support for special programs and services requires the overhead of a public health system. Having a credible plan for public health practice improvement would justify requests to finance the foundations of the system. Building financial support is a responsible way to sustainably develop the public health system at the foundation of successful vertical programs" (Bellagio District Public Health Workshop Participants 2017).

While such a strategy could work well for control programs, eradication programs are likely to face their deepest challenges in places where public health services have been deeply neglected for political reasons—as in the case both on the Afghanistan–Pakistan border and in northern Nigeria. Areas of the world with poor health services are also likely to be areas where governments will not put forward credible plans for health service improvement.

That said, the areas where eradication programs will have problems are predictable. Adequate public health infrastructure is among the "constellation of conditions" that make disease eradication possible (Dowdle and Cochi 2011). Feasibility analyses of eradication programs tend to focus on biological feasibility and cost-benefit analyses, neglecting analyses of where public health infrastructure is failing. But, it would certainly be possible, using a metric like that suggested in chapter 3 of this volume, to identify areas of inadequate public health infrastructure *prior* to undertaking an eradication program and to develop plans to strengthen that infrastructure.

The trust borne of community involvement; the foundations of good health provided by nutrition, sanitation, and basic health services; the power of intersectoral action; and the engagement of skilled, committed health workers are all critical to successful single-disease initiatives. When these health system functions are in place, not only is disease elimination possible, but disease-specific interventions often provide additional health system benefits. The model of comprehensive PHC outlined at Alma-Ata and Astana is the foundation, not the antithesis, of successful vertical programs.

REFERENCES

Aylward, Bruce. 1997. "Strengthening routine immunization services in the Western Pacific through the eradication of poliomyelitis." *J Infect Dis* 175 (Suppl. 1): S268–S271.

Bellagio District Public Health Workshop Participants. 2017. *Public health performance strengthening at districts: Rationale and blueprint for action.* www.who.int/alliance -hpsr/bellagiowhitepaper.pdf.

Bhutta, Zulfiqar Ahmed. 2002. "Children of war: The real casualties of the Afghan conflict." *BMJ* 324 (7333): 349–352.

Brilliant, Lawrence B. 1985. *The management of smallpox eradication in India.* Ann Arbor: University of Michigan Press.

Cavalli, Anna, Sory Bamba, Mamadou Traore, Marleen Boelaert, Youssouf Coulibaly, Katja Polman, Marjan Pirard, and Monique Van Dormael. 2010. "Interactions between global health initiatives and country health systems: The case of a neglected tropical diseases control program in Mali." *PLoS Negl Trop Dis* 4 (8): e798.

Closser, Svea, Kelly Cox, Thomas M. Parris, R. Matthew Landis, Judith Justice, Ranjani Gopinath, Kenneth Maes, Hailom Banteyerga Amaha, Ismaila Zango Mohammed, Aminu Mohammed Dukku, Patricia A. Omidian, Emma Varley, Pauley Tedoff, Adam D. Koon, Laetitia Nyirazinyoye, Matthew A. Luck, W. Frank Pont, Vanessa Neergheen, Anat Rosenthal, Peter Nsubuga, Naveen Thacker, Rashid Jooma, and Elizabeth Nuttall. 2014. "The impact of polio eradication on routine immunization and primary health care: A mixed-methods study." *J Infect Dis* 210 (Suppl. 1): S504–S513.

Closser, Svea, Rashid Jooma, Emma Varley, Naina Qayyum, Sonia Rodrigues, Akasha Sarwar, and Patricia Omidian. 2016. "Polio eradication and health systems in Karachi: Vaccine refusals in context." *Glob Health Commun* 1 (1): 1–9.

Closser, Svea, Anat Rosenthal, Judith Justice, Kenneth Maes, Marium Sultan, Sarah Banerji, Hailom Banteyerga Amaha, Ranjani Gopinath, Patricia Omidian, and Laetitia Nyirazinyoye. 2017. "Per diems in polio eradication: Perspectives from community health workers and officials." *Am J Public Health* 107 (9): 1470–1476.

Closser, Svea, Anat Rosenthal, Kenneth Maes, Judith Justice, Kelly Cox, Patricia A. Omidian, Ismaila Zango Mohammed, Aminu Mohammed Dukku, Adam D. Koon, and Laetitia Nyrazinyoye. 2016. "The global context of vaccine refusal: Insights from a systematic comparative ethnography of the Global Polio Eradication Initiative." *Med Anthropol Q* 30 (3): 321–341.

Closser, Svea, Anat Rosenthal, Thomas Parris, Kenneth Maes, Judith Justice, Kelly Cox, Matthew A. Luck, R. Matthew Landis, John Grove, Pauley Tedoff, Linda Venczel, Peter Nsubuga, Jennifer Kuzara, and Vanessa Neergheen. 2012. "Methods for evaluating the impact of vertical programs on health systems: Protocol for a study on the impact of the Global Polio Eradication Initiative on strengthening routine immunization and primary health care." *BMC Public Health* 12 (1): 728.

Cueto, Marcos. 2004. "The origins of primary health care and selective primary health care." *Am J Public Health* 94 (11): 1864–1874.

de Quadros, Ciro. 1997. "On towards victory." In *Polio*, edited by Thomas Daniel and Frederick Robbins, 181–198. Rochester, NY: University of Rochester Press.

———. 2009. "The whole is greater: How polio was eradicated from the Western Hemisphere." In *The practice of international health: A case-based orientation*, edited by Daniel Perlman and Ananya Roy, 54–69. Oxford: Oxford University Press.

Dowdle, Walter R., and Stephen L. Cochi. 2011. "The principles and feasibility of disease eradication." *Vaccine* 29 (S4): D70–D73.

Foege, William H. 2011. *House on fire: The fight to eradicate smallpox*. Berkeley: University of California Press.

Frenk, Julio. 2006. "Bridging the divide: Global lessons from evidence-based health policy in Mexico." *Lancet* 368 (9539): 954–961.

Global Polio Eradication Initiative. 2013. *Polio eradication and endgame strategic plan 2013–2018*. Geneva: World Health Organization.

Global Technical Consultative Group for Poliomyelitis Eradication. 2000. *Global eradication of poliomyelitis*. Geneva: World Health Organization.

Gunnala, Rajni, Ikechukwu U. Ogbuanu, Oluwasegun J. Adegoke, Heather M. Scobie, Belinda V. Uba, Kathleen A. Wannemuehler, Alicia Ruiz, Hashim Elmousaad, Chima J. Ohuabunwo, Mahmud Mustafa, Patrick Nguku, Ndadilnasiya Endie Waziri, and John F. Vertefeuille. 2016. "Routine vaccination coverage in Northern Nigeria: Results from 40 district-level cluster surveys, 2014–2015." *PLoS One* 11 (12): e0167835.

Hampton, Lee. 2009. "Albert Sabin and the coalition to eliminate polio from the Americas." *Am J Public Health* 99 (1): 34–44.

Henderson, D. A. 2009. *Smallpox: The death of a disease; The inside story of eradicating a worldwide killer*. Amherst, NY: Prometheus Books.

Kew, Olen M., Roland W. Sutter, Esther M. de Gourville, Walter R. Dowdle, and Mark A. Pallansch. 2005. "Vaccine-derived polioviruses and the endgame strategy for global polio eradication." *Annu Rev Microbiol* 59 (1): 587–635.

Levine, Ruth. 2007. *Case studies in global health: Millions saved*. Sudbury, MA: Jones and Bartlett.

Needham, Cynthia, and Richard Canning. 2003. *Global disease eradication: The race for the last child*. Washington, DC: ASM Press.

Omer, Saad B., Walter A. Orenstein, and Jeffrey P. Koplan. 2013. "Go big and go fast—Vaccine refusal and disease eradication." *N Engl J Med* 368 (15): 1374–1376.

Packard, Randall M. 2016. *A history of global health: Interventions into the lives of other peoples*. Baltimore: Johns Hopkins University Press.

Pan American Health Organization. 1995. *The impact of the expanded program on immunization and the polio eradication initiative on health systems in the Americas: Final report of the "Taylor Commission."* Washington, DC: Pan American Health Organization.

Rotary Foundation. 1985. "PolioPlus Programme: Criteria for funding of polio immunization programmes." *Assignment Children* 69–72:187–192.

Rushton, Simon. 2011. "Global health security: Security for whom? Security from what?" *Political Studies* 59 (4): 779–796.

Storeng, Katerini T. 2014. "The GAVI Alliance and the 'Gates Approach' to health system strengthening." *Glob Public Health* 9 (8): 865–879.

Suleri, Abid Qaiyum. 2013. "Insecurity breeds insecurity." In *Development Challenges Confronting Pakistan*, edited by Anita Weiss and Saba Gul Kattak, 57–69. Sterling, VA: Kumarian Press.

Taylor, Carl E. 1978. "Development and the transition to global health." *Med Anthropol* 2 (2): 59–70.

World Health Organization. 1978. "Declaration of Alma-Ata." In *International Conference on Primary Health Care*. Alma-Ata, USSR. https://www.who.int/publications/almaata_declaration_en.pdf

———. 2002. *Polio eradication in the Western Pacific Region*. Manila: World Health Organization.

Continuity between Comprehensive Primary Health Care and Sustainable Development Goals

MELISSA SHERRY AND DAVID BISHAI

Acting on the principles of primary health care (PHC) stated at the Alma-Ata Conference in 1978 will further the Sustainable Development Goals (SDGs) of 2015. The SDGs are seventeen targets covering social development, the environment, and economic progress (United Nations 2015). Reaching the SDGs depends on recognizing the interconnectedness of different sectors. Responsibility for achievement of the SDGs lies with national governments and global stakeholders across the world, and will require multisectoral partnerships to achieve change (United Nations 2015).

The Alma-Ata Declaration called for multisectoral, community-engaged responses to locally defined challenges that remain at the core of public health practice. The term *primary health care*, which continues to define the legacy of Alma-Ata, refers to the combined realization of accessible primary (medical) care services and multisectoral public health practice. This chapter details the importance of strengthening public health practice at the national and district levels because strong public health practice supports *all* of the SDGs—not just the health-related goals. This chapter reviews evidence linking progress on improving public health practice worldwide as called for in the Alma-Ata Declaration with achievement of the SDGs.

Drawing on evidence from around the world, this chapter documents how strengthening the public health component of PHC can create stronger communities and healthier environments in support of each of the SDGs.

Introduction

In 2015, the United Nations General Assembly adopted a resolution called "Transforming Our World: The 2030 Agenda for Sustainable Development" (United Nations 2015). The new framework for development outlined seventeen universal goals with 169 targets crossing three main domains: social development, the environment, and economic progress (GBD 2015 SDG Collaborators 2016; Gostin and Friedman 2015; United Nations 2015). As compared to the Millennium Development Goals (MDGs), the SDGs are substantially broader and seek to align efforts in all policies to attain goals that expand on the MDG agenda to accelerate global progress in achieving a singular strategy for a healthier people and planet (Gostin and Friedman 2015).

This chapter first describes the SDGs and then defines public health and the essential public health functions (EPHFs) as nonnegotiable features of PHC. The articles of the Alma-Ata Declaration described a vision of PHC that entailed an evidence-based, data-driven, multisectoral response to community-engaged problem-solving. The public health profession has historically developed a code of practice to do exactly that. Over the past several decades, the profession has repeatedly defined a set of EPHFs that flesh out executable details of the vision of PHC outlined by the Alma-Ata Declaration.

The chapter then shows how PHC's public health arm contributes to the specific SDG indicators across the seventeen goals and explains how a focus on improving PHC's public health contribution creates a framework for achievement of these indicators. We describe a path forward to achieve not only the health indicators outlined by the SDGs but also for improved partnerships and multisector action to achieve all SDGs.

Overview of Sustainable Development Goals, Primary Health Care, and Essential Public Health Functions

A key element of "development" is the ability of a society to identify and solve collective problems. The concept of development underlying the SDGs requires that multiple sectors work together to carry out cycles of monitoring, reviewing, and acting to solve problems facing both nations and people.

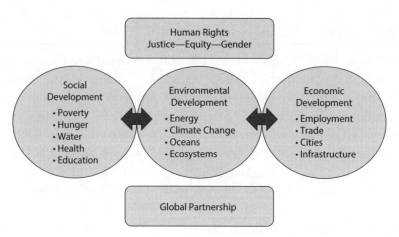

Figure 5.1. Sustainable Development Goals Framework.

Brief Summary of SDGs

The SDGs aim for progress in three domains: social, environmental, and economic development. As shown in figure 5.1, the SDGs are concerned with the interconnectedness of development efforts across these domains, as well as a human rights and equity lens that overlays each of these areas. Figure 5.1 lists these goals at a very high level. They are listed in more detail in the first column of table 5.1 (United Nations 2015).

Primary Health Care Depends on Essential Public Health Functions

The Institute of Medicine (2013) defines public health as "what we as a society do collectively to assure the conditions in which people can be healthy" (xi). PHC as defined in the Alma-Ata Declaration aspires to achieve the exact same goal through collective activity. The EPHFs define a core set of activities that should be carried out in every community. These core activities are carried out by entire systems and involve a variety of public and private health providers, nongovernmental organizations (NGOs), and government officials from health, education, public works, law enforcement, and social services. The multisectorality and inclusivity stem from the orientation of public health to address upstream root causes of poor health. The population-level focus was embodied in the full articulation of PHC at the Alma-Ata Conference. In 2016, World Health Assembly Resolution 69.1 called for United Nations member states to strengthen public health governance through increased public health capacity and focus on the delivery of the EPHFs.

EPHFs are the activities that governments and their people need to undertake to create healthy communities. They protect populations from disease, injury, and environmental threats, and are the cornerstone of health systems' ability to promote health and prevent illness. EPHFs provide the framework through which populations are protected from illness and injury, provided with sanitary and safe living conditions, and given the knowledge necessary to maintain optimal health. When public health is done well, nobody notices because health crises do not occur. When public health is poorly performed, common problems include the following:

- epidemics go undetected and unchecked,
- communities resist healthy behaviors,
- sanitary laws are not enforced,
- safety is compromised, and
- hospitals and clinical services do not maintain quality and access.

The whole health system is compromised when public health is not sufficiently carried out, creating a burden on hospitals and clinics, and threatening the health and well-being of communities.

While lists of EPHFs vary slightly by region, one set of EPHFs, according to J. M. Martin-Moreno and colleagues (2016), appears as follows:

Assessment Functions
1. Monitoring Health Status to Identify Community Health Problems
2. Diagnose and Investigate Health Problems and Health Hazards in the Community

Policy Development and Multi-Sector Action Functions
3. Inform, Educate, and Empower People about Health Issues
4. Develop Policies and Plans That Support Individual and Community Health Efforts
5. Mobilize Community Partnerships to Identify and Solve Health Problems

Assurance Functions
6. Enforce Laws and Regulations That Protect Health and Ensure Safety
7. Link People to Personal Health Services
8. Assure a Competent Health Workforce
9. Evaluate and Assure Effectiveness, Accessibility, and Quality of Preventive Health Services
10. Research for New Insights and Innovative Solutions to Health Problems
11. Disaster Preparedness

Together, the EPHFs support the multi-stakeholder cycle of "assessment, policy development, assurance." Progress on the SDGs requires public health units to work with communities to collect data, develop policy responses, and convene multiple groups and agencies to respond to identified health challenges. The assessment functions are monitoring and surveillance functions that provide information necessary for carrying out health assessments; preparing for epidemic and disaster warning systems, planning policy and intervention, and resource allocation; and measuring progress. The policy development functions cover concepts of coordinated actions to support and protect health, as well as partnerships for identification and remediation of health problems. These are cornerstone activities for action on the SDGs (Martin-Moreno et al. 2016). The remaining assurance functions represent action functions necessary to carry out public health practice.

The Role of Public Health and Primary Health Care in Achieving Sustainable Development Goals

At the core of public health practice are functions that represent the actions necessary for all SDGs to be achieved, including data collection for informing action, creating policy, convening communities and stakeholders across sectors to address issues, and enabling functions that ensure the effectiveness of public health actions across communities. When performed together, the package of EPHFs become a platform for improvements in health as well as environmental and social development.

However, while the monitoring and surveillance and enabling of functions carried out by public health departments are important, the element of public health practice most relevant to sustainable development is really the policy development component.

Participatory Policy Development

The Alma-Ata Declaration called for multisectoral, community-engaged responses to locally defined challenges. Rising to this challenge, many public health practitioners have set out to convene and enable communities. The EPHFs listed under the heading "Policy Development" describe the critical actions needed to create the community platforms from which the SDGs can be achieved. Simply tracking health-related data and threats does not change outcomes. Political support to address public health problems arises differently in different contexts. Convening affected communities and political stakeholders to make use of data can help them achieve shared understanding, which can lead to coherent action in many settings. The link between the policy development functions and progress toward SDGs is highlighted in the following section.

Inform, Educate, and Empower People about Health Issues

The importance of health promotion to support health, well-being, and equity has long been recognized, and is prominent in the Alma-Ata Declaration, the Ottawa Charter, the Commission on Social Determinants, and many other global health movements (World Health Organization 1978; Commission on Social Determinants of Health 2008; Lawn et al. 2008; Rohde et al. 2008). Research linking health promotion activities to health outcomes, reductions in domestic violence, and improved nutrition demonstrates the importance of health promotion in the achievement of many of the SDGs (International Union for Health Promotion and Education 2000; Gilson et al. 2007). More specifically, health promotion programs improve health- and non-health-related indicators across the human life course. Past studies have shown:

1. In early childhood: Health promotion can help prevent neonatal deaths in developing countries and may help improve health behaviors, prevent tobacco use, and reduce injuries later in life. Community-level health promotion interventions targeted at young children can also improve long-term mental health outcomes (Guyer et al. 2009; Gogia and Sachdev 2010; Petersen et al. 2016).
2. In childhood: Health promotion programs can improve children's amount of physical fitness and healthy nutrition, as well as lower smoking rates and the incidence of being bullied (Langford 2015). Health promotion programs based in schools have also been shown to improve mental health outcomes (Petersen et al. 2016).
3. In adolescence: Health promotion programs that include community and multisectoral approaches to improving adolescent health can result in improved sexual health, reduced incidence of being bullied, fewer teen pregnancies, and improved school attendance (International Union for Health Promotion and Education 2000; Shackleton et al. 2016).
4. In adulthood: Health promotion interventions in the workplace can impact physical activity, dietary behavior, and healthy weight, as well as absenteeism, sick leave, and mental health outcomes (Kaspin et al.

2013; Rongen et al. 2013; Petersen et al. 2016; White et al. 2016). Community health promotion programs can improve heart health and diet quality, and reduce injury-related morbidity and deaths (International Union for Health Promotion and Education 2000).

5. In old age: Health promotion programs can improve the ability of the elderly to self-manage their health and improve their well-being (Goetzel et al. 2007).

DEVELOPING POLICIES AND PLANS THAT SUPPORT INDIVIDUAL AND COMMUNITY HEALTH EFFORTS

While public health actions such as health promotion and policy development are often thought to be focused only on the health sector, execution of these public health functions has been the basis for multisectoral action for decades, given the significant role that other sectors play in contributing to health (World Health Organization 2013a, 2013c). Policies to alter the con-

---

Case Study: Health Promotion

One example of how health promotion initiatives from the health sector can lead to improvements in multiple other areas of development is a case study from India, where, starting in 1992, the All India Institute of Hygiene and Public Health worked with the World Health Organization to gather data on human immunodeficiency virus (HIV) prevalence among sex workers and promote treatment, condom promotion, and health education in this population. As public health workers began working closely with women to promote health and improved hygiene practices, it became evident that changing health outcomes would also require a broader approach that addressed education, social contexts, and human rights activism. Subsequently, the program, called the Sonagachi HIV/AIDs Intervention Project (SHIP), launched a multisector approach to addressing the needs of sex workers by implementing interventions such as vaccination and treat-ment of services for children of sex workers, literacy classes, political activism for workers' rights, advocacy action with political leaders and law enforcement, community mobilization, microcredit schemes, and cultural programs. The sex workers were able to create their own membership organization, the Durbar Mahila Samanwaya Committee, and successfully improved occupational health standards for sex workers, upgraded living conditions and literacy rates, and reduced rates of HIV infections and rates of sexually transmitted infections in Sonagachi. The SHIP organization expanded to include forty red light districts across West Bengal. This demonstrates how health promotion can lead to multisector actions and policies. Plans that cross sectors improve social and economic conditions along with health outcomes (Durbur Mahila Samanwaya Committee Theory and Action for Health Research Team 2007).

---

tribution of the social determinants of health cannot be addressed by the health sector alone (Commission on Social Determinants of Health 2008; Bert et al. 2015).

The Health in All Policies (HiAP) approach asks multiple sectors of government to seek and find synergy and complementarity in their goals. All government sectors are designed to promote well-being of the population, and well-being includes many facets beyond health. Rather than stipulate that health goals supersede all other interests, HiAP asks for cooperation to find areas of complementarity and to avoid creating policies with harmful human impact (World Health Organization 2013c). The HiAP approach has been widely used in various contexts, with many examples of initiatives demonstrating the effectiveness of this approach (World Health Organization 2011a, 2013a, 2013c, 2014a; Perrier and Shankardass 2011; Howard and Gunther 2012; Kickbusch and Gleicher 2012; McQueen et al. 2012; Rudolph et al. 2013). Some impactful examples of the HiAP approach include reductions in fatal road crashes in Sweden, progress on environmental issues, lower tobacco use and related mortality in Brazil, and improvements in the structural environments that support improved fitness and nutrition in Mexico, among others (World Health Organization 2011b, 2014a).

Public health's facilitation of HiAP creates partnership platforms from which the SDGs can be addressed, which fulfills SDG 17. These partnerships also address the root causes of health that relate directly to the other SDGs, ranging from hunger and poverty to sustainable development and healthy environments. Public health can play a critical role of convening and participating in multisectoral partnerships for development of policies that maximize the likelihood of achieving health- and non-health-related SDGs.

MOBILIZE COMMUNITY PARTNERSHIPS TO IDENTIFY AND SOLVE HEALTH PROBLEMS

The HiAP approach provides a platform by which communities can begin to address the complex, interconnected nature of the SDGs; however, the implementation of such approaches often relies on community trust, organization, and mobilization to effect change. One of the key public health functions is the engagement and mobilization of community platforms for health, which are the partnerships formed with communities and other stakeholders in order to assess and assure population health (Sherry et al. 2017). These community platforms adapt interventions to the local context and execute their delivery so that the community is engaged and the actions are community centered (Sherry et al. 2017).

Case Study: Health in All Policies

In 2009, the Ecuadorian National Plan for Good Living (NPGL) was developed in an effort to coordinate across sectors to build policies, strategies, and programs that included a rights-based, social justice–oriented perspective for social policy (Pan American Health Organization 2015). The NPGL defined health broadly and focused on a social determinants of health approach to set goals organized through the Development Coordinating Ministry, which oversees the Ministries of Health, Labor, Education, Inclusion, Migration, and Housing (World Health Organization 2014). Based on the National Development Plan that served as the road map for development and implementation of social policies, regional and local governments were able to develop their own plans, tailored to meet local needs. Between 2006 and 2011, when the program was implemented, income inequality fell 12% and social investment increased two and a half times. Sanitation improved, with the proportion of urban households with toilets and sewer systems increasing by 7% and improvements in rural households with access to waste collection increasing from 22% to 37% (Pan American Health Organization 2015). Further, investments in justice-related initiatives increased fifteenfold, public investment and credits for agriculture doubled, and medical consultations in health services increased (Pan American Health Organization 2015). Overall, health and development indicators related to multiple Sustainable Development Goals improved as the result of a Health in All Policies approach to creating healthier living environments.

Literature on community platforms for health shows that building platforms for community participation and mobilization can lead to improved outcomes across a range of health and development outcomes (Rifkin 1996, 2014; McCoy et al. 2012; Kenny et al. 2013; Edmunds and Albritton 2015; George et al. 2015). Community participation in health improves health knowledge, service quality, and health-related outcomes in communities (Russell et al. 2008; Kenny et al. 2013). Best practices in community engagement include power sharing, collaborative partnerships, bidirectional learning, and the use of multicultural health workers for intervention delivery (Cyril et al. 2015). Public health policies that pursue these partnerships will build trust within communities (Blas et al. 2008). Communities that trust their leaders and one another are the foundation of sustainable development.

Evidence for the impact of mobilizing communities to address health and its social determinants generally covers multiple pathways to community engagement (Rifkin 1996; Draper et al. 2010; UKAID and DFID Human Resource Development Centre 2011; Meier et al. 2012; Kenny et al. 2013; Tiwari et al. 2014; Beracochea 2015; George et al. 2015). Studies show that

Case Study: Mobilizing Communities

Achieving the Sustainable Development Goals (SDGs) requires partnership across multiple sectors and necessitates the need for strong community platforms for achievement of health and social gains. One example of how community platforms for health and development can translate Health in All Policies (HiAP) approaches into action at the local level was the experience of the Gerbangmas movement in Lumajang district in East Java, Indonesia. Starting in 2005, the district health office of the Lumajang district created "enriched health posts," which were designed to promote community education, empowerment, and services related to health issues as well as education (World Health Organization 2011). Because of the initial success of these health posts, the district health office expanded the posts to become platforms for communities, public health, and other government sectors to work together to achieve twenty-one indicators crossing health, development, and economic priorities (Commission on Social Determinants of Health 2008).

The Gerbangmas movement relied on community volunteers to conduct needs assessments, discuss problems in the community, create action plans for health, and monitor and evaluate activities, with the support and partnership of the district health office, religious institutions, and other government sectors such as industry and trade, public works, and agriculture (Blass et al. 2008; Siswanto 2009). In 2011, the program was relaunched to address newly defined indicators and aimed to focus beyond public health to issues such as the environment, the role of women, and economic development. The precedent set by the Gergbanmas movement continues to inform policy and development in Indonesia (Nugroho 2016; Sururi 2013).

The Gerbangmas movement led to improvements across fourteen indicators for human development, one indicator for the economy, and six indicators for the household environment, and serves as an example of how public health leadership to engage and mobilize partnerships with other sectors can help achieve the SDGs (Commission on Social Determinants of Health 2008).

---

convening community platforms can improve a range of health outcomes, improve institutional trust, and enhance effectiveness of policies and interventions (McCoy et al. 2012; Lassi and Bhutta 2015; Jack et al. 2017). Community platforms are the vehicle by which the policies and interventions designed to achieve development goals are customized to local context and adopted by communities.

LINKING POLICY DEVELOPMENT FUNCTIONS OF PUBLIC HEALTH TO SUSTAINABLE DEVELOPMENT GOALS

The participatory policy development component of public health can contribute to the achievement of both health- and non-health-specific SDGs. The following lists examples of supporting literature for the effects of health promotion, policy development, and community engagement efforts on non-health-specific SDGs.

- *SDG 2 (zero hunger)*: Studies of community-based food and nutrition programs found that highly visible and persuasive educational campaigns related to nutrition and food security, combined with multisectoral community engagement, successfully improved a variety of nutritional indicators (International Union for Health Promotion and Education 2000; Ismail et al. 2003; Tontisirin and Bhattacharjee 2008).

- *SDG 4 (quality education)*: School-based health promotion programs, in particular those that engage with communities, have shown positive effects in reducing body mass index, smoking, and incidence of being bullied, as well as increasing physical activity, fitness, and fruit and vegetable intake among children and adolescents: outcomes that may lead to better attendance and school performance (International Union for Health Promotion and Education 2000; Beets et al. 2009; Li et al. 2011; Langford et al. 2015).

- *SDG 5 (gender equality)*: Health promotion programs, in particular, those that engage with schools and communities and include interventions such as economic incentives, can reduce teenage pregnancy, bullying and victimization, and incidence of adolescent marriages, and improve sexual health outcomes: all factors that help keep women in school and improve gender equality indicators (International Union for Health Promotion and Education 2000; Shackleton et al. 2016).

- *SDG 8 (working conditions and economic growth)*: Several reviews show that workplace health promotion interventions, in particular, when coupled with additional occupational health and safety approaches, can improve physical health and health behaviors as well as psychosocial outcomes, and reduce injuries among workers (Rongen et al. 2013; Cooklin et al. 2016). Workplace health promotion reduces illness-related absenteeism, increases productivity and competitiveness, and is an important component of modern economic and industrial policy (International Union for Health Promotion and Education 2000).

- *SDG 10 (reducing inequalities)*: Health promotion programs can narrow health disparities by addressing risks in vulnerable groups, such as individuals with mental health challenges, at-risk youth, individuals with disabilities, and marginalized populations such as indigenous groups (Barry et al. 2013; Heller et al. 2014; McCalman et al. 2014; Petersen et al. 2016).

- *SDGs 11–13 (sustainable cities and communities, responsible consumption and production, and climate change)*: Responsible stewardship of common-pool resources requires public health practices that promote shared understanding of the system's interrelatedness (Ostrom et al. 1994). Community engagement to address the complexities of the animal-human ecosystem can have major implications for human health, especially in the face of climate change (Bowen and Ebi 2015). "One health" approaches relying on strong public health surveillance, policy, and partnerships with communities have improved outcomes ranging from human zoonotic disease burden to livestock illness to economic outcomes (Baum et al. 2017).

- *SDG 16 (peace, justice, and strong institutions)*: Literature on health promotion, policy development, and community engagement shows that when these public health functions are strong, marginalized groups gain a voice, violence is reduced, working conditions become safer, women's health and well-being can improve, educational opportunities can increase, hunger can diminish, and the sustainability of the environment can be addressed (Rifkin 1996, 2014; International Union for Health Promotion and Education 2000; Ismail et al. 2003; Commission on Social Determinants of Health 2008; Tontisirin and Bhattacharjee 2008; Beets et al. 2009; Li et al. 2011; World Health Organization 2011b, 2014a; McCoy et al. 2012; Barry et al. 2013; Institute of Medicine 2013; Kenny et al. 2013; Rongen et al. 2013; Heller et al. 2014; McCalman et al. 2014; Bowen and Ebi 2015; Edmunds and Albritton 2015; George et al. 2015; Langford et al. 2015; Newman et al. 2015; Cooklin et al. 2016; Petersen et al. 2016; Shackleton et al. 2016).

- *SDG 17 (partnerships for the goals)*: Public health functions related to community mobilization and policy development across sectors represent partnerships for sustainable development (Gilson et al. 2007). These functions embody the targets of SDG 17.

Monitoring and Assuring Functions

Monitoring and assuring functions that enable and execute policies, programs, and systems designed also contribute to community well-being in an essential way. Evidence for each of these EPHFs has important implications for achieving health- and non-health-related SDGs.

SURVEILLANCE AND MONITORING

In order to facilitate success in carrying out policy development functions as described earlier, monitoring and surveillance must also be performed. Collection of data is recognized as a central tenet of achieving the 2030 Sustainable Development agenda, not only for monitoring the SDGs but also for driving action (Durand 2015). The surveillance and monitoring functions ensure that the data needed for measurement of health status, quality of life, health inequalities, disease burden (including infectious disease warnings), and the social and environmental determinants of health that contribute to health outcomes across communities are captured and monitored over time. Surveillance and monitoring systems created and maintained by public health departments provide the information needed for quantifying and tracking the magnitude of threats to health that cross many of the SDGs. Data are typically gathered locally at the community and facility levels but can be aggregated at district, state, and national levels to track SDG progress (Thomas et al. 2016). Measurement and monitoring systems are the basis for measuring progress and developing action plans to achieve SDGs through carrying out policy development functions (World Health Organization 2015).

Surveillance systems built for health can be modified to collect and identify health threats across the range of SDGs, from bioterrorism risks to domestic violence incidents to climate change, in addition to tracking health-related outcomes such as maternal and child mortality. Improving surveillance systems to include measures for climate change, sustainability, water and sanitation, poverty, hunger, and disease information results in systems that can be actionable for both health- and non-health-related SDGs (Pan American Health Organization 2001; Bravata et al. 2004; South Africa Every Death Counts Writing Groups 2008; World Health Organization 2015; Moulton and Schramm 2017).

ASSURANCE FUNCTIONS OF PUBLIC HEALTH

The remaining EPHFs are those that enable and assure that policies, programs, and systems are effectively carried out and functioning in ways that protect and ensure health. These functions include enforcement of laws and regulations that protect public health, ensuring equitable access to health services; guaranteeing a strong public health workforce and assuring effectiveness, accessibility, and quality of primary care and other preventive services. Evidence for each of these EPHFs has important implications for achieving health- and non-health-related SDGs.

More specifically, public health laws and regulations contribute to many SDGs by protecting the environment, ensuring industry regulation of pollutants, helping prevent morbidity and premature death, reducing injury-related morbidity and deaths, and also promoting sustainable environments, reducing violence, and creating safer neighborhoods (Wang et al. 2014; Slovic et al. 2015; Sabel et al 2016). The SDG agenda specifically calls for universal health coverage (SDG 3.8) to achieve stronger health systems, and the actions needed to ensure equitable access to services contributes to this goal as well as to the achievement of non-health-specific SDG targets, from SDG 1 and 2 (no poverty and no hunger) to SDG 5 (gender equality), SDG 10 (reduced inequalities), and SDG 17 (partnerships for the goals) (Rantala et al. 2014; Baum et al. 2009). SDG 3c specifically focuses on substantially increasing the recruitment, development, training, and retention of the health workforce, and achievement of this target must include training a strong public health workforce; it cannot be limited to clinical context alone for the SDG agenda to be successful (Schmidt et al. 2015; World Health Organization 2014b). Public health departments that develop strong working relationships with personal health care service delivery organizations can improve resource efficiency in the delivery of preventive services, which contributes significantly to SDG 10 (reducing inequalities), in addition to SDG 3 (health and well-being for all) (Boelen 2000). Preparing for disasters is an assurance function with the potential to reduce impacts including morbidity, mortality, and damage resulting from disasters, and is critical to the achievement of SDGs ranging from 6 (clean water and sanitation) to 11 (sustainable cities and communities) to 16 (peace, justice, and strong institutions) (Norris et al. 2008; Gursky et al. 2012; Lumpkin et al. 2013; Gil-Rivas et al. 2016; Jha et al. 2016; Skryabina et al. 2017). Together, the assurance functions of public health are critical for success in policy development and mobilization of communities while also contributing to success in achieving many of the other SDGs.

Parallels and Overlap between the Sustainable Development Goals and Primary Health Care's Public Health Contribution

The public health component of PHC is responsible for monitoring, reviewing, and facilitating action on the factors that affect health based on local epidemiology, capabilities, and political feasibility. Each one of the tasks of public health is represented in the seventeen SDGs. Public health practice requires partnerships to make progress on issues as complex as these. Its progress comes from connecting communities, NGOs, vertical health programs, and non-health-sector actors, such as development agencies, departments of transportation and urban planning, environmental agencies, and others that seek solutions for addressing the determinants of health (Centers for Disease Control and Prevention 2014; 69th World Health Assembly 2016; Martin-Moreno et al. 2016).

At a more granular level, we can enumerate the SDGs to show how public health can address each of them (table 5.1).

Differences between the Sustainable Development Goals and the Direct Responsibilities of Public Health

The SDGs are broad and cover many domains that are outside of public health's direct realm of responsibility. While some SDGs explicitly address health goals, others that were not specifically related to health still have indicators that relate directly to the actions of public health. Some SDGs, such as SDG 4 ("Ensure inclusive and equitable quality education and promote lifelong learning opportunities for all"), have no measures that are directly linked to health, per se (United Nations 2015). Nevertheless, public health still plays a role in these functions. For example, child health is a predictor of school attendance and educational opportunities; therefore, public health actions that improve child health and well-being can still lead to improvements in this SDG, even without measurement of health-specific indicators within this SDG (Suhrcke and de Paz Nieves 2011).

If PHC is functioning well in a community, there would be capacity in collecting epidemiological data on health and its determinants, and there would be efforts in building cross-community partnerships and offering advocacy for measures to protect human flourishing. A high-functioning public health department is integral to PHC and as such can be a valuable contributor to all SDGs, including those that are only secondarily related to health. One of the key messages of the SDG agenda is that multisector action

Table 5.1. Linking Sustainable Development Goal (SDG) indicators to strong essential public health functions

SDG	*How Better Public Health Practice Advances This Goal*
1. End poverty in all forms everywhere	Proper public health practice must convene a community—breaking down class barriers that perpetuate poverty.
2. End hunger, achieve food security and improved nutrition, and promote sustainable agriculture	Public health has a proven track record of identifying food-insecure households and addressing root causes.
3. Ensure healthy lives and promote well-being for all ages	Life course perspective taken by public health guides collection of data and policy formation to maximize health and well-being.
4. Ensure inclusive and equitable quality education and promote lifelong learning opportunities for all	Health influences learning outcomes and school attendance. Health promotion in communities and schools can help keep kids healthy to attend school and can help children develop healthier lifestyles.
5. Achieve gender equality and empower all women and girls	Whole population perspective. Historically, public health actions taken on maternal and child health concerns evolve into inclusion and equality for women and girls.
6. Ensure availability and sustainable management of water and sanitation for all	Ensuring safe water and sanitation are core services of public health.
7. Ensure access to affordable, reliable, sustainable, and modern energy for all	Public health specialists have data and expertise to keep energy solutions environmentally sustainable.
8. Promote sustained, inclusive, and sustainable economic growth, full and productive employment, and decent work for all	Public health expertise in occupational health and safety assures that workplaces are decent.
9. Build resilient infrastructure, promote inclusive and sustainable industrialization, and foster innovation	Public health should be consulted as infrastructure and industry develop through a Health in All Policies approach to ensuring development efforts promote health and well-being in communities.
10. Reduce inequality within and among countries	Public health interventions use data to target those who are more vulnerable in order to reduce disparities.
11. Make cities and human settlements inclusive, safe, resilient, and sustainable	Cities without public health functions are uninhabitable. From controlling vermin to violence and involving residents in solutions, public health is key to "one health" solutions that address the intersection of animal human ecosystem health.

Continued

Table 5.1. continued

SDG	How Better Public Health Practice Advances This Goal
12. Ensure sustainable consumption and production patterns	Public health engages communities in understanding and addressing how sedentary lifestyles and overconsumption threaten health.
13. Take urgent action to combat climate change and its impacts	Public health experts help communities form and execute preparedness planning for extreme weather events unleashed by climate change.
14. Conserve and sustainably use the oceans, seas, and marine resources for sustainable development	Public health can educate communities on their role in ocean conservation and sustainability, and can address local human and environmental conflicts that undermine ocean conservation through convening communities for problem-solving and action.
15. Protect, restore, and promote sustainable use of terrestrial ecosystems, sustainably manage forests, combat desertification, and halt and reverse land degradation and halt biodiversity loss	Public health convenes communities and creates platforms from which "One Health" initiatives that protect animals, humans, and the environment can be mobilized.
16. Promote peaceful and inclusive societies for sustainable development, provide access to justice for all, and build effective, accountable, and inclusive institutions at all levels	Because proper public health practice must build circles of inclusive community engagement, it uses a universally shared concern for health as a springboard for accountability in other sectors.
17. Strengthen the means of implementation and revitalize the global partnership for sustainable development	Public health community is a global platform for sharing best practices in implementing all of the aforementioned ways to achieve the SDGs.

is essential to achievement of each of the goals. While each SDG does not explicitly call for public health action, empowering public health departments to collect data, convene partnerships, and mobilize communities to act creates a platform from which all SDGs can be strengthened.

This keystone role for public health in PHC was envisioned by the authors of the Alma-Ata Declaration. Article VII of the declaration stipulates that "primary health care reflects and evolves from the economic conditions and sociocultural and political characteristics of the country and its communities and is based on the application of the relevant results of social, biomedical and health services research and public health experience." It demands the coordination of efforts across agriculture, animal husbandry, food, industry, education, housing, public works, communications, and other sectors. Moreover, the public health component of PHC promotes "maximum community and individual self-reliance and participation in the planning, organization, operation and control of primary health care" (World Health Organization 1978, 2).

Conclusions: Linking Sustainable Development Goals to Public Health Improvement

The leaders who met in Alma-Ata in 1978 saw "health for all" as emerging from communities' ability to continuously adapt to achieve harmonious co-existence of humans and their planet. Although the label *primary health care* might mislead some to think only of medical services, the detailed Alma-Ata goals are as large as the fullest aspirations of the authors of the SDGs. This chapter has fleshed out the details of PHC in terms of the EPHFs that were developed in the 1990s as a benchmarking system. The broad scope of public health practice allowed this chapter to show a point-by-point alignment between stronger public health practice and achieving each one of the seventeen SDGs.

The need for a focus on public health strengthening has never been greater. Achieving the SDG agenda, minimizing the harms of the next pandemic, and responding to a coming century of preventable noncommunicable diseases (NCDs) are all compelling reasons to make the public health workforce more capable. This chapter shows that while there may not be a global blueprint for achieving the SDGs, there is a way for each community to find local solutions to their own sustainable development by improving public health workers' ability to perform each of the EPHFs. The public health workforce is already on site. They need to be coached toward recognizing and improving their performance as local conveners and leaders of sustainable development.

Ensuring that all people have access to high-quality public health practice–oriented services is essential to achieving the SDGs. Public health agencies, which are capable of collecting and using data to drive health promotion campaigns, are a basic necessity for improvements in health- and non-health-related indicators. The ability of public health units to convene communities and work collectively with other sectors to carry out health promotion and education campaigns, to develop HiAP approaches, and to create strong community platforms from which interventions can be delivered can significantly improve indicators that relate to both health- and non-health-specific SDGs (Rifkin 1996, 2014; International Union for Health Promotion and

Education 2000; Ismail et al. 2003; Commission on Social Determinants of Health 2008; Tontisirin and Bhattacharjee 2008; Beets et al. 2009; Li et al. 2011; World Health Organization 2011b, 2014a; McCoy et al. 2012; Barry et al. 2013; Institute of Medicine 2013; Kenny et al. 2013; Rongen et al. 2013; Heller et al. 2014; McCalman et al. 2014; Bowen and Ebi 2015; Edmunds and Albritton 2015; George et al. 2015; Langford et al. 2015; Newman et al. 2015; Cooklin et al. 2016; Petersen et al. 2016; Shackleton et al. 2016). Public health has the potential to improve indicators that cross each of the seventeen SDGs.

There is a clear financial, as well as a moral, case for strengthening public health. Public health strengthening can prevent the expensive and growing burden of NCDs. As the medical sector grows, the expense of every case of illness grows and the savings from prevention get bigger every year. New financial arrangements have led to global cost-sharing of the financial burden of disease. Further, the threat of NCDs, which the World Health Organization estimates will account for 80% of global mortality by 2020, requires strong leadership by public health to deliver on EPHFs to impact determinants of NCDs (Mathers and Loncar 2006; World Health Organization 2013b).

Strengthening public health practice supplies communities, districts, and nations with critical capabilities needed for SDG attainment. Linking public health strengthening to SDGs allows for a clearer picture of the role strong public health systems can play in achieving development targets across sectors and provides support for the need to launch a new global strategy that empowers public health departments worldwide to deliver leadership in EPHFs in support of the SDG agenda.

REFERENCES (SEE PAGE 341 FOR FULL CITATIONS FOR BOXED TEXT)

Barry, M. M., A. M. Clarke, R. Jenkins, and V. Patel. 2013. "A systematic review of the effectiveness of mental health promotion interventions for young people in low and middle income countries." *BMC Public Health* 13:835.

Baum, F. E., M. Begin, T. Houweling, and S. Taylor. 2009. "Changes not for the fainthearted: Reorienting health care systems toward health equity through action on the social determinants of health." *Am J Public Health* 99 (11): 1967–1974.

Baum, S. E. M., Catherine Machabala, Peter Daszak, Robert Salerno, and William Karesh. 2017. "Evaluating one health: Are we demonstrating effectiveness?" *One Health* 3:5–10.

Beets, M. W., B. R. Flay, S. Vuchinich, F. J. Snyder, A. Acock, K. K. Li, K. Burns, I. J. Washburn, and J. Durlack. 2009. "Use of a social and character development program to prevent substance use, violent behaviors, and sexual activity among elementary-school students in Hawaii." *Am J Public Health* 99 (8): 1438–1445.

Beracochea, E. 2015. *Improving aid in global health.* New York: Springer.

Bert, Fabrizio, Giacomo Scaioli, Maria Roasara Gualano, and Roberta Sillquini. 2015. "How can we bring public health in all policies? Strategies for healthy societies." *Journal of Public Health Research* 4 (1): 393.

Blas, E., Lucy Gilson, Michael P. Kelly, Ronald Labonté, Jostacio Lapitan, Carles Muntaner, Piroska Östlin, Jennie Popay, Ritu Sadana, Gita Sen, Ted Schrecker, and Ziba Vaghri. 2008. "Addressing social determinants of health inequities: What can the state and civil society do?" *Lancet* 372 (9650): 1684–1689.

Boelen, C. 2000. *Towards unity for health: Coordinating changes in health services and health professions practice and education.* Geneva: World Health Organization.

Bowen, Kathryn, and Kristie Ebi. 2015. "Governing the health risks of climate change towards multi-sector responses." *Curr Opin Environ Sustain* 12:80–85.

Bravata, D., Kathryn McDonald, Wendy Smith, Chara Rydzak, Herbert Szeto, David Buckeridge, Corinna Haberland, and Douglas Owens. 2004. "Systematic review: Surveillance systems for early detection of bioterrorism-related diseases." *Ann Intern Med* 140 (11): 910–922.

Centers for Disease Control and Prevention. 2014. "The public health system and the 10 essential public health services." Accessed October 21, 2016. http://www.cdc.gov/nphpsp/essentialservices.html.

Commission on Social Determinants of Health. 2008. *Closing the gap in a generation: Health equity through action on the social determinants of health.* Geneva: World Health Organization.

Cooklin, A., N. Joss, E. Husser, and B. Oldenburg. 2016. "Integrated approaches to occupational health and safety: A systematic review." *Am J Health Promot* 31 (5): 401–412.

Cyril, S., B. J. Smith, A. Possamai-Inesedy, and A. M. Renzaho. 2015. "Exploring the role of community engagement in improving the health of disadvantaged populations: A systematic review." *Glob Health Action* 8:29842.

Draper, A. K., G. Hewitt, and S. Rifkin. 2010. "Chasing the dragon: Developing indicators for the assessment of community participation in health programmes." *Soc Sci Med* 71 (6): 1102–1109.

Durand, M. 2015. "Getting the measure of the Sustainable Development Goals." *OECD Observer* 303:16–17.

Durbur Mahila Samanwaya Committee Theory and Action for Health Research Team. 2007. "Meeting community needs for HIV prevention and more: Intersectoral action for health in the Sonagachi red light area of Kolkata."

Edmunds, Margo, and Ellen Albritton. 2015. *Global public health systems innovations: A scan of promising practices.* Academy Health and Robert Wood Johnson Foundation. https://www.academyhealth.org/files/AH2015GlobalPublicHealthReport.pdf.

GBD 2015 SDG Collaborators. 2016. "Measuring the health related Sustainable Development Goals in 188 countries: A baseline analysis from the Global Burden of Disease Study 2015." *Lancet* 388:1813–1850.

George, A., K. Scott, S. Garimella, R. Mondal, R. Ved, and K. Sheikh. 2015. "Anchoring contextual analysis in health policy and systems research: A narrative review of contextual factors influencing health committees in low and middle income countries." *Soc Sci Med* 133:159–167.

Gil-Rivas, V., and R. P. Kilmer. 2016. "Building community capacity and fostering disaster resilience." *J Clin Psychol* 72 (12): 1318–1332.

Gilson, Lucy, Jane Doherty, Rene Loewenson, and Victoria Francis. 2007. *Challenging inequality through health systems.* World Health Organization Commission on Social Determinants of Health. https://www.who.int/social_determinants/resources /csdh_media/hskn_final_2007_en.pdf.

Goetzel, Ron, David Shechter, Ronald Ozminkowski, David Stapleton, Pauline Lapin, J. Michael McGinnis, Catherine Gordon, and Lester Breslow. 2007. "Can health promotion programs save Medicare money?" *Clin Interv Aging* 2 (1): 117–122.

Gogia, S., and H. S. Sachdev. 2010. "Home visits by community health workers to prevent neonatal deaths in developing countries: A systematic review." *Bull World Health Organ* 88 (9): 658B–666B.

Gostin, L. O., and E. A. Friedman. 2015. "The Sustainable Development Goals: One-health in the world's development agenda." *JAMA* 314 (24): 2621–2622.

Gursky, E. A., and G. Bice. 2012. "Assessing a decade of public health preparedness: Progress on the precipice?" *Biosecur Bioterror* 10 (1): 55–65.

Guyer, Bernard, Sai Ma, Holly Grason, Kevin Frick, Deborah Perry, Alyssa Sharkey, and Jennifer McIntosh. 2009. "Early childhood health promotion and its life course health consequences." *Acad Pediatr* 9 (3): 142–149.

Heller, T., D. Fisher, B. Marks, and K. Hsieh. 2014. "Interventions to promote health: Crossing networks of intellectual and developmental disabilities and aging." *Disabil Health J* 7 (1 Suppl.): S24–S32.

Howard, Rob, and Stephen Gunther. 2012. *Health in All Policies: An EU literature review 2006–2011 and interview with key stakeholders.* http://chrodis.eu/wp-content /uploads/2015/04/HiAP-Final-Report.pdf.

Institute of Medicine. 2013. *Public health linkages with sustainability: Workshop summary.* Washington, DC: National Academies Press.

International Union for Health Promotion and Education. 2000. *The evidence of health promotion effectiveness: Shaping public health in New Europe.* Luxembourg: European Commission.

Ismail, Suraiya, Maarten Immink, Irela Mazar, and Guy Nantel. 2003. *Community-based food and nutrition programmes: What makes them successful.* Food and Agriculture Organization of the United Nations. http://www.fao.org/3/a-y5030e .pdf.

Jack, H. E., S. D. Arabadjis, L. Sun, E. E. Sullivan, and R. S. Phillips. 2017. "Impact of community health workers on use of healthcare services in the United States: A systematic review." *J Gen Intern Med* 32 (3): 325–344.

Jha, A., R. Basu, and A. Basu. 2016. "Studying policy changes in disaster management in India: A tale of two cyclones." *Disaster Med Public Health Prep* 10 (1): 42–46.

Kaspin, L. C., K. M. Gorman, and R. M. Miller. 2013. "Systematic review of employer-sponsored wellness strategies and their economic and health-related outcomes." *Popul Health Manag* 16 (1): 14–21.

Kenny, Amanda, Nerida Hyett, John Sawtell, Virginia Dickson-Swift, Jane Farmer, and Peter O'Meara. 2013. "Community participation in rural health: A scoping review." *BMC Health Serv Res* 13 (64). https://bmchealthservres.biomedcentral.com/articles /10.1186/1472-6963-13-64.

Kickbusch, Ilona, and David Gleicher. 2012. *Governance for health in the 21st century*. World Health Organization. http://www.euro.who.int/__data/assets/pdf_file/0019/171334/RC62BD01-Governance-for-Health-Web.pdf?ua=1.

Langford, Rebecca, Christopher Bonell, Hayley Jones, Theodora Pouliou, Simon Murphy, Elizabeth Waters, Kelli Komro, Lisa Gibbs, Daniel Magnus, and Rona Campbell. 2015. "The World Health Organization's Health Promoting Schools framework: A Cochrane systematic review and meta-analysis." *BMC Public Health* 15 (130): https://bmcpublichealth.biomedcentral.com/articles/10.1186/s12889-015 -1360-y.

Lassi, Z. S., and Z. A. Bhutta. 2015. "Community-based intervention packages for reducing maternal and neonatal morbidity and mortality and improving neonatal outcomes." *Cochrane Database Syst Rev* (11): CD007754.

Lawn, J. E., J. Rohde, S. Rifkin, M. Were, V. K. Paul, and M. Chopra. 2008. "Alma-Ata 30 years on: Revolutionary, relevant, and time to revitalise." *Lancet* 372 (9642): 917–927.

Li, K. K., I. Washburn, D. L. DuBois, S. Vuchinich, P. Ji, V. Brechling, J. Day, M. W. Beets, A. C. Acock, M. Berbaum, F. Synder, and B. R. Flay. 2011. "Effects of the Positive Action programme on problem behaviours in elementary school students: A matched-pair randomised control trial in Chicago." *Psychol Health* 26 (2): 187–204.

Lumpkin, J. R., Y. K. Miller, T. Inglesby, J. M. Links, A. T. Schwartz, C. C. Slemp, R. L. Burhans, J. Blumenstock, and A. S. Khan. 2013. "The importance of establishing a national health security preparedness index." *Biosecur Bioterror* 11 (1): 81–87.

Martin-Moreno, J. M., M. Harris, E. Jakubowski, and H. Kluge. 2016. "Defining and assessing public health functions: A global analysis." *Annu Rev Public Health* 37: 335–355.

Mathers, C. D., and D. Loncar. 2006. "Projections of global mortality and burden of disease from 2002 to 2030." *PLoS Med* 3 (11): e442.

McCalman, Janya, Tsey Komla, Roxanne Bainbridge, Kevin Rowley, Nikki Percival, Lynette O'Donoghue, Jenny Brands, Mary Whiteside, and Jenni Judd. 2014. "The characteristics, implementation and effects of Aboriginal and Torres Strait Islander health promotion tools: A systematic literature search." *BMC Public Health* 14 (712): https://bmcpublichealth.biomedcentral.com/articles/10.1186/1471-2458-14 -712.

McCoy, D. C., J. A. Hall, and M. Ridge. 2012. "A systematic review of the literature for evidence on health facility committees in low- and middle-income countries." *Health Policy Plan* 27 (6): 449–466.

McQueen, David V., Matthias Wismar, Vivian Lin, Catherine M. Jones, and Maggie Davies. 2012. *Intersectoral governance for Health in All Policies: Structures, actions, and experiences*. Copenhagen: World Health Organization.

Meier, Benjamin Mason, Caitlin Pardue, and Leslie London. 2012. "Implementing community participation through legislative reform: A study of the policy framework for community participation in Western Cape province of South Africa." *BMC International Health and Human Rights* 12 (15). https://bmcinthealthhumrights .biomedcentral.com/articles/10.1186/1472-698X-12-15.

Moulton, A. D., and P. J. Schramm. 2017. "Climate change and public health surveillance: Toward a comprehensive strategy." *J Public Health Manag Pract* 23 (6): 618–626.

Newman, L., F. Baum, S. Javanparast, K. O'Rourke, and L. Carlon. 2015. "Addressing social determinants of health inequities through settings: A rapid review." *Health Promot Int* 30 (Suppl. 2): ii126–ii143.

Norris, F. H., S. P. Stevens, B. Pfefferbaum, K. F. Wyche, and R. L. Pfefferbaum. 2008. "Community resilience as a metaphor, theory, set of capacities, and strategy for disaster readiness." *Am J Community Psychol* 41 (1–2): 127–150.

Nugroho, J. S., and D. Sriyantini. 2016. "Political Reconstruction Law Society Building Policy Action Alert Healthy Prosperous and Dignified in Making Healthy Generation of Gold in the District Lumajang." IOSR *J Humanities Soc Sci* 21 (11): 10–14. http://iosrjournals.org/iosr-jhss/papers/Vol.%2021%20Issue11/Version-4/C2111041014.pdf.

Ostrom, E., R. Gardner, and J. Walker. 1994. *Rules, games, and common-pool resources.* Ann Arbor: University of Michigan Press.

Pan American Health Organization. 2001. *Experiences with the inclusion of sexual violence indicators in the health information and surveillance systems of Bolivia, Ecuador, and Peru.* Washington, DC: World Health Organization.

———. 2015. *Health in all policies: Case studies from the region of the Americas.* Washington, DC: World Health Organization.

Perrier L., and K. Shankardass. 2011. *Getting started with Health in All Policies: A resource pack.* https://pdfs.semanticscholar.org/9fe8/31a0209bf8a8d36e6290cc1a6e8 0687a8b14.pdf?_ga=2.215866007.1870300363.1568036952-1993406079 .1568036952.

Petersen, I., S. Evans-Lacko, M. Semrau, M. M. Barry, D. Chisholm, P. Gronholm, C. O. Egbe, and G. Thornicroft. 2016. "Promotion, prevention and protection: Interventions at the population- and community-levels for mental, neurological and substance use disorders in low- and middle-income countries." *Int J Ment Health Syst* 10:30.

Rantala, R., M. Bortz, and F. Armada. 2014. "Intersectoral action: Local governments promoting health." *Health Promot Int* 29 (Suppl. 1): i92–i102.

Rifkin, S. B. 1996. "Paradigms lost: Toward a new understanding of community participation in health programmes." *Acta Tropica* 61 (2): 79–92.

———. 2014. "Examining the links between community participation and health outcomes: A review of the literature." *Health Policy and Planning* 29 (Suppl. 2): ii98–i106.

Rohde, J., S. Cousens, M. Chopra, V. Tangcharoensathien, R. Black, Z. A. Bhutta, and J. E. Lawn. 2008. "30 years after Alma-Ata: Has primary health care worked in countries?" *Lancet* 372 (9642): 950–961.

Rongen, A., S. J. Robroek, F. J. van Lenthe, and A. Burdorf. 2013. "Workplace health promotion: A meta-analysis of effectiveness." *Am J Prev Med* 44 (4): 406–415.

Rudolph, Linda, Julia Caplan, Connie Mitchell, Karen Ben-Moshe, and Lianne Dillon. 2013. *Health in All Policies: Improving health through intersectoral collaboration.* Institute of Medicine of the National Academies. https://www.phi.org/uploads /application/files/q79jnmxq5krx9qiu5j6gzdnl6g9s41l65co2ir1kz0lvmx67to.pdf.

Russell, Nancy, Susan Ingras, Nalin Johri, Henrietta Kuoh, Melinda Pavin, and Jane Wickstrom. 2008. *The Active Community Engagement Continuum.* USAID, ACQUIRE Project. http://www.acquireproject.org/fileadmin/user_upload/ACQUIRE /Publications/ACE-Working-Paper-final.pdf.

Sabel, C. E., R. Hiscock, A. Asikainen, J. Bi, M. Depledge, S. Van Den Elshout, R. Friedrich, G. Huang, F. Hurley, M. Jantunen, and S. P. Karakitsios. 2016. "Public health impacts of city policies to reduce climate change: Findings from the URGENCHE EU-China project." *Environ Health* 15 (Suppl. 1): 25.

Schmidt, Harald, Lawrence O. Gostin, and Ezekiel J. Emanuel. 2015. "Public health, universal health coverage, and Sustainable Development Goals: Can they coexist?" *Lancet* 386 (9996): 928–930.

Shackleton, N., F. Jamal, R. M. Viner, K. Dickson, G. Patton, and C. Bonell. 2016. "School-based interventions going beyond health education to promote adolescent health: Systematic review of reviews." *J Adolesc Health* 58 (4): 382–396.

Sherry, Melissa, Abdul Ghaffar, and David Bishai. 2017. "Community platforms for public health interventions." In *Disease control priorities: Improving health and reducing poverty*, 3rd edition, edited by Dean T. Jamison, Hellen Gelband, Susan Horton, Prabhat Jha, Ramanan Laxminarayan, Charles N. Mock, and Rachel Nugent, 267–284. Washington, DC: World Bank.

69th World Health Assembly. 2016. *Strengthening essential public health functions in support of the achievement of universal health coverage*. World Health Assembly, May 27.

Skryabina, Elena, Gabriel Reedy, Richard Amlot, Peter Jaye, and Paul Riley. 2017. "What is the value of health emergency preparedness exercises? A scoping review study." *Int J Disaster Risk Reduct* 21:274–283.

Slovic, Anne Dorothée, Maria Aparecida de Oliveira, João Biehl, and Helena Ribeiro. 2015. "How can urban policies improve air quality and help mitigate global climate change: A systematic mapping review." *J Urban Health* 93 (1): 73–95.

South Africa Every Death Counts Writing Groups. 2008. "Every death counts: Use of mortality audit data for decision making to save the lives of mothers, babies, and children in South Africa." *Lancet* 371 (9620): 1294–1304.

Suhrcke, Marc, and Carmen de Paz Nieves. 2011. *The impact of health and health behaviours on educational outcomes in high-income countries: A review of the evidence*. Copenhagen: WHO Regional Office for Europe.

Sururi, Nazarus, Heru Ribawanto, and Mochammad Rozikin. n.d. "Movement of building healthy communities as innovation in health care in villages Citrodiwangsan Lumajang Subdistrict." *J Public Adm* 1 (2): 238–247.

Thomas, J. C., E. Silvestre, S. Salentine, H. Reynolds, and J. Smith. 2016. "What systems are essential to achieving the Sustainable Development Goals and what will it take to marshal them?" *Health Policy Plan* 31 (10): 1445–1447.

Tiwari, Reena, Marina Veronica Lommerse, and Dianne Smith. 2014. *M2 models and methodologies for community engagement*. Singapore: Springer.

Tontisirin, K., and L. Bhattacharjee. 2008. "Community based approaches to prevent and control malnutrition." *Asia Pac J Clin Nutr* 17 (Suppl. 1): 106–110.

UKAID and DFID Human Resource Development Centre. 2011. *Helpdesk report: Community engagement in health service delivery*. http://www.heart-resources.org/wp-content/uploads/2011/11/Community-Engagement-in-Health-Service-Delivery-November-2011.pdf.

United Nations. 2015. *Sustainable Development Knowledge Platform*. https://sustainabledevelopment.un.org/index.html. Accessed January 12, 2017.

Wang, S., J. Xing, B. Zhao, C. Jang, and J. Hao. 2014. "Effectiveness of national air pollution control policies on the air quality in metropolitan areas of China." *J Environ Sci (China)* 26 (1): 13–22.

White, M. I., C. E. Dionne, O. Wärje, M. Koehoorn, S. L. Wagner, I. Z. Shultz, C. Koehn, K. Williams-Whitt, H. G. Harder, R. Pasca, R; V. Hsu, L. McGuire, W. Shulz, D. Kube, and M. D. Wright. 2016. "Physical activity and exercise interventions in the workplace impacting work outcomes: Stakeholder-centered best evidence synthesis of systematic reviews." *Int J Occup Environ Med* 7:61–74.

World Health Organization. 1978. "The Alma Ata Conference on primary health care." *WHO Chronicle* 32:409–430.

———. 1978. *Alma-Ata Declaration on primary health care, Article VII*. Geneva: World Health Organization. https://www.who.int/publications/almaata_declaration_en.pdf.

———. 2011a. *Global status report on noncommunicable diseases 2010*. https://apps.who.int/iris/bitstream/handle/10665/44579/9789240686458_eng.pdf?sequence=1.

———. 2011b. *Social determinants approaches to public health: From concept to practice*. https://www.who.int/social_determinants/tools/SD_Publichealth_eng.pdf.

———. 2013a. *Demonstrating a health in all polices analytic framework for learning from experiences. Based on literature reviews from Africa, South-East Asia and the Western Pacific*. https://apps.who.int/iris/bitstream/handle/10665/104083/9789241506274_eng.pdf;jsessionid=63ABA64847E96FE510F5BE9E733CA0F6?sequence=1.

———. 2013b. *Global Action Plan for the Prevention and Control of NCDs 2013–2020*. https://apps.who.int/iris/bitstream/handle/10665/94384/9789241506236_eng.pdf?sequence=1.

———. 2013c. *Health in All Policies: Seizing opportunities, implementing policies*. http://www.euro.who.int/__data/assets/pdf_file/0007/188809/Health-in-All-Policies-final.pdf?ua=1.

———. 2014a. *Health in All Policies: Helsinki Statement. Framework for Country Action*. https://apps.who.int/iris/bitstream/handle/10665/112636/9789241506908_eng.pdf?sequence=1.

———. 2014b. *Health in All Policies (HiAP) framework for country action*. https://www.who.int/cardiovascular_diseases/140120HPRHiAPFramework.pdf.

———. 2015. *Health in 2015 from MDGs, the Millennium Development Goals to SDGs, Sustainable Development Goals*. https://apps.who.int/iris/bitstream/handle/10665/200009/9789241565110_eng.pdf?sequence=1.

CHAPTER SIX

Four Principles of Community-Based Primary Health Care

Support, Appreciate, Learn/Listen, Transfer (SALT)

Marlou De Rouw, Alice Kuan, Philip Forth, Rituu B. Nanda, and Luc Barrière Constantin

Is it possible to imagine a world where individuals and communities recognize and respect their common humanity and live out their full potential to contribute to society as a whole?
—*The Constellation (2016)*

When communities take ownership of their health challenges, they take action to overcome them. Ownership drives action that will not be dependent on external stimulus; it is the foundation of sustainability.

In various priority issues, such as maternal and child health or the human immunodeficiency virus/acquired immunodeficiency syndrome (HIV/AIDS), the global health agenda emphasizes the importance of communicating and building partnerships with the communities affected by these issues. This community-based focus could generate solutions where community members participate in a health intervention, and this is often exemplified by the recruiting and training of community health workers to perform safe practices and promote health within their social circles. The term *community*, therefore, is used generously in delineating its significance to health program interventions. However, while global health stakeholders have used the term to a seemingly infinite extent, truly comprehending its meaning is a major challenge. Understanding who is considered part of a community and how they are bound together is a complex task due to the layers of nuanced history and evolution that shape how community members thrive as a group.

There are aspects of communities that can be clearly observed and delineated. On the most basic level, communities are made up of people who are geographically close to one another. They live in the same location and are thus affected by the same issues impacting a certain area. Through daily proximity and interaction, community members build relationships with one another, naturally amplifying their mutual trust, recognition of shared concerns, and ability to work together to solve shared problems. Community members can build on each other's ability to create effective, realistic solutions that are aligned with the structures of their governance, culture, and values.

Stories of communities in this chapter exhibit a fluid definition of the term. Community boundaries vary depending on countless contextual factors regarding the identity of peoples who share common values, trust, and concerns in their daily lives. However, all the communities we discuss have undergone a learning process that enabled them to be more effective in using their own assets to create solutions. They illustrate community engagement as a participatory process in a cycle of problem-solving. These stories demonstrate how empowerment means community members realizing and acting on their potential to take ownership of challenges that they face collectively. Owning challenges brings responsibility to articulate their root causes and then to work toward solving the challenges with collective strengths to meet collective needs.

The approach we describe and illustrate here has been shown to be helpful across a wide spectrum of issues including child health, maternal health, nutrition, cholera, diabetes, Ebola, AIDS, malaria, poliomyelitis, water, sanitation and hygiene, palliative care, sexual and reproductive health, drugs, suicide prevention, and aging with dignity. Combined, these reflect a continuum of comprehensive, community-engaged, primary health care (PHC), as fully articulated in both the Alma-Ata and Astana Declarations. It is precisely in PHC where communities have an inevitable role to play—a role that is often forgotten but must now resurface as a recognized driving force in defining priorities, co-managing health facilities, creating demand, and engaging people to uptake needed health services to achieve PHC.

Truly successful PHC requires internal and central trust-building that begins with the people themselves, giving them the ability, the voice, and the equal playing field to become a part of the solution. The issues communities face every day are direct reflections of what needs to be improved in health systems. Their struggles are direct demonstrations that they should be included in designing the solutions to their problems, because they have lived with them and therefore have personal knowledge of what should be done about the problem. As a result, an inevitable link forms between PHC and communities that benefit from it.

We present three case studies in which communities have taken ownership of their health challenges. These case studies stress two principles that underpin the development of the community as it takes ownership of its challenge. The first principle asserts that *we appreciate strengths rather than analyze weaknesses.* When a community comes to appreciate its strengths, it can act based on those strengths to improve its situation. That improvement can become the basis for systematic action that moves the community toward its shared objective. The second principle asserts that *a community can take sustainable action only when its members recognize that they have a shared interest in a better future.* This recognition *comes through dialogue.* Dialogue requires that the many voices of the community are heard and listened to. The dialogue can produce coherent community action when all members of the community feel that their concerns have been recognized in the plans that the community makes.

Ownership, Appreciation, and Coherence

Ownership means that the community decides on the action it wishes to take and that it takes this action. Ownership does not mean the rejection of resources that outside organizations can bring to support the individual and the community. However, there is a world of difference between outside experts telling people what they need to do and people asking for the resources and expertise they need to execute their own plans.

Ownership is not the definition of *empowerment*, though it is certainly an aspect of empowerment. Ownership implies more than consultation and engagement. Figure 6.1 develops the path to ownership in the context of Arnstein's (1969) ladder of participation: The ladder makes the point that there are gradations in participation in the depth and range of redistribution of power. Ownership goes beyond consultation, engagement, and empowerment. This understanding dates back to Article VII of the Alma-Ata Declaration, which states: "Primary health care . . . requires and promotes maximum community and individual self-reliance and participation in the planning, organization, operation and control of PHC, making fullest use of local, national and other available resources; and to this end develops through appropriate education the ability of communities to participate."

The communities take ownership using a learning cycle. In this cycle, groups think about the actions that they intend to take, take those actions, and then reflect on the outcome of those actions with a view to improvement.

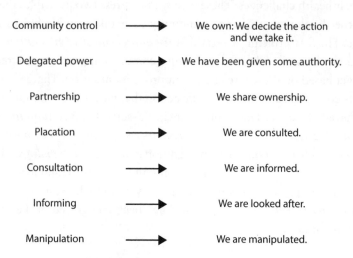

Rungs on the Arnstein Ladder		The Path to Community Ownership
Community control	⟶	We own: We decide the action and we take it.
Delegated power	⟶	We have been given some authority.
Partnership	⟶	We share ownership.
Placation	⟶	We are consulted.
Consultation	⟶	We are informed.
Informing	⟶	We are looked after.
Manipulation	⟶	We are manipulated.

Figure 6.1. Arnstein's model of community participation. Source: Arnstein 1969

One early implementation of the learning cycle was through the Deming Cycle (plan, do, study, act), which is now widely used in industry after its introduction in Japan after the World War II (Deming 1967). Applications of the learning cycle have spread beyond industry in a variety of forms (see, e.g., Kolb and Fry 1975).

Collison and Parcell (2004) recognized that an essential aspect of any form of learning cycle was the conversation that supported each stage in the cycle. If the learning cycle is no more than a mechanical process or executed by a narrow subgroup on behalf of the community, it will fail. At each step in the learning cycle, one objective is to bring together the different perspectives that are found in all communities. The dialogue that is part of each step in the cycle seeks to establish a coherent view within the community that is an essential element of sustained progress. Broadening the participation in the learning cycle expands the portfolio of community assets to confront the challenges.

When a community appreciates the strengths that it already has, these strengths can be the basis of further actions. The advantages of the strengths-based approach in comparison with a more traditional, deficit-based approach has been called appreciative inquiry (Cooperrider and Srivastva 1987). Appreciating one's strength is a better spur to action than seeing only deficit.

When a community begins to use this form of a learning cycle, it needs the support of a facilitator who is experienced with the approach. In addition to helping the community apply the steps of the learning cycle, the facilitator supports the dialogue that develops a coherent view within the community and encourages the community to appreciate its own strengths. As time goes by, these skills develop within the community, and the need for an external facilitator fades away.

The Community Life Competence Process and SALT

In this chapter, we present three examples in which communities have used a learning cycle approach to improve their health situation in Botswana (HIV control), India (increase in the uptake of immunization), and Guinea/Liberia (restoring trust between communities and health care workers after Ebola).

Figure 6.2 shows the steps of the learning cycle that have been used in the examples. A precondition is becoming motivated by knowing that action can result in a healthier and more prosperous place to live. Many people live lives of resignation. They do not know or do not believe that anything can improve their community. Ownership of the knowledge and belief in possibility precedes moving into action. The purpose of the first steps is to stimulate that ownership and the ensuing actions. The steps in the learning cycle are preceded by a Step 0, in which the community must come together to establish a common identity grounded in mutual humanity. This augmented learning cycle is referred to in this chapter as the Community Life Competence Process (CLCP). Augmenting the learning cycle with an initial step of unification of shared identity is critical to achieve coherence in the formation and execution of the action plan.

In Step 1 of the CLCP, the community defines a "shared dream": the common objective for which the community will work.

In Step 2, the community defines its current position through a self-assessment. This is effective in stimulating productive dialogue within the community as members discuss their current position (Parcell and Collison 2009).

In Step 3, the community creates an action plan to move from its current situation to its desired situation.

In Step 4, the community carries out its action plan.

In Step 5, the community reflects on the progress that it has made to prepare for the next cycle. The community explores the lessons it has learned and the material that it can share with its peers to help them to progress.

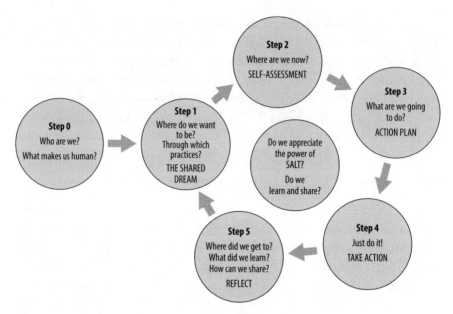

Figure 6.2. The community life competence process. SALT = support, appreciate, learn/listen, and transfer.

The style of facilitation reinforces the possibility that the community will take action. A challenge for the facilitator is to bring together a broad cross section of voices from within the community, many of which are rarely heard and even more rarely listened to. The discussion that arises within the structure of CLCP offers new perspectives. When these diverse perspectives are listened to with respect, this dialogue produces a broader view of the community challenge. We do not pretend that the community becomes united and takes action. Rather there is a coherence to the community perspective that opens the door to an agreed-upon set of actions, and the coherence can develop with those actions.

Botswana: Communities Acting Together to Control HIV

ALICE KUAN (JOHNS HOPKINS), MARLOU DE ROUW AND
RITUU B. NANDA (THE CONSTELLATION), WITH INPUT FROM
NAHPA BOTSWANA AND UNAIDS BOTSWANA

Communities Acting Together to Control HIV (CATCH) encourages citizens of Botswana to put their own strengths and resources toward the health and social issues they are facing.

Four Principles for Greater Community Ownership

Here we describe how facilitators support the community as it applies the Community Life Competency Process (CLCP) to face its challenges. The approach is based on four main principles: it *supports* the community, *appreciates* its strengths, *learns* from the community, and *transfers* what it learns to its peers.

The SALT Approach

SALT is an acronym that describes the mental model that facilitators use when they accompany communities through the CLCP, and it stands for support, appreciate, learn, and transfer. Traditional modes of education emphasize a passive receptive learner receiving knowledge from a teacher. Collaborative learning stresses discovery of a latent human ability to analyze problems and to find solutions to those problems. The SALT approach challenges everyone to leave the mind-set of teachers versus learners behind and to appreciate and develop strengths.

A central role of the facilitator in the CLCP is to ask questions that allow community members to recognize their strengths and achievements and to use them to take further action. Communities are usually only too well aware of their weaknesses; however, they are frequently unaware of their strengths.

The facilitator in the CLCP makes the community aware that it is not alone in working in this way on similar challenges and can make the links between communities so that they can share their experiences, their hopes, and their concerns with each other and learn from one another. Those links may be between neighboring villages, but with technology the links can be half a world away.

There are several contrasts between facilitation that is expert-led and facilitation that is based on the SALT acronym:

- Experts rely on their own expertise, while the SALT approach to facilitation focuses on the strengths of people and communities to respond.
- Experts rely on specialists to define the problem and offer the solution to the problem, while SALT facilitation reveals strengths so a community can come together to find solutions.
- Experts instruct and advise, while SALT facilitation emphasizes learning and sharing.

SALT facilitation supports the community as it moves toward ownership of its challenge.

Lamboray (2016) provides more details on the development of the SALT approach in his book *What Makes Us Human*. The Constellation website provides further discussion of the approach (https://www.communitylifecompetence.org/our-approach.html).

Although CATCH emerged from a concern for HIV, the community saw HIV in a broader light, helping them implement actions reaching far beyond the disease itself. Two success factors contributed to the enthusiasm of participants and the growth of the communities: (1) the involvement of traditional leaders and (2) a common tracking system.

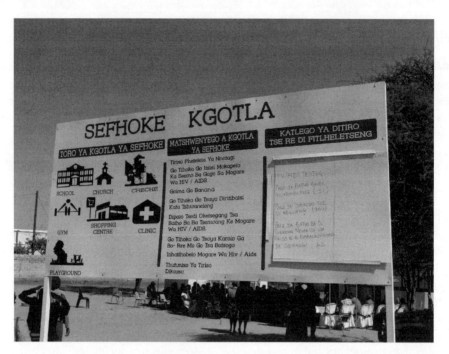

Figure 6.3. A CATCH dashboard in the Sefhoke Ward in Tlokweng, a village in the South-East District of Botswana. Source: National AIDS and Health Promotion Agency

At the start of CATCH, communities shared concerns over the proliferation of HIV/AIDS; they had not yet organized ownership of their behaviors and potential to tackle relevant problems. Throughout the process of CATCH, not only were they able to take ownership of the problem, but they also became active learning communities that defined their actions based on lessons received from one another. In CATCH, communities capture their own progress on so-called dashboards—painted billboards that are set up strategically within the locality. The boards are their way of expressing ownership of the actions toward their vision, showing the communities' dreams, action plans, progress, and achievements.

Participating communities revealed untapped ability to spread trust of the medical system through peer communication, and this had spillover effects beyond merely promoting HIV testing—defeating one obstacle often leads to overcoming other issues it has caused, as well as other related obstacles. Buy-in from the traditional leaders was crucial in forming strategic alliances to improve HIV screening and referral, and these alliances can evolve to serve other purposes. Some of the villages responded to CATCH in unexpected ways. Their stories illustrate the fruits of the communities' intrinsic strengths, their unified spirit, and what happens when they take control of their own health as a contribution to successful PHC.

Background: HIV/AIDS in Botswana

Botswana's people continue to confront a severe HIV epidemic, with 20.3% of adults aged 15–49 years old living with HIV (UNAIDS 2018). According to the National AIDS and Health Promotion Agency (NAHPA), many factors contribute to the epidemic, including multiple and concurrent sexual partnerships, intergenerational sex, alcohol and high-risk sex, stigma and discrimination, and gender-based violence (US President's Emergency Plan for AIDS Relief 2016).

Community-Based Strategy

CATCH was designed to expand grassroots HIV responses under traditional leadership and community-engaged planning and action. It exemplifies the CLCP approach of figure 6.2 to convene community members to identify local challenges and solutions. CATCH facilitators started with inclusion of community leaders, followed by introducing CATCH to communities. Facilitators undertook a series of home visits to appreciate individual hopes and concerns, and they scheduled community-wide conversations where villagers developed a common vision, identified collective issues and strengths, and planned and implemented activities toward the vision.

During every step in this process, CATCH opened the space for community members to trust one another and share information, creating a vital, community-specific dialogue—a core aspect of progressing toward effective PHC. In the Tlokweng and Ba-Ga-Malete communities, the top three strengths that communities discovered in themselves through active listening and conversation were knowledge about HIV, openness to discussion, and shared desire to see a positive change in behavior (The Constellation 2016). When they put those strengths to work, common actions implemented by the villagers themselves included community member promotion of HIV testing, the organization of health and wellness days, condom distribution, and the building of a youth center. As better systems of youth engagement and materials distribution arose out of local leadership in CATCH, communities also contributed an insistence to sustain the gains they made. During the process, the *kgosis*, the traditional village leaders, took on a leading role. Facilitators asked the simple but deep question "What are you proud of?"—and to respond, the kgosis rediscovered their assets as leaders and applied them to build enduring solutions.

Pogiso Botlhole, a traditional leader of Khudiring Ward in the Southeast District, was trained with seventy-four other chiefs in 2017. He recalled that at the outset not everyone in the community supported the CATCH project. Sometimes, villagers had questions about whether there were any personal benefits rather than shared benefits from participating in CATCH. To solve this, the Southeast District community and NAHPA hosted a knowledge share fair, in which villagers explored many initiatives regarding HIV and general health that had been started, led, and sustained by communities. Through this learning exchange, they came to appreciate and experience the SALT and CLCP methods by themselves, acknowledging the value of collective spirit and dialogue. After some time, Botlhole and other traditional leaders gained the support and trust of families for implementing this bottom-up approach. "SALT forms a bond with the people we visit; they may not change overnight but over time they will change," Botlhole remarked. "As per an old saying . . . it takes the whole village to raise a child" (Botlhole 2017).

When CATCH first started, Botlhole realized that the problem at hand was not merely the HIV epidemic. "When a person is diagnosed with HIV," Botlhole explains, "he or she often instantly defaults on expensive treatment because underlying problems may remain untouched! Many abuse drugs and alcohol." Along with this, each community faced issues rooted in gender-based violence, teen pregnancy, and lack of prenatal care. Botlhole describes how they made SALT visits to the homes of people, particularly those who had ailments or difficulties such as drug abuse and HIV:

> We did not visit once, we came back several times. These people now felt that they were not alone, they were supported. Through appreciation they realised that though they had major medical issues, their life had not come to an end. This increased their self-confidence. They started appreciating their own selves. We invited these people to dream together about the future of their village. Their dreams were like "Our children will not get infected by HIV" or "Our children will not use drugs." "There will be a school in the village" was another one. Through this dream building the issues became a community thing and was no longer an individual issue. This, I think, encouraged them to take action. (Botlhole 2017)

The community conversations, during the self-assessment phase of the learning cycle, in which members reflect on their current position, helped bring those issues forward. Botlhole now counts the results: some people stopped brewing alcohol illegally, and some admitted that they were defaulting on treatment.

Monitoring Progress

Communities promoted monitoring and accountability on a "CATCH dashboard," which was a painted billboard set up by the communities with the support of local artists (see fig. 6.3 on page 134). The board informed villagers on unfolding progress while also communicating events to "outsiders." Dashboards mirrored community challenges and achievements by detailing three sections, each illustrating different information gathered by community members to monitor community-level issues, prioritize goals, envision solutions, and implement activities. The content of these sections was elaborated by the community through joined envisioning, self-assessment, and action.

The first section shows various illustrations detailing the community members' common vision and main goals. The second section reviews challenges that the community believes should be prioritized for immediate action, by themselves. The final section highlights accomplishments of the community in light of the most urgent issues described in section 2. As a result, the billboard has the ability to mobilize community members for action.

The effects of the dashboard continue to be transformative. Communities use it to positively change each other's attitudes toward health problems. Community members who see the dashboard become interested in the displayed issues, often inspiring their devotion to address them; they soon recognize, as a result, that they own not only these problems but also the solutions. This helps inform more villagers about the issues, mobilize neighboring communities to connect and coordinate with one another, and encourage agreement on their innate abilities to innovate. The process of taking ownership incites the transformation of communities from identifying a problem to working together to generate shared solutions, aligning with the goals of PHC and helping them become active learning communities. Botlhole (2017) describes the experiences they have had with the dashboard:

> We have been fairly successful in reducing consumption of alcohol through [the] SALT process in Botswana. Our villages have dashboards where they share their dreams, hopes and concerns, self-assessment and action points. Where alcohol was an issue, villagers made action plans like bars would close between 12 pm [and] 8 am. The community members took their

dreams and action points to the authorities like police or people who issue bar license[s]. Community members were able to convince the authorities. We see that funding for churches and schools in the villages has increased and for bars has reduced in the areas where we are working.

Assam, India: Improving Immunization Coverage through Villages Taking Ownership of the Challenge

Philip Forth and Rituu B. Nanda (the Constellation)

There is a growing body of literature showing that demand-side interventions lead to significant improvement in childhood vaccination coverage in low- and middle-income countries (Oyo-Ita et al. 2012). With this growing realization that community-level factors influence vaccination uptake, more recent strategies to increase vaccination coverage have attempted to focus on community-based interventions. Existing community engagement programs, however, mostly focus on communication activities that do not actively involve communities in planning, monitoring, and surveillance activities (Sabarwal et al. 2015).

Despite a long-standing national program for immunization in India since 1985, only 65.2% of 12- to 23-month-old children are fully immunized (UNICEF India 2015). In 2015, the organization 3ie awarded a grant to the Constellation and the Public Health Foundation of India to implement and evaluate the SALT approach, which seeks to go beyond information and engagement to encourage communities to take ownership of the challenge of immunization. A study protocol for evaluation is described in Pramanik and colleagues' 2018 article "Impact evaluation of a community engagement intervention in improving childhood immunization coverage: A cluster randomized controlled trial in Assam, India."

The communities were supported by facilitators from the Centre for North East Studies in Bongaigaon and the Voluntary Health Association of Assam in Udalguri and Kamrup as they worked through the CLCP. The communities at stake here are defined as groups of people from the same location, sharing relationships or trust or interest: they live in the same village and neighborhood and are facing the same challenges. A team of three facilitators and a supervisor worked with the thirty communities in each of the three districts. During the year, the Constellation worked with the facilitators to develop their skills in the execution of the steps of the CLCP with the SALT approach.

As with CATCH in Botswana, facilitators identified and supported local champions in the communities to maintain the continuity of the process within the communities and to provide links between the facilitators and the community. The local champions were able to advise, for example, when flooding made access to a particular village difficult or when busy times in the fields made a visit inappropriate.

During the early stages of the intervention (Step 0 of the CLCP in figure 6.2), each facilitator visited individuals and small groups to discuss their hopes and concerns for the health of their children. As interest increased, the facilitators found that it was more effective to work as a team of three to lead the community through steps of the cycle. As the experience and confidence of the facilitators grew, they became skilled at documenting each step of the process for the community and then using that documentation in the succeeding steps.

In every village, there is an accredited social health activist (ASHA) who has the responsibility to create awareness of health, to mobilize the community, and to increase the use of existing health services. In doing so, ASHAs ensure greater access and participation of the communities' members in the delivery of these basic essential health care services. In Assam, the burden placed on the shoulders of ASHAs is large. ASHAs have remarked that more people are coming to them to find out the immunization schedule. In Kadamguri, Udalguri District, mothers now meet regularly, and their action plan has motivated some women to take on the responsibility of informing others about the immunization schedule. Nikunja Damaria, ASHA for Kadamguri, remarked: "The village is very large and I am not able to cover all houses and inform the mothers of the vaccination. I don't have time to go to each and everyone [sic]. My workload has been reduced because communication about immunization has been taken up by women from the community." In a similar vein, Alpana Chakravarty, ASHA of Gaurajhar village, said: "The SALT process has made our job easy. Earlier we had to give constant reminders to the community on the immunization schedule, but now the community . . . itself is keeping contact . . . with us to know the immunization schedule."

Amrit Rabha, a facilitator in Udalguri, has noticed some deeper changes. The women have come to realize that they have some common concerns. This has brought them together, and a network is developing. The ASHA tells two or three women about the immunization schedule, and the network shares the information. Such empowerment brings the community to another level, whereby people are taking action together, solving their problems, and learning from what they are doing. Sonashi Mishra, a young mother, follows up with those who miss the vaccination. Anita Dumari, another mother, noted: "I should let other mothers know about immunization. Every child in my village should be healthy; it is my moral responsibility to help others." "These meetings are a learning opportunity," says a young mother. "I [have] never missed a schedule of vaccination but never bothered to ask why it was given. If everyone learns about this, no one will miss an immunization schedule of their babies."

A second indicator of change is that as the community begins on the second cycle of the CLCP, the challenges that the community wishes to deal with often widen. The concern of the village broadens beyond the health of children to include the cleanliness of the village and the quality of the water supply to induce community ownership of other elements of PHC. People begin to ask, "If we can do something about immunization, why can't we do something about the cleanliness of our village or the quality of our water supply?" Those issues strongly relate with the health and well-being of the population; these are elements of disease prevention that have direct impact on access and service delivery by reducing utilization of facilities. It also increases the social acceptance of proven methods and technologies for the improvement of health and well-being of the communities. A young woman in Jongakholi Village in Kamrup said: "We realized through collective discussion that the water supply problem could only be solved if we c[a]me together. So far, we have been working in twos and threes." Communities have also started to take action around the Anganwadi centers: These are rural child care centers that were set up by the Government of India in 1985. In Batabari Village, their center had been washed away by floods, and through dialogue the community recognized that they did not have to wait for the government to rebuild the center. In another village, the center had not provided any food for the children for a year, so one lady began to cook in her home and bring it to the center in order to provide the children with a hot meal.

When a community begins to take ownership of their challenges, there is the potential for tension between those who seek to take ownership and those who feel that they currently have ownership. The tension can be an indicator that change is taking place. An important role of the facilitator is to support and to encourage the dialogue within the community so that these tensions are resolved and the community can move forward together in a coherent way. While these tensions have not been severe in Assam, they have been present. In Assam, the challenge for the facilitator is to work with the ASHA so that she does not see the SALT approach as a threat or an implicit criticism of her work but rather as an approach that supports her and makes her job easier. Over time, the ASHA and the auxiliary nurse midwife in Udalguri began to understand that this approach does not threaten their position or status and that it can ease their workload. The ASHA of a village of Udalguri affirms that it is important that this kind of community conversation and action is replicated in other villages. She affirmed, "My work burden has been shared by the community; the vaccination rate is going up. I want other villages to also adopt this approach of coming together, talking to each other. Therefore, today I have invited the ASHA of village Batabari Number 2 to come here so that she can learn what we are doing so that this can be done in her village."

Toward the end of the year of implementation of the SALT/CLCP approach, the communities came together to share what they had learned with one another and with representatives of the broader community in Assam. There was a daylong event in each of the three districts: the events were attended by forty-one, sixty-four, and forty-five community members in Udalguri, Bongaigaon, and Kamrup, respectively. A state-level event was held in Guwahati on the fourth day, at which the communities were represented by fifteen communities from the three districts. At each of these events, communities shared their experiences with their peers, and officials listened to the achievements of the communities. At one level, this was an opportunity for groups to learn from one another and to understand that others were facing and finding answers to the same challenges that they were facing. At another level, community members were stimulated to further action by the recognition that what they had done and what they had learned was of interest and importance to others. These events play a vital role in sustaining communities as they work to improve their situation.

The facilitators of the process needed to change the way they approached communities. Many facilitators have become comfortable with an approach where they offer something to the community, perhaps a commodity or money. With the SALT approach, they have nothing to offer, and it takes courage to approach the community empty-handed. One facilitator in Kamrup was particularly doubtful about this approach, but he came to recognize the power of appreciation and is now an enthusiastic supporter of the approach. "Every letter in SALT is powerful. Appreciation and learning are important for me. Appreciation has the power to create a comfortable environment. When we start to appreciate, it opens up doors for communication, and we become more approachable. In other projects I have worked on, we didn't listen to people." Now he receives invitations to work with other villages in Kamrup. Similar changes in the behavior of facilitators who use the SALT approach have been documented by Zachariah and colleagues (2018).

Community and individual ownership of health concerns is not a challenge to existing systems. Rather, community ownership can be the basis for a partnership that opens the possibility of leveraging existing resources to deliver better results for essential health care delivery and other related areas in PHC at lower costs.

Guinea/Liberia: Restoring Trust between Community Health Care Workers and Health Care Post-Ebola

Luc Barrière Constantin (the Constellation)
and Alice Kuan (Johns Hopkins)

Short Summary

In early 2016, three Ebola-affected countries—Guinea, Liberia, and Sierra Leone—held open space conferences organized with the support of the German Institute for Medical Mission (and the Deutsche Gesellschaft für Internationale Zusammenarbeit). The goal was to hear communities and various actors of that region address the question of how the respective national health systems could be improved and what contributions communities could make to support government efforts. A serious loss of confidence of the population vis-à-vis health care providers was pointed out as a major detrimental effect of the outbreak of Ebola. The Regional Confidence Project (RCP) aimed at restoring relationships and trust between communities and health facilities on both sides of the border between Liberia and Guinea. Between September 1, 2016, and August 31, 2017, the project cooperated with seven health facilities and sixteen villages or communities. The RCP, as a whole, had three arms for action. The community mobilization arm aimed to empower communities to find solutions to health challenges with their own strength using the SALT/CLCP approach (Papkalla et al. 2017).

The purpose was to restore a constructive dialogue between communities and the health staff in a way that allows for greater participation and support of the community members to the health infrastructures. Such participation aimed at increasing access and utilization through demand creation for sound and socially acceptable health care. The facilitators were able to organize and execute community discussions with all actors, including health staff and health authorities. These meetings were designed to reveal and rely on the strengths of each member, and to rebuild confidence between the various actors. Through the various steps of the CLCP cycle, communities managed to identify where they wanted to be in the near future and to mobilize local actors and energy for simple but effective actions. Practical collaboration such as maintenance and cleaning of health facilities and comanagement of the health system helped to reduce tensions, discomfort, and mistrust that were the source of reduced use of the health system. Communities decided to collaborate in a more practical way with health staff and also started to develop and implement their own activities in their context.

Between June 2016 and June 2017, there were very positive changes in both countries in the use of health services. Utilization has increased dramatically, especially in smaller health facilities at outpatient departments as well as in antenatal clinics (Papkalla et al. 2017). However, even though the confidence of the communities was restored through open and frank dialogue with health staff and health authorities, there is a need to point out that such renewed attendance could not have happened without improvements in the health services themselves. The complementarity of the community dialogue with the health system, on the one hand, and the improvements in health infrastructure, on the other, produced positive results. Improvements also came from the other arms of the same project. The combination of renewed and facilitated dialogue and the strengthening of the health infrastructures was critical to rebuilding confidence among communities.

Communities developed simple action plans that were doable with local resources. For example, after being guided by the community facilitator during discussions related to health issues, communities realized the potential of such practice to tackle other burning issues related to the life of their villages. Therefore, in addition to the results the project had envisaged, almost all villages made plans for the regular cleaning of public places and for increasing the number of public latrines. Some villages decided to create dumping sites, while others built cemeteries outside the village. They were able to manage access to clean water and more effective use of mosquito nets (Papkalla et al. 2017). As we consider a broader definition of health, the issues tackled by communities (those defined here as well as groups of people living in the same village and neighborhood and facing the same challenge) are strongly related to PHC. They became practical and socially acceptable when they were discussed and accepted, and owned by community members. The most important result of the project, however, was that it allowed people to have goal-oriented conversations and made communication between communities and health facilities constructive. It is important to remember that these results were obtained after only ten months of intervention.

Purpose of the Interventions following the Ebola Virus Epidemic

At the end of the open space conferences held from February to March 2016, one of the recommendations made by the representatives from the three countries (Sierra Leone, Liberia, and Guinea) was to restore the population's confidence in health workers and overall health services. Emphasis was put on comanagement of health infrastructures as well as the inclusion of Ebola survivors in management and increase of preparedness of communities toward epidemic outbreaks. The participation of community members in the management of health facilities is a powerful way to ensure people's acceptance, uptake, and accessibility to essential health care.

In that regard, partners of the project proposed the SALT/CLCP approach to be applied in a systematic and large-scale manner to further open communities' discussions on a lengthier time frame. This strength-based approach allowed community members to define the relevant actors; their vision of effective, acceptable, and accessible health services delivery; and how they would be able to contribute to that vision. Community facilitators who were trained to reveal and nurture people's strengths accompanied the various discussions and interactions within communities and with the actors to ensure practical implementation of the decisions made during these discussions.

Population-Level Responses

Dialogue included community members as well as health staff and health authorities. District and prefecture authorities were also involved in order to institutionalize the dialogue. Two facilitators per community were identified among community members according to simple criteria, the most important being the need for the facilitator to be from the community and to be accepted as a facilitator by the community members themselves. They started to stimulate conversations with the support of community chiefs. Although there were some significant differences between communities, the facilitators organized at least one meeting every two weeks, and they also arranged to meet with specific groups in between. Facilitators initiated a mapping of the villages' public health assets so they could be seen at a glance. With additional social mapping, community members analyzed how specific community members were affected by ill health, which risks exist, and which social groups are important for strengthening healthy behavior and practices. Together, they discussed and prioritized factors promoting and endangering health such as behavior, cultural rites, or social rules. There was broad attendance, including the chiefs, women, youth, and other specific groups during these community conversations. It is an important element of the SALT/CLCP approach to ensure proper and holistic representation of the community members so that everyone feels part of the proposed solutions.

With all this information, the community was able to shape its vision of what kind of community it wants to be, and where it finds itself on the path toward its vision. This paved the way to plan community actions that were needed to improve cleanliness and ensure regular meetings between health facilities and community members. During the SALT visits in which health staff usually participated, conflicts between health facilities and villagers were addressed and solved. In both countries, the health authorities of the counties or prefectures were part of the team and were involved in the emerging new dialogue between health facilities and communities.

One example of SALT's impact is encompassed in developing support for the Agape Health Clinic in Liberia. The clinic imposed high fees for their health services, rising even higher than prices for the same services from public dispensaries. SALT generated the needed conversations where both the faith-based health care provider and the villagers could voice their concerns and needs. The result was an agreement on the new fee for services and the building of a new consultation room at the clinic for antenatal care. The district authorities also agreed on the support of a part-time midwife (Papkalla et al. 2017). This not only benefited women who needed services but also encouraged villagers and district authorities to give their support to the clinic once again. The SALT/CLCP approach allowed for a frank discussion to occur between actors instead of unilateral decisions being made by the health staff and the faith-based personnel. It deliberately included women.

Rosaline Gamy, of Baala (Guinea), said: "Our village was very dirty because of the pigs. They dragged their defecations everywhere in the village. In addition, when you forget . . . food outside, they put their mouths [o]n it. After several meetings from September to November, it is at the beginning of December 2017 that all pig holders have agreed to put the pigs behind fences. Any pork found outside will be shot by young people chosen for the cause. So today, all pigs are [behind] fences. At least one step [has been] taken in the cleanliness of the village" (Papkalla et al. 2017).

Although the official project ended in August 2017, facilitators, communities, and health staff continued their dialogue for the improvement of various issues related to their action plans and the general life of the communities. Community members realized the opportunity to have a constructive dialogue, opening possibilities to take action using their local resources. That ownership of actions decided together during the process makes them sustainable. Nongovernmental organization facilitators (the trainers) have continued to ensure the support of community facilitators, months after the closure of the project. Local authorities have also requested expansion to other communities.

Conclusion

The foundation of a sustainable response to health challenges can occur through ownership of those challenges at an individual and a community level. Ownership means that the community decides on the action that it wishes to take, and that it takes that action. Ownership means that the community asks for support that it knows it needs rather than relying on outsiders to give them what they think they need. It means that the community uses its own people's innovation, communicate what they want, and great change ensues. Ownership means increasing the demand on health services through increased participation of beneficiaries in the management of the health system. Finally, ownership means adapting the services to the needs of nearby communities—in particular, for essential care.

We presented three examples where communities have applied a modified learning cycle called the CLCP to allow them to take ownership of their particular challenges. The learning cycle alone will rarely lead to the sense of ownership and responsibility necessary for a sustainable response. Four factors under the acronym SALT (support, appreciate, learn/listen, and transfer) were a critical part of the facilitation that governed the learning cycle.

One factor critical for sustainable community action is that a wide cross section of a community's members recognize that they have a shared interest in a better future. This critical element of the community concept is reinforced along with the implementation of the SALT/CLCP approach as people are taking action together—solving problems—and are learning from their actions. At each step in the learning cycle, facilitators bring together the different voices that are found in the community and support a dialogue that seeks to establish a coherent view within the community. A second critical factor to sustain action is that the community appreciates the strengths that it already has so that these can be the foundation of further action. The facilitator works so that communities recognize their current strengths and can begin to take action based on those strengths.

The communities in Botswana, Assam, and Liberia/Guinea described in this chapter illustrate that when communities have recognized that they have shared interests and appreciate their strengths, they will take action on a broad front.

Community Responses Extend beyond the Specific Challenge to the Root of Health Problems

When the community dialogue in Botswana was opened, people discussed their dream for their village and the obstacles that stood in the way of that dream. Because trust was built during home visits, many villages felt confident to voice their hopes and concerns during community gatherings, and because the approach puts appreciation consciously at the center, these voices were now also being heard. From the open exchange between community members, it became clear that underlying causes of HIV, such as drug and alcohol abuse, needed to be addressed if the response was to be effective. In contrast with traditional disease-siloed programs that are often less flexible and only leave room for antiretroviral interventions, this time HIV was addressed in a holistic way, with communities themselves working on the roots of their problems. Community funds go to schools rather than bars. Communities' ownership is beautifully expressed in the centrally placed billboards where progress is measured and celebrated.

The Community Response Has Spread to Cover a Range of Issues beyond the Initial Concern

The Liberia-Guinea example illustrates how communities develop ownership of the approach itself. With good facilitation, community members take an appreciation mode of interaction that carries them on to tackle other issues. The spillover effect of SALT/CLCP goes far beyond the entry point (in this case, the issue with the health system) but reinforces the participation aspect of the PHC through related scientifically sound and socially acceptable methods and actions for improving the health and well-being of the population. It is also a way toward sustainability of the activities.

The Community Response Has Supported and Strengthened the Formal System Rather Than Challenged It

Assam showed a collaboration between ASHAs (the representatives of the formal state system of care) and the community. In Assam, ASHAs invited their peers from nearby communities to see what was going on in their community in hopes of spreading this idea of ownership. The crucial insight that this approach reduces the burden on the traditional system is beginning to spread without any formal intervention on the part of the facilitators. It would be shortsighted to see the SALT/CLCP approach as antithetical to the narrow system of health care service provision. These cases show an approach that supports the formal system and reduces the burden on that system.

The Alma-Ata Declaration of 1978 and the Astana Declaration of 2018 have placed the community, as the owners of their health, at the heart of PHC. The capacity of individuals and communities to organize themselves and to take effective action in service of their health is as critical to public health practice as epidemiology, policy-making, hygiene, and sanitation; indeed, an engaged community is essential to a sustained response. However, neither the Alma-Ata Declaration nor the Astana Declaration provide a blueprint to create, to support, and to sustain an engaged community. This chapter, using on-the-ground examples from three different countries, has provided and demonstrated the successful use of a methodology to carry out these important tasks that are at the core of PHC.

REFERENCES

Arnstein, Sherry R. 1969. "A ladder of citizen participation." *J Am Plan Assoc* 35 (4): 216–224.
Botlhole, Pogiso. 2017. "Traditional leaders and bottoms up approach for effective HIV response." *Community Life Competence* (blog), November 2, 2017. https:// aidscompetence.ning.com/profiles/blogs/involve-traditional-leaders.
Collison, Chris, and Geoff Parcell. 2004. *Learning to fly.* Chichester: Wiley.
———. 2016. "CATCH Dashboard Sefhoke Launch News Article." *CATCH SE News.* https://aidscompetence.ning.com/profiles/blogs/sefhoke-on-the-move.
Cooperrider, D. L., and S. Srivastva. 1987. "Appreciative inquiry in organizational life". In *Research in Organizational Change and Development*, vol. 1, edited by R. W. Woodman and W. A. Passmore, 129–169. Stamford, CT: JAI Press.
Deming, W. Edwards. 1967. "What happened in Japan?" *Industrial Quality Control* 24 (2): 89–93.
Kolb, David A., and Ronald E. Fry. 1975. "Towards an applied theory of experiential learning." In *Theories of group processes*, edited by Gary L. Cooper, 33–58. New York: Wiley.

Lamboray, Jean-Louis. 2016. *What makes us human?* Balboa Press.

Oyo-Ita, M., C. E. Nwachukwu, C. Oringanje, and M. M. Meremikwu. 2012. "Cochrane Review: Interventions for improving coverage of child immunization in low- and middle-income countries." *Evidence-Based Child Health* 7 (3): 959–1012.

Papkalla, Ute, George Maxwell, Sanoh Yomba, and Luc Barrière Constantin. 2017. *With new confidence into a healthy future.* https://www.communitylifecompetence.org/uploads/6/3/7/1/63712543/en_difaem_results_rcp_liberia.pdf.

Parcell, Geoff, and Chris Collison. 2009. *No more consultants.* Chichester: Wiley.

Pramanik, S., A. Ghosh, R. B. Nanda, M. de Rouw, P. Forth, and S. Albert. 2018. "Impact evaluation of a community engagement intervention in improving childhood immunization coverage: A cluster randomized controlled trial in Assam, India." *BMC Public Health* 18 (534): https://bmcpublichealth.biomedcentral.com/articles/10.1186/s12889-018-5458-x.

Sabarwal, S., R. Bhatia, B. Dhody, S. Perumal, H. White, and P. Jyotsna. 2015. *Engaging communities for increasing immunization coverage: What do we know?* Scoping Paper 3. New Delhi: 3ie.

UNAIDS. 2018. "Botswana 2018." http://www.unaids.org/en/regionscountries/countries/botswana.

UNICEF India. 2015. *Rapid Survey on Children (2013–2014).* https://wcd.nic.in/sites/default/files/RSOC%20National%20Report%202013-14%20Final.pdf.

US President's Emergency Plan for AIDS Relief. 2016. "Botswana: Country Operational Plan (2016) Strategic Direction Summary." https://www.pepfar.gov/documents/organization/257359.pdf.

Zachariah, B., E. E. de Wit, J. D. Bahirat, and J. F. G. Bunders-Aelen. 2018. "What is in it for them? Understanding the impact of a 'support, appreciate, listen team' (SALT) based suicide prevention peer education program on peer educators." School of Mental Health. https://doi.org/10.1007/s12310-018-9264-5.

PART TWO

Country Case Studies
of Primary Health Care at Scale
and the Way Forward

Bangladesh's Health Improvement Strategy as an Example of the Alma-Ata Declaration in Action

TAUFIQUE JOARDER AND FERDOUS ARFINA OSMAN

Bangladesh, a densely populated lower-middle-income country of 165 million, with gross domestic product (GDP) per capita of US$1,516.51 as of 2017, has achieved considerable progress in health over the past few decades. There was a twenty-seven-year rise in life expectancy and the total fertility rate fell from more than 7 to 2.1 since Bangladesh's independence in 1971 (World Bank 2017).

The country has recently been applauded as an "exceptional" health performer and credited for achieving "good health at low cost" (Koehlmoos et al. 2011). Bangladesh, despite its relatively lower health expenditure compared to neighboring countries, has made exceptional progress in reducing both fertility and mortality compared to most other countries in South Asia (Balabanova, Mills, and Conteh 2013; Das and Horton 2013). Bangladesh spends three percent of GDP or US$37 per capita on health per year. In contrast, India, Sri Lanka, and Nepal spend 4.7%, 3.5%, and 5.8% of GDP (as of 2014), respectively (Government of Bangladesh 2018b). Despite its low level of health costs, Bangladesh has attained sustained health gains over the past few decades (table 7.1).

This sustained progress in health can be attributed to several factors inside and outside the health sector. The most important among them is that the country, since its independence, gave primary health care (PHC) the topmost priority in health policy. Soon after the Alma-Ata Declaration in 1978, Bangladesh incorporated the concept of PHC in its policy documents, and since then it has been regarded as one of the key strategies for achieving "Health for All." With a view to attain this goal, the government has developed a countrywide network of health infrastructure and aimed the policy

Table 7.1. Improvement of health status in Bangladesh (1970s–2015)

Indicators	1971	1980	1990	2000	2010	Latest
Population growth rate (in %)	2.09	2.78	2.47	1.96	1.12	1.05 (2017)
Infant mortality rate (per 1,000 live births)	148.6	133.6	99.7	64	39.1	28.2 (2016)
Under-5 mortality rate (per 1,000 live births)	222.7	198.6	143.8	87.4	49.4	34.2 (2016)
Maternal mortality ratio (per 100,000 live births)	3,000[1]	1,330[2]	569	399	194[3]	176 (2015) 196[4] (2016)
Life expectancy at birth (in years)	47.14	53.48	58.40	65.32	70.20	72.49 (2016)
Total fertility rate (birth per women aged 15–49 years)	6.94	6.36	4.49	3.17	2.33	2.10 (2016)
Delivery care by trained personnel (in %)	2[2]	5[5]	8[6]	11.6[7]	27.8[8]	42.1[9]
Percentage of fully immunized children (12–23 months)	2[2]	75[5]	66[6]	60.4[7]	86. 0[8]	83.8[9]

Source: Most information is from the World Databank of the World Bank (World Bank 2017), except numbered notes.

[1] First Five-Year Plan of Bangladesh (Government of Bangladesh 1973).

[2] Second Five-Year Plan of Bangladesh (Government of Bangladesh 1980).

[3] Bangladesh Maternal Mortality and Health Care Survey 2010 (NIPORT, MEASURE Evaluation, and icddr,b 2012).

[4] Bangladesh Maternal Mortality and Health Care Survey 2016 (NIPORT, icddr,b, and MEASURE Evaluation 2017).

[5] Fourth Five-Year Plan of Bangladesh (Government of Bangladesh 1990).

[6] Fifth Five-Year Plan of Bangladesh (Government of Bangladesh 1997).

[7] Bangladesh Demographic and Health Survey 1999–2000 (NIPORT, Mitra and Associates, and ORC Macro 2001).

[8] Bangladesh Demographic and Health Survey 2011 (NIPORT, Mitra and Associates, and ICF International 2013).

[9] Bangladesh Demographic and Health Survey 2014 (NIPORT, Mitra and Associates, and ICF International 2015).

focus on the vulnerable sections of the population living in rural areas: the poor, women, and children. Governments irrespective of political regime have largely demonstrated considerable policy continuity and commitment to improve health conditions through PHC. Yet, amid these positive trends, the health system also has many challenges and shortcomings. The current chapter presents Bangladesh's experience of improving its health indicators by giving emphasis on PHC as described in the Alma-Ata Declaration. It examines the application of the concept of PHC in Bangladesh across the principles of the declaration. We start this chapter by reviewing the operation of the entire health system with a special focus on the social and political background of PHC as a series of sectoral reforms and the functional features of the health system of Bangladesh. In the second part, we present empirical data collected from Bangladeshi communities who were asked to share perspectives on comprehensive PHC.

Sociocultural, Political, and Economic Background of Primary Health Care in Bangladesh

Colonial Legacy of the Health System in Bangladesh:
What Did the British Put into Place?

The history of therapeutics in the region of present-day Bangladesh dates to when Ayurveda and Unani medicine were in practice throughout the Indian subcontinent. The Western medical system was introduced formally in 1714, with the introduction of Indian medical services by the British colonial government. In 1938, the Indian National Congress formed the National Health Subcommittee under the aegis of the National Planning Committee. This committee, popularly known as the Sokhey Committee, under the chairmanship of Colonel S. Sokhey, emphasized maintenance of the health of the people by the state and integration of preventive and curative health services all over India. Another milestone in the history of health services of India was the publication of the Bhore Committee report in 1946, which recommended radical reform of the entire health system for providing community-oriented care for the entire population. The Bhore Committee extensively studied the population health status and health system of India and recommended an integrated public health service amalgamating both curative and preventive services. To achieve broad community coverage, the committee recommended establishing rural health centers and ensuring equity and community participation. Thus, the concepts of preventive care, community participation, social justice, and equity were discussed in the Indian context well ahead of the Alma-Ata Declaration. However, the Bhore Committee report was not acted on because immediately after its publication, the British rule in the Indian subcontinent was terminated. Thus, the British ultimately left a curative, urban-biased, and elite-controlled health care system in India.

In 1947, with the independence of British India, India and Pakistan were founded, with present-day Bangladesh referred to as East Pakistan. The postrevolutionary Pakistan regime did not take immediate steps to indigenize the health care system, whereas India's founders made health a priority. Pakistan in the 1950s gave no consideration to implementing the Bhore Committee report and continued with the curative, urban-biased, elite-dominated health care system until the epidemics of diseases like malaria, small pox, and cholera became a serious concern. In 1961, the Pakistani government attempted to implement the Bhore Committee report and designed a rural health center scheme, which was approved in 1967. The scheme required the establishment of a thirty-one-bed thana health complex (THC) in each rural thana (now *upazila*, or the subdistrict) to provide primary-level care (both inpatient and outpatient) to the rural population. By 1970, in then East Pakistan, now Bangladesh, 140 THCs were built. These hospitals are the predecessors of present-day upazila health complexes (UpHCs).

Impact of Liberation War on Health System

In 1971, Bangladesh gained independence from Pakistan, and the health system that the country inherited from Pakistan was still largely urban biased and curative despite the pilot introduction of THCs. The health system was extremely limited in terms of health infrastructure, workforce, and public health measures such as sanitation and nutrition (Osman 2004). The inherited health infrastructure of the country, inhabited by nearly seventy million people, included eight medical colleges, one postgraduate medical institute, thirty-seven tuberculosis clinics, 151 rural health centers, and ninety-one maternal and child welfare centers. As a result, in the initial years after independence, the health sector policy focus was on building the required health infrastructure, particularly in rural areas, so that the majority of the population could be served. The first national long-term five-year plan (1973–1978) laid emphasis on building a network of THCs. Accordingly, the THC scheme was approved by the government in 1976.

Alongside this, Chowdhury and colleagues (2013) noted that the liberation war led to the beginning of a social transformation process. This process was characterized by social mobilization, institutional pluralism, and civil dynamism, creating space for multiple stakeholders including government, nongovernmental organizations (NGOs), informal providers, international donors, and commercial enterprises. In health service delivery, all these stakeholders collaborated to pursue a pro-equity strategy, concentrating direct action on high-priority health issues such as family planning, immunization, oral rehydration therapy, tuberculosis, vitamin A supplementation, and others.

Historical Evolution of Primary Health Care in Bangladesh since the 1970s

In 1978, Bangladesh became a signatory to the Alma-Ata Declaration and committed to achieving Health for All by 2000. One year later, Bangladesh started piloting PHC in six upazilas (also known as thana at different times), each inhabited by about 250,000 people. The second national long-term five-year plan (1980–1985), being closely influenced by the Alma-Ata Declaration in 1978 and the local context of increased prevalence of communicable diseases, adopted PHC as a policy strategy to ensure Health for All. Building health infrastructure was the key strategy to achieve this goal, with a key focus on constructing one THC in each thana and one union health and family welfare center (UHFWC) in each union by 1985. Conversely, since independence, international donors had been identifying overpopulation, malnutrition, and a high incidence of communicable diseases as the major problems related to the health status of the population of the country. Accordingly, external funds were devoted to address many of these issues. The country, thus, embraced the selective PHC strategy, with a focus on vertical programs including maternal and child health and family planning services, immunization against major infectious diseases, and prevention and control of endemic diseases. These selective programs produced impressive results in maternal and child health.

The 1970s and 1980s saw a trend of growing private sector and NGO participation in health service provision in response to the growing demand for health services that outpaced government investments in new health care resources. In 1982, the government relaxed restrictions on private laboratories, clinics, and hospitals, spurring even faster growth in private sector health care services (Khan 1996). Since the 1980s, the private sector has flourished, and in recent years the country has been experiencing a proliferation of private sector health services, which include mostly clinical services.

The first evaluation of the national Health for All strategy was conducted in 1986, identifying important bottlenecks in implementing PHC in Bangladesh. According to the report, inadequacy in managerial processes, lack of adequate resources, bias toward curative medicine, and a lack of coordination and community involvement were the hindrances to translating PHC into action. Based on the recommendation of the report, the Government of Bangladesh initiated the Intensified PHC Program in two upazilas in two districts, and this method was gradually extended across the country.

A shift of focus took place in late 1990s, from infrastructure building to governance issues and from a programmatic approach to institutional reform designed to ensure efficiency and effectiveness of health services. In 1998, PHC was redefined as the essential service package (ESP) in order to prioritize delivery of cost-effective services to the most vulnerable communities. The ESP is built on the commitment to the PHC approach and includes: reproductive health care, including family planning; child health care; communicable disease control; limited curative care; and behavior change communication. Concomitant attempts were undertaken to establish community clinics (CCs) at the grassroots level to provide ESP services such as a one-stop service center, which would replace the long-practiced domiciliary services that had been customary for the rural people.

But in 2001, the newly elected government, led by the Bangladesh Nationalist Party (BNP), abandoned the idea of having CCs established by the previous government, led by the Awami League (AL), partly due to political differences and partly due to the "not-so-positive" outcome of the new initiative. CCs were actually launched at the tail end of the AL regime in 1998 without having the ground ready for implementation, leading to poor performance in the initial days. A study (Osman 2005) found widespread confusion and misunderstanding among the field-level health workers about their roles at the CCs after transitioning from their traditional roles visiting households. Such confusion along with the resentment of the high officials of the Directorate General of Family Planning (DGFP) against the government's decision to unify health and family planning operations eventually triggered noncooperation of the family planning workers at the field level. This, in turn, culminated into the withdrawal of domiciliary services by the field workers, soon after the initiation of operations at the CCs. The noncooperation of these field workers seriously affected family planning services and behavior change communication activities. From 1996/97 to 2003, many health indicators (total fertility rate and life expectancy) remained stagnant or unchanged while others did not show any significant improvement (Government of Bangladesh 2003; Streatfield 2003). The third service delivery survey report 2003 also found that utilization of government health services decreased from 13% in 1999 to 10% in 2003 (CIET 2003). The new government, led by the BNP, blamed the slow progress of health indicators on the introduction of CCs and the erosion of long-practiced domiciliary services. All these factors were placed by the BNP government as justifications for leaving the CCs and restoring domiciliary services in 2003. Different studies even demonstrated an improvement of health indicators after the restoration of domiciliary services in later years. Comparison of figures between the Maternal Health Services and Maternal Mortality Survey 2003 (NIPORT et al.

2003) and the Bangladesh Demographic and Health Survey 2007 (NIPORT et al. 2007) reveals that total fertility rate was slightly reduced, from 3.3 in 2003 to 2.7 in 2007, and life expectancy at birth increased from 66.9 years in 2003 to 68.4 in 2006 (World Bank 2017). The infant mortality rate and the maternal mortality ratio also saw a declining trend during that period. However, with the AL back in power in 2009, CCs were reinstated and revitalized, and both domiciliary and CC-based static services were allowed to continue operating side by side.

National policies (National Health Policy 2000 and 2011) and programs also upheld the concept of ESP and expressed commitments to PHC by making it one of the key policy strategies for ensuring health care for all. The National Health Policy 2011 also reiterates the commitment toward PHC. One of the specific goals of the policy is "ensuring primary health and emergency care for all."

From time to time, the government has also undertaken various programs/initiatives that support the principles of PHC. For instance, in 2004, in order to reduce the financial barriers faced by poor women in accessing maternal health care and to increase utilization of maternal health services, government, with support from the World Health Organization (WHO), piloted the Maternal and Child Health Voucher Scheme, a demand-side financing initiative that, in 2007, formally launched and scaled up in a large number of districts. Currently, the program is being implemented in fifty-three upazilas of forty-one districts (Government of Bangladesh 2016). The voucher entitles its holder to specific free-of-charge health services including antenatal and postnatal care, safe delivery, treatment for complications including caesarian section, transportation costs, and laboratory tests (Government of Bangladesh 2013). Additionally, the Directorate General of Health Services (DGHS) has been implementing a community-based skilled birth attendant (CSBA) training program since 2003 in order to address the shortage of skilled manpower human resources in remote areas to provide obstetric care. Under the program, community-based health workers, including family welfare assistants (FWAs), women health assistants, and similar health workers in NGOs and the private sector, are provided with midwifery training. The CSBAs are trained to conduct normal deliveries at home and to identify the complicated cases to be referred to the nearby health facilities where comprehensive emergency obstetric and neonatal care services are available (Government of Bangladesh 2013). The CSBA training program is now organized in 465 upazilas of 64 districts (Government of Bangladesh 2016).

A Pluralistic Approach to Primary Health Care

The health system of Bangladesh includes four major stakeholders: the government health system, private providers, NGO providers, and a donor community (Ahmed et al. 2013). The government sector has a mandate to not only set policies and regulate them but also to provide comprehensive health services. The fast-growing private sector offers profitable high-end services for the rich but also includes a vast informal economy of frontline providers retailing services among the poor. The NGO sector focuses on the health needs of the poor, as part of a broader array of development interventions (World Bank 2005). Finally, the donor community exercises disproportionate weight in determining policy and programmatic priorities while orchestrating technical assistance and directing delivery strategies. Altogether, these stakeholders must work together to deliver PHC, though coordination remains difficult.

Organization of Bangladesh's Public Sector Services

The country is composed of eight divisions, 64 districts, 490 upazilas, 4,553 unions, and 40,977 wards (figure 7.1) (Government of Bangladesh 2018c). The Ministry of Health and Family Welfare is responsible for delivering PHC services through its two wings—the DGHS and the DGFP (figure 7.1). PHC services of both directorates begin at the ward level,* through a set of community-based health staff, with supervisory staff located at the union level (the lowest administrative unit) and referral primary care facilities located at the union and upazila levels (World Bank 2010).

CCs, located at the ward level, are the lowest level of health facility (Government of Bangladesh 2018c), providing PHC services to rural people. CCs are built on a public-private partnership arrangement where community members donate a piece of land on which the government builds the clinic and then provides logistics, human resources, and medicine to make it functional. As per the government policy, for every six thousand rural residents, there should be one CC located within thirty minutes' walking distance. As mentioned before, these clinics are one-stop service centers that provide basic primary health and family planning services. The CCs also represent the first contact and entry point to the health referral system. While providing treatment for simple ailments, CCs also identify complicated cases and establish a referral linkage with the higher facilities at the union and upazila levels (i.e., the UHFWCs and

---

*Constituent unit of a union. A union consists of nine wards.

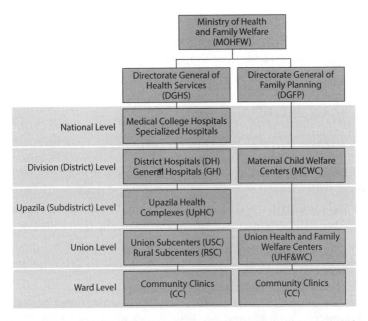

	Ministry of Health and Family Welfare (MOHFW)	
	Directorate General of Health Services (DGHS)	Directorate General of Family Planning (DGFP)
National Level	Medical College Hospitals Specialized Hospitals	
Division (District) Level	District Hospitals (DH) General Hospitals (GH)	Maternal Child Welfare Centers (MCWC)
Upazila (Subdistrict) Level	Upazila Health Complexes (UpHC)	
Union Level	Union Subcenters (USC) Rural Subcenters (RSC)	Union Health and Family Welfare Centers (UHF&WC)
Ward Level	Community Clinics (CC)	Community Clinics (CC)

Figure 7.1. Public sector health service structure in Bangladesh showing bifurcated parallel tracks.

the UpHCs). One community health care provider provides health care services at the CCs six days a week. One health assistant, appointed by DGHS, and one FWA, appointed by DGFP, provide service at CCs three days a week, alternating while they provide services at the household level on the remaining three days. Community health care providers and health assistants are appointed by the DGHS while FWAs are appointed by the DGFP.

At the union level, DGHS operates 87 UHFWCs, while DGFP runs 3,860 UHFWCs, of which 1,500 have been upgraded and are now allowed to provide primary and outpatient care (World Bank 2010). Not all the UHFWCs have medical doctors. Notwithstanding the provision that there should be a medical doctor in each UHFWC, the facilities typically are manned by paramedics and community-level staff, including one subassistant community medical officer, one family welfare visitor, one family planning inspector, one pharmacist, and one office assistant. Family welfare visitors and family planning inspectors are appointed by the DGFP, while others are appointed by the DGHS.

At the upazila level—the apex of the network of PHC facilities—there are thirty-one-bed and fifty-bed hospitals called UpHCs[†] that provide both out-

†UpHCs were formerly known as thana health complexes (THCs).

patient and inpatient care to an area with a population of about 250,000. PHC in rural Bangladesh has been organized around UpHCs. UpHCs are run by physicians, nurses, and other support staff, the number of which varies depending on the number of beds. For instance, for thirty-one-bed UpHCs there are nine sanctioned posts for physicians, while for fifty-bed UpHCs there are twenty-one physician posts.

PRIVATE SECTOR ROLE IN PRIMARY HEALTH CARE

Currently, the majority of health care in Bangladesh is delivered by the private sector, with a formal sector comprising qualified practitioners serving the affluent and an informal sector serving the poor. Formal private sector providers are typically urban and draw staff from public sector personnel who hold dual jobs, working in both public sector and private sector practices simultaneously (Gruen et al. 2002; Bloom et al. 2011). Informal providers lack formal qualifications and are unregistered.

Publicly staffed services at CCs are physically accessible and located within a few kilometers of most rural villagers, but public health facilities remain mostly underutilized due to the perceived low quality of service (Nornmand et al. 2012). Non-availability of physicians, drugs, and other basic amenities could be cited as the prime reasons for low utilization. The public sector employs about 30.5% of all registered doctors in Bangladesh (Government of Bangladesh 2018c). However, many of these doctors do not go to their job locations. This means that these doctors are available on paper but not in reality in the place of their posting. This phenomenon is described by Chaudury and Hammer (2003) as "ghost doctors." As a result of insufficient services at public facilities, there has been increased utilization of private formal and informal sector health facilities. According to Bangladesh Health Watch (2007), the "unqualified practitioners" in the private sector are responsible for providing 60% of treatment services in rural Bangladesh. The standards of their services are not effectively regulated, which puts the quality of service in question.

Informal drug sellers are in practice as the frontline care providers for many, particularly the poor, operating in mostly unregulated ways. Unregulated drug selling and consultation by these untrained informal providers exacerbate the already poor health of this vulnerable population. This situation has resulted in high health care expenditures and catastrophic health outcomes (Democracy Watch 2010). The Government of Bangladesh (2018b) noted that both drug vendors and village doctors (informal providers without medical degrees practicing in a rural setting) stock and retail domestically produced modern drugs, the sales of which account for about 69.3% of out-of-pocket health expenditures.

It is difficult to bring informal drug sellers into an accountability framework, as there is no formal mechanism to track these informal, unregistered providers. Moreover, the regulatory mechanism for the production, marketing, and use of drugs is controlled by the Drugs Act of 1940 (and the rules made under it in 1946) and the Drugs (Control) Ordinance of 1982 (Government of Bangladesh 2018a). Reforming the mechanisms for the marketing of drugs is a formidable challenge, as it may affect the interests of powerful stakeholders. Informal monitoring or consumer awareness could also help reduce the vulnerability of the poor to be victimized by this inappropriate use of drugs. Low literacy and low awareness of risks are barriers to achieving accountability through citizen monitoring of service quality (Wolf et al. 2005).

Nongovernmental Organizations as a Multisectoral Approach to Primary Health Care

NGOs began to emerge immediately after liberation to provide relief and rehabilitation to the war-affected population. Gradually, the size and scope of NGOs saw expansion into other areas, spanning from microfinance, education services, social safety-net programs, agricultural extension, environmental protection, water and sanitation provision, disaster management, and legal and human rights education to capacity-building. In addition to service delivery, NGOs have also rediversified the commercial sector, launching the operation of commercial banks, telecommunications, and more. Ahmed Mushtaque Raja Chowdhury and colleagues (2013) explain the rationale for this as "partly to lessen dependence on donors during a period of economic downturn and develop an independent source of internally generated revenue" (1736). Due to their multisectoral character, NGOs have been able to provide effective services to address community needs. Various innovative efforts have been undertaken by NGOs, including projects to provide water, sanitation, and housing, and to improve child survival, early childhood development, nutrition, health, and community-building (Afsana and Wahid 2013). However, provision of health services has been the second most common area of service activity after microcredit, with nearly 60% of NGOs providing health care–related services (World Bank 2005).

In response to the low quality of government services and the high cost involved in formal private sector services, a vibrant and large NGO sector emerged in the 1980s as a growing alternative to provide quality services to the poor and marginalized who are underserved by the public and private sectors. Many NGOs focus on smaller geographical areas to provide mainly preventive care. The larger national NGOs (Bangladesh Rural Advancement Committee [BRAC], Gonoshasthaya Kendra, Grameen Bank) have strong organizational and management capacity to provide both preventive and curative services. These NGOs are well equipped with training and research facilities and information management systems, and are mostly financed by donor agencies. Cooperation between NGOs and the government in service provision is quite common in Bangladesh. Recognizing the effectiveness of NGOs in reaching the community since the 1980s, various government and NGO partnership initiatives for delivering basic PHC services, including immunization, family planning, tuberculosis control, distribution of oral rehy-

---

Urban Primary Health Care: An Example of GO-NGO Partnership

In the 1990s, in urban areas, government expanded its scope of partnership with nongovernmental organizations (NGOs) through complete outsourcing/contracting out public sector services to NGOs. Under this arrangement, the Ministry of Local Government, Rural Development and Cooperatives manages primary health care (PHC) services in urban areas through contractual partnership among urban local bodies and NGOs with financial support from development partners. Two public-private partnership projects have emerged influential with regard to making contributions to urban PHC in Bangladesh. First, the Urban Primary Health Care Service Delivery Project (the successor of the Urban Primary Health Care Project launched in 1998) aims to provide basic PHC services to the urban poor in big cities in Bangladesh. The project provides health care for the urban poor, offering varied service packages free of cost. The project covers more than ten million urban population in the country (Ahmed et al. 2015). Second, the NGO Health Service Development Program, started in 1997, supports the delivery of essential service packages through a national network of NGOs. These NGOs are operating 330 clinics that serve about twenty-three million people, almost 15% of Bangladesh's population (USAID 2015). As an outcome of the program, NGO facilities have become the most commonly available health service provider, as 58% of slum and 53% of nonslum communities have an NGO facility within one kilometer (National Institute of Population Research and Training, International Center for Diarrheal Disease Research Bangladesh, and MEASURE Evaluation 2013).

---

dration solution, and urban PHC programs, have been launched. Such "GO-NGO" partnerships have produced a significant number of success stories in health service delivery.

Multiple Counterparts (Auxiliary Workers)

The health system of Bangladesh consists of multiple cadres of health care providers employed by the public, private, and NGO sectors who serve the population. The public sector employs physicians and a large number of auxiliary and mid-level staff that include subassistant community medical officers, sanitary inspectors, health inspectors, midwives/nurses, and health technicians. In addition to these, the government also employs a large pool of field workers—one for every five to six thousand people at the ward or village level. Field workers are the key agents providing PHC services in Bangladesh. There are different categories of field workers at the union, ward, and village levels, all of which are community-based, regular government health workers assigned to deliver domiciliary health and family planning services. NGOs also employ and train a large number of community health workers, but the exact number of this workforce is not available. The government has a positive attitude toward community health workers (CHWs) employed by NGOs. NGOs have even partnered with the government to supply village/ward-level workers to temporarily fill critical job vacancies. For example, Save the Children's Integrated Safe Motherhood, Newborn Care and Family Planning Project (2009–2013) temporarily filled vacant FWA posts in the area covered by their program.

Along with a large number of physicians, the private sector also employs nurses and technologists, who actually serve the majority of the population of the country. As mentioned before, private sector health services are also delivered by a large number of qualified and unqualified practitioners of traditional medicine (including village doctors and *kobiraj*—a type of traditional healer—drug sellers, faith healers, etc.) known as alternative private providers. Among others, the informal providers—the "village doctors" and drug vendors, who are often the same people—are the main source of health care available to the poor, especially in rural areas. This group forms the largest group of health care providers in Bangladesh. Bangladesh Health Watch (2007) reported that there were around twelve village doctors and eleven sales people at drug retail outlets providing diagnosis and treatment per ten thousand population. A study by Ahmed and colleagues (2013) noted that more than seventy thousand unregistered drug retailers (and village doctors) are the first contact for most people in rural areas. Despite being the largest group of providers, the government does not have any clear policy guidance regarding these informal health service providers.

BOTTOM-UP, COMMUNITY-ENGAGED PLANNING, ORGANIZATION, AND CONTROL

Community-engaged planning is a significant health policy focus of the Government of Bangladesh. To facilitate the engagement of community members in local-level health plans, both the government and NGOs have various structures/initiatives. NGOs have made key contributions in identifying unique opportunities for meaningful interfaces between the government and communities, and working to institutionalize those models of engagement at district and national scales (Hunter et al. 2015). In general, NGOs provide support to the government structures for community engagement and also develop and implement their own model for community capacity-building and community-led behavior change communication. Community health programs of BRAC, CARE, Save the Children, and so forth are leading examples. It is worth noting that BRAC community health workers, known as the Shasthya Kormis and Shasthya Shebikas, have made notable contributions to improving health awareness and capacity of the community to address diarrhea and tuberculosis.

Both rural and urban local government institutions have built-in structures for community engagement in health planning at the local level. The lowest tier of rural local government, called the Union Parishad (UP), has thirteen standing committees to deal with local development issues, among which one deals with health and family planning services. Additionally, in urban areas, City Corporation (local government institution in large cities) has a standing committee on health, although municipalities (local government institutions in small towns) do not have any such committees.

Each level of the PHC service network in rural areas—from the CCs to the UpHCs—also has community representative committees to encourage community engagement in decision-making. The CCs at the ward level have two committees to ensure community engagement in health service delivery:

1. A thirteen-to-seventeen-member community group, headed by the member of UP representing the concerned ward,[‡] with the UP chair

‡Union Parishad is a directly elected, local government body at the union level consisting of a chairman and twelve members, among whom nine are male and three must be female. Nine male members must be directly elected by the local people, while the female members are elected in reserved seats and may be directly (by the local people) or indirectly (by the

and the CC staff and members of the community as the members, is responsible for supporting the day-to-day management of the CC, preparing local-level plans, including fund generation, use and maintenance, and monitoring and evaluation of performance of the CCs. This committee is supposed to make the CC staff accountable to the UP.

2. A thirteen-to-seventeen-member community support group (CSG) composed of beneficiaries and other community members, with at least one-third women. In the catchment area of each CC, there will be three CSGs, each comprising thirteen to seventeen members. The CSG is responsible for creating health awareness among the beneficiaries about the services provided by the CC especially. The model for these CSGs was adapted from CARE's community support system and the Narsingdi Model, the Japanese International Cooperation Agency's (JICA) successful community mobilization model.

Although UHFWCs do not have their own oversight committees, there are three other community committees at the union and ward levels that have representatives from UPs, along with the staff of UHFWCs, the CCs, and finally the community people as members. There is a seven-to-nine-member family planning committee at the ward level; a five-to-six-member UP standing committee on education, health, and family planning, as mentioned earlier; and a twenty-to-twenty-five-member UP family planning committee. These committees are supposed to meet periodically to review the nature and status of services provided by the facilities concerned.

Similarly, at the UpHC, two such committees exist:

1. A twenty-one-member Upazila Hospital Management Committee headed by the local Member of Parliament and upazila chairman, vice chairman, upazila health and family planning officer, and representatives of the community as members, responsible for monitoring health service conditions at the upazila.

2. A five-member Upazila Health and Family Welfare Committee (one of seventeen upazila committees formerly known as standing committees) headed by the upazila vice chairman, with upazila health and family planning officer as member secretary and the local elites as members, responsible for overseeing health and family planning services at the upazila.

male members) elected. Nine male members represent each of the constituent wards of the parishad (numbering nine), while each female member represents three wards.

Although the committees offer the promise of a wide range of community-engaged, bottom-up planning, in reality, they have been largely nonfunctional in terms of ensuring citizen control over services. Most importantly, the poor, who constitute the majority of the service users, often remain underrepresented in the committees. A study on CSG members found that the committee members were generally drawn from the village elite, with significantly higher levels of both education and income than the majority of the clinic users and frequently with strong connections to local power structures (Mahmud 2004). Besides, as Osman and colleagues (2015) observed, the committees do not meet regularly, the members are often unaware of their responsibilities, and in many cases, they merely exist on paper. More importantly, they do not have any executive power over the services they monitor. Such a combination of factors, including underrepresentation of the service users, lack of executive authority of the committees, and reluctance on the part of the members to make the committees effective, has contributed to limiting their effectiveness in mobilizing collective action.

However, despite the fact that the committees have yet to achieve the expected level of performance in ensuring community engagement, their effectiveness in increasing the level of awareness and demand for services among the community has been evident. An increase in facility-based deliveries, from only 27% in 2010 to 47% (14% public, 29% private) in 2016, as reported by the 2016 Bangladesh Maternal Mortality and Health Care Survey, bears testimony to this (National Institute of Population Research and Training, International Center for Diarrheal Disease Research Bangladesh, and MEASURE Evaluation 2017).

Apart from having the aforementioned committees, having CCs at the ward level is another deliberate attempt by the government to improve community engagement. The fourth sector-wide program (2017–2022) currently being implemented by the Government of Bangladesh has stressed the importance of improving community engagement through the CCs. Furthermore, a recent study reveals that proximity of CCs (1–1.5 km distance) to community members has also made health services easily accessible to rural people, removing the physical barriers to access (Osman and Bennett 2018).

A Community's Perspective on Bangladesh's Comprehensive Primary Health Care

To gather community-level perspectives on PHC in Bangladesh, we conducted a mixed-methods study on UpHCs (i.e., the hub of the PHC network in Bangladesh) in 2010–2011. The study consisted of three distinct phases. The first phase of the study comprised key informant interviews and document review to understand the historical evolution of PHC in Bangladesh. The second phase was quantitative, with a cross-sectional survey of twenty UpHCs of Bangladesh stratified with ten UpHCs from Dhaka and ten from the remote district of Barishal. WHO's Health System Performance Assessment guideline was adapted for the Bangladeshi context and applied to rank the twenty UpHCs based on their performance. The "highest-performing" and the "lowest-performing" UpHCs were selected for further in-depth study. This in-depth study included qualitative observation of the UpHC facilities and a household survey in a randomly selected village within the catchment area of the UpHCs. The qualitative study involved observation of UpHC operations for fifteen days; in-depth interviews with local government leaders, physicians, subassistant community medical officers, paramedics, field staff, and purposively selected inpatient and outpatient patients. Finally, participatory rural appraisal sessions in study villages (i.e., the villages where a household survey was conducted) included thirty people from different socioeconomic strata who met for facilitated discussion.

Population-Level Responses
SUPPLY OF SAFE WATER AND BASIC SANITATION

During in-depth interviews, patients expressed satisfaction with the availability of safe drinking water, sanitary latrines, and the spread of handwashing. They also reported that the Ministry of Health and Family Welfare's responsibilities focus on providing health education concerning water and sanitation and occasional inspection of sanitary latrines during diarrheal disease outbreaks. The interviews aligned with the organizational structure of government services providing safe water and sanitation. In Bangladesh, the responsibility of providing safe water and basic sanitation falls on the Department of Public Health Engineering of the Ministry of Local Government, Rural Development, and Cooperatives rather than on the Ministry of Health and Family Welfare. Many NGOs are involved in providing safe water and sanitation in association with the government, but there are no clear guidelines for collaboration and coordination, as reported by the key informants and physicians.

IMMUNIZATION

Our household survey results confirmed that vaccination coverage is succeeding in Bangladesh. In-depth interviews with subassistant community medical officers, paramedics, and field staff revealed good examples of collaboration among the government, NGOs, and the community. The EPI (Expanded Programme on Immunization) staff, most of which are recruited from the local community, were successfully informing the community where and when vaccination outreach events would take place. Prior to a vaccination event, they would organize courtyard meetings in the community and prepare a list of families who have unvaccinated children. If anyone from the list did not show up in the vaccination program, the EPI staff would go directly to their home and vaccinate the child. They also maintained a register of pregnant women in the community in order to give them tetanus toxoid. As CCs are being introduced, these rural facilities are being used as permanent locations for vaccination. Respondents of qualitative interviews from both the study areas (high performing and low performing) identified immunizations against the major infectious diseases to be the most important component of PHC.

Promotion of Food Supply and Proper Nutrition

An important finding was prevalent concern that promotion of food supply and proper nutrition was being neglected in the PHC system. The physician respondents noted that some vertical and temporary nutrition projects had been implemented without any follow-up or scaling-up mechanisms.

Community-Targeted Responses

Through qualitative observation, we found that an on-site "health education get-together" (*Shastho Shikkhar Ashor*) on the premises of the high-performing Dhamrai UpHC induced high satisfaction regarding health education there. It had high visibility, and its label itself attracted the attention of patients, creating high attendance at the early morning health education sessions conducted by trained health educators. A twenty-one-inch television was kept there to show documentaries covering various aspects of health and healthy living. Apart from the morning session, which takes place every day between 08:30 and 09:00 a.m., doctors are also instructed to provide relevant health education to patients. Five union subcenters are attached to the Dhamrai UpHC. These subcenters also arrange health education sessions and are instructed to maintain a register book to note the topics of discussion, the number of participants, and the name of the instructor at each session. Reflecting on the usefulness of health education programs, one health assistant (government community health worker) commented: "Previously people did not even know how to use [a] tooth brush. Now you see how commonly they brush their teeth. If you ask any school kid, he or she knows the proper way of brushing."

Respondents of the study suggested that information and communication materials can play a pivotal role in informing people of their health entitlements. Currently, these materials concentrate on health practices only. Respondents said that these materials can be developed in such a way that they can impart information regarding health entitlements and the facilities and resources available at nearby health centers. There is already a wide network of government health workers who are primarily responsible for disseminating health information. These workers can play a fundamental role by informing people about available services and the entitlement of the people in addition to their usual health education messages. A more active role of local government was recommended for community empowerment. A local government leader, during an in-depth interview, suggested that the local government authorities can organize regular community meetings where health issues can be discussed. These local government meetings can also pave the way for community members to express their complaints and experiences regarding their encounters with health facilities.

Our discussion on the sociocultural, political, and economic context of PHC in Bangladesh illustrates the importance of a pluralistic health system that included a focus on women's health, gender equity, and community inclusion. For instance, increased participation of women in economic activities, improved communications, and the government policy of encouraging female education helped improve maternal and child health indicators and increased life expectancy. Community-based approaches, such as the vast network of both government and NGO community health workers contributed to the country's achievements in the fields of family planning, immunization, oral rehydration, tuberculosis control, childhood nutrition, and so forth, to name a few.

It is well worth highlighting that women-focused health services contributed greatly to Bangladesh's strategy of improving health outcomes. Women determine many intrahousehold health behaviors regarding food, water, and health care seeking. Women's social networks spread norms of behavior that contribute to population control, primary health and nutrition, disease control, and so on. Another lesson is that a policy environment fostering collaboration between multiple government sectors and multiple stakeholders inside and outside of government services can achieve more.

Challenges Ahead

Amid the noteworthy PHC achievements in Bangladesh described thus far, there remain significant challenges including: (1) addressing inequity and social determinants of health; (2) curbing high out-of-pocket expenditures; (3) providing better services for noncommunicable diseases (NCDs), elderly, disabled, and psychiatric patients; (4) growing the health workforce; (5) improving quality of care; and (6) addressing environmental health threats from climate change. For all these challenges, the platforms used for comprehensive PHC remain quite powerful.

Failure to Address Social Determinants of Health Resulting in Inequity

Bangladesh's health progress has yet to be fully inclusive—inequity is still a serious concern. The successive health sector plans of Bangladesh have stated aims to channel resources to vulnerable groups including women, children, and the poor, but in reality public expenditure continues to favor the rich relative to the poor. Health care expenditure of the Ministry of Health and Family Welfare at different levels shows that 27% of the primary-level health care allocation is going to the richest quintile and 21% to the poorest quintile (Huque et al. 2012). Out-of-pocket health expenditure is one of the highest in the world (67%), with private health expenditure being almost exclusively out of pocket (93%) (Joarder et al. 2019).

In rural Bangladesh, PHC services appear to be inequitable across significant measures such as access, treatment, and outcome. Various studies show a large disparity in use of maternal care between the rich and the poor (Chowdhury et al. 2006; Anwar et al. 2008). Particularly, the use of antenatal care, skilled birth attendants, and institutional delivery is substantially low in the three lower socioeconomic quintiles (Collin et al. 2007). Facility-based deliveries also show a disparity between the rich and the poor. Wealthier rural residents tend to use facilities for delivery care more than their poor counterparts, with a ratio of six to one (Kamal et al. 2016). Only 15% of pregnant women from the lowest wealth quintile households delivered their babies in a health facility compared to 70% for the richest quintile (National Institute of Population Research and Training, Mitra and Associates, and ICF International 2015). Additionally, in urban areas, a recently conducted Bangladesh Urban Health Survey (2013) reported an improvement in key health indicators of the slum population over the previously conducted survey in 2006. However, despite the improvement in the health status, a wide disparity in health of slum and nonslum areas is still evident. For instance, between 2006 and 2013, the percentage of women using medically trained providers for delivery has increased from 18% to 37% for slums and from 56% to 68% for nonslums (National Institute of Population Research and Training, International Center for Diarrheal Disease Research Bangladesh, and MEASURE Evaluation 2013).

Special Care for Elderly, Disabled, and Psychiatric Patients

According to the key informants and the physician respondents of the study just described, there was no special care or facility for the elderly or the disabled, except for informal individual benevolence of the providers. NCDs have only recently attracted attention. The government has begun to offer training for doctors on the care of NCDs. There was no facility in the Up-HCs to deal with cardiovascular diseases, cerebrovascular diseases, diabetes mellitus, psychiatric disorders, and several other NCDs, which occupy top positions in terms of the current burden of disease in Bangladesh. Inadequate services for NCDs are still found throughout the country.

Shortage of Human Resources and Compromised Quality of Care

Despite the presence of multiple cadres of auxiliary workers, access to PHC services is hampered by a dire shortage of support staff/auxiliary workforce in the health sector and an inappropriate skills mix. Severe shortages of sub-assistant community medical officers, nurses, and paramedics—particularly in rural areas—affects accessibility to PHC services. Bangladesh has about eight health workers per ten thousand population (Bangladesh Health Watch 2007), while WHO estimated that countries with fewer than twenty-three physicians, nurses, and midwives per ten thousand population generally fail to achieve adequate coverage rates to attain the health-related Millennium Development Goals (World Health Organization 2006).

The inappropriate ratios of doctors to nurses and doctors to technologists have remained another critical problem inhibiting a smoothly functioning team. Particularly, in the current context of PHC provision through ESPs from one-stop centers, an inappropriate skill mix is a great barrier to effective service delivery. Numbers of nurses, paramedics, pharmacists, and dentists are too low compared to that of doctors, whose work they are meant to complement. Currently, doctors make up 70% of the total registered professional workforce, and the remaining 30% are support staff (Government of

Bangladesh 2013). According to a recent estimate (Ahmed et al. 2011), there were about five physicians and two nurses per ten thousand population, while the ratio of nurses to physicians was 0.4 (i.e., 2.5 times more doctors than nurses).

Conversely, the increase in the number of unqualified allopathic providers during the past decade has been phenomenal compared to the growth of qualified or semiqualified allopathic providers. This proliferation indicates the prevalence of a weak regulatory system. These unqualified providers compromise quality of services (Cockcroft et al. 2007).

Addressing Environmental Health Threats from Climate Change

Bangladesh is one of the most vulnerable countries regarding environmental degradation and climate change. An estimated 70% of the population lives in a flood zone and 26% in a cyclone zone. The high population density of the country (1,265 per square kilometer, according to World Bank, 2017) results in a higher risk of mortality and morbidity. Over the past decades, Bangladesh has earned a reputation for managing to limit the devastation of environmental calamities during and shortly after a natural disaster (Cash et al. 2013). Yet, much needs to be done in terms of health systems resilience and long-term preparedness and disaster response.

Conclusion

Overall, Bangladesh is a role model for good health at a low cost. One of the critical determinants of its sustained success is the importance given by its health policymakers to the principles and practices of PHC from the beginning. Since Bangladesh's independence in 1971, it embraced some of the guiding principles of PHC, such as preventive care, community participation, social justice, and equity. Prior dissemination of the landmark reports by the Sokhey and Bhore Committees had set the stage. Right after gaining independence, Bangladesh directed its focus toward building health infrastructure in rural areas, where the majority of the population lived. As an avid supporter of the Alma-Ata Declaration and the Health for All movement, Bangladesh intensified its PHC endeavor during the successive decades. However, it did not shy away from some of the selective PHC programs addressing maternal and child health, family planning, immunization, nutrition, and so on.

In the 1990s, policymakers shifted the focus of the health system from a mere expansionary approach to building systematic institutional reforms in order to improve efficiency and effectiveness of health services. CCs were emphasized as a one-stop health solution for every six thousand rural population. The NGO sector also joined hands with the government to provide mostly preventive services to marginalized populations. Overall, the community focus and community-based approach of service delivery has been one of the most effective strategies for achieving health gains in Bangladesh.

PHC in Bangladesh, provided by the government and NGOs, is traditionally characterized by cooperation (not competition) between these two sectors, including multisectoral engagements, community centeredness, and pluralistic service provision (i.e., involvement of various types of service providers working in different capacities, modalities, and locations). These initiatives have resulted in some appreciable outcomes, especially in supply of safe water and basic sanitation, substantial vaccination coverage, and social and behavior change communication, among others.

However, some challenges remain, both at the policy and implementation levels. For example, in many areas, community-level health committees are nonfunctioning. Intersectoral collaborations often falter due to a lack of clear guidelines. Promotion of food supply and basic nutrition is still done using a vertical approach and is widely neglected. Inequity persists in terms of the economy (poor versus rich), geography (rural versus urban), location (slum versus nonslum). The shortage of human resources for health—including inappropriate skill mix, absolute shortage, insufficient training, and lack of regulation—are perpetuating challenges.

At the same time, the new millennium came with its own challenges. The epidemiological transition caused a shift in the traditional disease pattern and the need for response to the increased prevalence of NCDs and injuries. The country was urbanizing at an unprecedented pace, the private sector flourished within an unregulated health market, and out-of-pocket payments crippled health service seekers. With a legacy of admirable success in tackling the communicable disease problems, the country must make a transition to using its PHC platform to address the current health landscape.

We recommend that the fragmented approaches that remain in some aspects of health services (e.g., promotion of food supply and proper nutrition) should be brought further under a comprehensive PHC framework. More robust guidelines for intersectoral collaboration and community participation (and eventually empowerment) need to be devised at the policy level and implemented rigorously. Regulatory frameworks should be reviewed, updated, and strengthened against rapid and unregulated privatization, and resulting high out-of-pocket health expenditures. Policymakers should consult with researchers and experts and support local evidence generation in response to newer health challenges (e.g., NCDs, mental health, urbanization, environmental health) in order to keep pace with the burden of these additional health issues.

REFERENCES (SEE PAGE 341 FOR FULL CITATIONS FOR BOXED TEXT)

Afsana, Kaosar, and Syed Shabab Wahid. 2013. "Health care for poor people in the urban slums of Bangladesh." *Lancet* 382 (9910): 2049–2051.

Ahmed, Syed Masud, Bushra Binte Alam, Iqbal Anwar, Tahmina Begum, Rumana Huque, Jahangir A. Khan, Herfina Nababan, and Ferdous Arfina Osman. 2015. *Health Systems in Transition*, Vol. 5, No. 3, *Asia Pacific Observatory on Health Systems and Policies, World Health Organization.*

Ahmed, Syed Masud, Timothy G. Evans, Hilary Standing, and Simeen Mahmud. 2013. "Harnessing pluralism for better health in Bangladesh." *Lancet* 382 (9906): 1746–1755.

Ahmed, Syed Masud, Md Awlad Hossain, Ahmed Mushtaque Raja Chowdhury, and Abbas Uddin Bhuiya. 2011. "The health workforce crisis in Bangladesh: Shortage, inappropriate skill-mix and inequitable distribution." *Hum Resourc Health* 9 (1): 3.

Anwar, I., M. Sami, N. Akhtar, M. E. Chowdhury, U. Salma, M. Rahman, and M. Koblinsky. 2008. "Inequity in maternal health-care services: Evidence from home-based skilled-birth-attendant programmes in Bangladesh." *Bull World Health Organ* 86 (4): 252–259.

Balabanova, Dina, Anne Mills, and L. Conteh. 2013. "Good health at low cost 25 years on: Lessons for the future of health system strengthening." *Lancet* 381 (9883): 2118–2133.

Bangladesh Health Watch. 2007. *Health workforce in Bangladesh: Who constitutes the healthcare system? The state of health in Bangladesh 2007.* Dhaka: James P. Grant School of Public Health.

Bloom, Gerald, Hilary Standing, Henry Lucas, Abbas Uddin Bhuiya, Oladimeji Oladepo, and David H. Peters. 2011. "Making health markets work better for poor people: The case of informal providers." *Health Policy Plan* 26 (Suppl. 1): i45–i52.

Cash, R. A., S. R. Halder, M. Husain, M. S. Islam, F. H. Mallick, M. A. May, M. Rahman, and M. A. Rahman. 2013. "Reducing the health effect of natural hazards in Bangladesh." *Lancet* 382 (9910): 2094–2103.

Chaudhury, Nazmul, and Jeffrey Hammer. "Ghost doctors: Absenteeism in Bangladeshi health facilities." Bangladesh: World Bank, 2003.

Chowdhury, Ahmed Mushtaque Raja, Abbas Uddin Bhuiya, Mahbub Elahi Chowdhury, Sabrina Rasheed, Zakir Hussain, and Lincoln C. Chen. 2013. "The Bangladesh paradox: Exceptional health achievement despite economic poverty." *Lancet* 382 (9906): 1734–1745.

Chowdhury, Mahbub Elahi, Carine Ronsmans, Japhet Killewo, Iqbal Anwar, Kaniz Gausia, Sushil Das-Gupta, Lauren S Blum, Greet Dieltiens, Tom Marshall, Sajal Saha, and Jo Borghi. 2006. "Equity in use of home-based or facility-based skilled obstetric care in rural Bangladesh: An observational study." *Lancet* 367 (9507): 327–332.

CIET. 2003. *Third service delivery survey report 2003: Health and population sector program 1998–2003.* Dhaka.

Cockcroft A., N. Andersson, D. Milne, M. Z. Hossain, and E. Karim. 2007. "What did the public think of health services reform in Bangladesh? Three national community-based surveys 1999–2003." *Health Res Policy Syst* 5:1.

Collin, Simon M., Iqbal Anwar, and Carine Ronsmans. 2007. "A decade of inequality in maternity care: Antenatal care, professional attendance at delivery, and Caesarean section in Bangladesh (1991–2004)." *Int J Equity Health* 6 (1): 9.

Das, Pamela, and Richard Horton. 2013. "Bangladesh: Innovating for health." *Lancet* 382 (9906): 1681–1682.

Democracy Watch. 2010. "Health problems of women living in slums: A situation analysis of three selected slums in Dhaka City." Dhaka. http://www.dwatch-bd.org/ggtp/Research Reports/health problem.pdf.

Government of Bangladesh. 1973. "The first five year plan 1973–1978." Dhaka. http://www.plancomm.gov.bd/site/files/e23192da-65a5-48c5-b91f-bb6456207d6c/-.

———. 1990. "The fourth five year plan 1990–1995." Dhaka. http://www.plancomm.gov.bd/site/files/9d7dc59d-d6f6-4959-87d1-5d9bc8599694/-.

———. 1997. "The fifth five year plan 1997–2002." Dhaka. http://www.plancomm.gov.bd/site/files/87d366f2-20ff-4d0f-8ee7-539b44f48f19/-.

———. 2003. "Health and Population Sector Programme (HPSP) evaluation by IMED of the Ministry of Planning." Dhaka.

———. 2013. "Health bulletin 2012." Dhaka. http://dghs.gov.bd/bn/licts_file/images/Health_Bulletin/HealthBulletin2012_full.pdf.

———. 2016. "Health bulletin." Dhaka. http://www.dghs.gov.bd/index.php/en/home/4821-health-bulletin-2016.

———. 2018a. "Background: Directorate general of drug administration." Directorate General of Drug Administration. 2018. http://www.dgda.gov.bd/index.php/downloads/background.

———. 2018b. "Bangladesh national health accounts 1997–2015." Dhaka. http://www.heu.gov.bd/pdf/BNHA-V%201997-2015.pdf.

———. 2018c. "Health bulletin 2017." Dhaka. http://www.dghs.gov.bd/images/docs/Publicaations/HealthBulletin2017Final13_01_2018.pdf.

Gruen, Reinhold, Raqibul Anwar, Tahmina Begum, James R. Killingsworth, and Charles Normand. 2002. "Dual job holding practitioners in Bangladesh: An exploration." *Soc Sci Med* 54 (2): 267–279.

Hunter, Erin C., Munia Islam, and Jennifer Callaghan-Koru. 2015. "Lessons from the ground: A collection of case studies." Dhaka. https://bangladesh.savethechildren.net/sites/bangladesh.savethechildren.net/files/library/Lessons from the Ground A Collection of Case Studies.pdf.

Huque, Rumana, Abul Barkat, and Nazme Sabina. 2012. "Public health expenditure: Equity, efficacy and universal health coverage." In *Bangladesh Health Watch report 2011: Moving towards universal health coverage*, 25–32. Dhaka: James P. Grant School of Public Health.

Joarder, T., T. Z. Chaudhury, and I. Mannan. 2019. "Universal health coverage in Bangladesh: Activities, challenges, and suggestions." *Adv Public Health* 2019 (4954095): 1–12.

Kamal, Nahid, Sian Curtis, Mohammad S. Hasan, and Kanta Jamil. 2016. "Trends in equity in use of maternal health services in urban and rural Bangladesh." *Int J Equity Health* 15 (1): 27.

Koehlmoos, Tracey Perez, Ziaul Islam, Shahela Anwar, Shaikh A. Shahed Hossain, Rukhsana Gazi, Peter Kim Streatfield, and Abbas Uddin Bhuiya. 2011. "Health transcends poverty: The Bangladesh experience." In *"Good health at low cost" 25 years on: What makes a successful health system?*, edited by Dina Balabanova, Martin Mckee, and Anne Mills, 47–81. London: London School of Hygiene and Tropical Medicine.

Mahmud, Simeen. 2004. "Citizen participation in the health sector in rural Bangladesh: Perceptions and reality." *IDS Bull* 35 (2): 11–18.

National Institute of Population Research and Training, MEASURE Evaluation, and International Center for Diarrheal Disease Research Bangladesh, and MEASURE Evaluation. 2012. "Bangladesh maternal mortality and health care survey 2010." Dhaka. https://www.measureevaluation.org/resources/publications/tr-12-87.

———. 2013. "Bangladesh urban health survey 2013 final report." Dhaka. https://www.measureevaluation.org/resources/publications/tr-15-117.

———. 2017. "Bangladesh maternal mortality and health care survey 2016: Preliminary report." Dhaka. https://www.measureevaluation.org/resources/publications/tr-17-218.

National Institute of Population Research and Training, Mitra and Associates, and ICF International. 2013. "Bangladesh demographic and health survey 2011." Dhaka. https://dhsprogram.com/pubs/pdf/fr265/fr265.pdf.

———. 2015. "Bangladesh demographic and health survey 2014: Key indicators." Dhaka. https://dhsprogram.com/pubs/pdf/FR311/FR311.pdf.

National Institute of Population Research and Training, Mitra and Associates, Measure DHS, and Macro International. 2007. "Bangladesh demographic and health survey 2007." Dhaka. https://dhsprogram.com/pubs/pdf/FR207/FR207[April -10-2009].pdf.

National Institute of Population Research and Training, Mitra and Associates, and ORC Macro. 2001. "Bangladesh demographic and health survey 1999–2000." Dhaka. http://dhsprogram.com/pubs/pdf/FR119/FR119.pdf.

National Institute of Population Research and Training, Mitra and Associates, ORC Macro, Johns Hopkins University, and International Centre for Diarrhoeal Disease Research. 2003. "Bangladesh Maternal Health Services and Maternal Mortality Survey 2001." Dhaka. https://dhsprogram.com/pubs/pdf/FR142/FR142.pdf http://www.measuredhs.com/pubs/pdf/%0AFR142/00FrontMatter00.pdf %0A.

Normand, C., M. H. Iftekar, and S. A. Rahman. 2012. "Assessment of the community clinics: Effects on service delivery, quality and utilization of services." Dhaka. https://assets.publishing.service.gov.uk/media/57a08c35ed915d3cfd001236/bang_comm_clinics_web_version.pdf https://assets.publishing.service.gov.uk/media/57a08c35ed915d3cfd001236/ba ng_comm_clinics_web_version.pdf.

Osman, Ferdous Arfina. 2004. *Policy making in Bangladesh: A study of the health policy process*. Dhaka: A. H. Development Publishing House.

———. 2005. "Implementation constrained by a lack of policy ownership: Evidence from Bangladesh." *Asia Pac J Public Admin* 27 (1): 19–36.

Osman, Ferdous Arfina, and Sara Bennett. 2018. "Political economy and quality of primary health service in rural Bangladesh and the United States of America: A comparative analysis." *J Int Dev* 30 (5): 818–836.

Osman, Ferdous Arfina, Jamie Boex, Mokshedul Hamid, and Abdul Hannan Shaikh. 2014. "An analysis of functional assignments in health and education in Bangladesh: The role of local governments and local administration." Dhaka: UNDP.

Streatfield, Peter Kim. 2003. "Health and population sector program 1998–2003, Bangladesh: Status of performance indicators 2002." Dhaka. https://www .researchgate.net/publication/290036932_Health_and_Population_Sector _Programme_1998-2003_Bangladesh_Status_of_Performance_Indicators_2002.

Wolf, Michael S., Julie A. Gazmararian, and David W. Baker. 2005. "Health literacy and functional health status among older adults." *Arch Intern Med* 165:1946–1952.

World Bank. 2005. "The economics and governance of nongovernmental Organizations in Bangladesh." Consultation draft. Washington, DC. http://documents.worldbank .org/curated/en/105291468207267279/pdf/382910BD0NGOre10also03586101PUB LIC1.pdf.

———. 2010. "Bangladesh health sector profile 2010." Washington, DC. http:// documents.worldbank.org/curated/en/239091467997274128/pdf/688850ESW0P113 0rofile0final0Dec028.pdf.

———. 2017. "Data bank." 2017. https://data.worldbank.org/country/bangladesh.

World Health Organization. 2006. *The world health report 2006: Working together for health*. Geneva. https://www.who.int/whr/2006/whr06_en.pdf?ua=1.

CHAPTER EIGHT

Ethiopia

*Expansion of Primary Health Care through the Health
Extension Program*

ZUFAN ABERA DAMTEW, MEIKE SCHLEIFF, KEBEDE WORKU,
CHALA TESFAYE CHEKAGN, SEBLEWENGEL LEMMA,
ONAOPEMIPO ABIODUN, MIGNOTE SOLOMON HAILE,
DENNIS CARLSON, AHMED MOEN, AND HENRY B. PERRY

The concept of primary health care (PHC) encapsulated in the 1978 Alma-Ata Declaration called for urgent action by all governments to protect and promote the health of all the people of the world (World Health Organization 1978). The challenge was accepted in Ethiopia since at that point the health system was dependent on a centralized, top-down approach that had failed to provide health services to 80% of the population in 1974 (Kloos 1998a). Furthermore, true community participation and appropriate strategies to address community needs were lacking. The health care system at that point was predominantly urban based and curative focused: In 1972, 92% of government expenditure on medical care was on hospitals, and the per capita government expenditure in the two largest cities (Addis Ababa and Asmara) was twenty times greater than for the rest of the country, which at that time was almost entirely rural (Kloos 1998a). Although the regime of Mengistu Haile Mariam (commonly referred to as the Derg), in power from 1974 to 1991, had its roots in socialist principles and formally committed itself to supporting the principles of the Alma-Ata Declaration, the reality was that the redistribution of resources to the periphery was limited for various reasons (Kloos 1998a). Worsening economic conditions, famine, and devotion of more than half of the government budget to military expenditures prevented the investment of funds needed for improvement of the PHC system.

With the overthrow of the Derg in 1991, the Transitional Government of Ethiopia began the arduous process of rebuilding its health system, which had been largely destroyed by civil war. The Transitional Government of Ethiopia's health policy emphasized and focused on reconstruction of health facilities and extension of service to the rural area (Kloos 1998a), but it took until 2003 for it to realize that a radical transformation of the health system would be required in order to implement the principles of Alma-Ata for the benefit of the population. Thus, Ethiopia did not properly respond to the call of Alma-Ata, but it finally did so in the early part of the twenty-first century.

This chapter reviews the past forty years of Ethiopian efforts to put community-based PHC front and center in the broader scope of its national health system. We note some of the successes and pitfalls encountered in implementation, such as the lack of skilled human resources, accessibility of health services and appropriate supervision, and bureaucratic administration, that have impacted Ethiopia's capacity to champion the fundamental principles of the Alma-Ata Declaration (Kloos, 1998b).

Ethiopia's Primary Health Care System before 2000

Throughout the 1960s and early 1970s, the government's policies, plans, and strategies focused on increasing coverage and utilization by decentralizing basic health services, but these services were unfortunately almost entirely limited to hospitals in urban settings, with the exception of one hundred or so health centers scattered throughout the country staffed by community nurses and health officers who had graduated from the Gondar College of Public Health. Only 20% of the population had access to PHC services in 1974 (Kloos, 1998a). Following the overthrow of Emperor Haile Selassie's government in 1974 and the takeover by the military leadership of the Derg regime, the health system was reorganized to give greater priority to the underserved rural population (Kitaw et al. 2007). The Derg regime introduced health policies and health administrative guidelines that were inspired by socialist principles and that were supported by the Alma-Ata Declaration on PHC. The regime required high school and university students to build rural health stations and conduct national literacy campaigns. Particular strengths in Ethiopia's implementation of PHC in the late 1970s and 1980s included the deployment of thousands of community health agents and volunteer health promoters as well as trained traditional birth attendants.

In 1991, the Ethiopian People's Revolutionary Democratic Front seized power from the Derg regime and formed the Transitional Government of Ethiopia (Balabanova 2013). At that time, health coverage was at a low level since many health facilities had been damaged or looted during the civil war and disease outbreaks had ravaged the country (Kloos 1998b). These facilities had low utilization rates, partly as a result of their physical inaccessibility to the largely rural population (Sebhatu 2008).

In 1993, a new health policy was established that emphasized democratization, fiscal and political decentralization, collaboration with neighboring countries, and promotion of the participation of the private sector in health care (Kloos 1998b). This policy also recognized that disease prevention and health promotion were fundamental for improving the health of the population. This prioritization of preventive and promotive care differed from past health strategies, which had focused on curative services and the construction of health facilities.

Ethiopia's Primary Health Care System Advances Beginning at the Turn of the Century

To articulate its long-term goals for population health, the government developed the Health Sector Development Plan (HSDP) beginning in 1997. Figure 8.1 outlines major health system development events since then. In the early twentieth century, the government embraced the viewpoint that health development is an essential component of social and economic development (Balabanova 2013). The HSDP had four (HSDP I to IV) consecutive phases, which were implemented using the cycle of five years, starting in 1996/97. The first HSDP (1997/98–2001/02) was based on critical reviews of prevailing national health problems and a broader awareness of newly emerging health problems in the country. During the HSDP II (2002/03–2004/05), the health extension program (HEP) of Ethiopia was initiated for the implementation of a basic health package and to improve access for health services. To further consolidate the gains from the HEP and enhance community engagement and inclusiveness in health, the Federal Ministry of Health launched the Women's Development Army (WDA) in 2011. As part of the government's long-term plan, in 2015 the Federal Ministry of Health developed the Health Sector Transformation Plan, which covers July 2015 to June 2020.

The HSDP was a twenty-year strategy that was implemented on a rolling basis in four phases, each implementation period lasting five years (World Health Organization 2015). The PHC approach was given due attention in all of these plans. The government also ensured that the Health Sector Development Programs (I-III/1997–2010) were in line with its Plan for Accelerated and Sustained Development to End Poverty (PASDEP) (Balabanova 2013). PASDEP is a strategic framework that guided all development activities including those in the health sector. PASDEP was operative for the five-

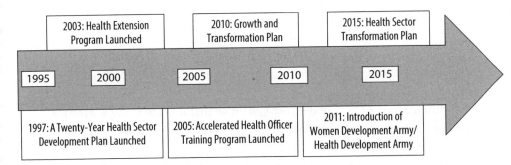

Figure 8.1. Timeline for the health sector and other development initiatives in Ethiopia.

year period between 2005/2006 and 2009/2010 as a midterm plan to achieve the United Nations Millennium Development Goal (MDG) targets to be achieved by 2015 along with the government's vision for Ethiopia's development (Federal Democratic Republic of Ethiopia 2010). The main objectives of the health sector components of PASDEP were to reduce child mortality, improve maternal health, and combat the spread and prevalence of HIV/AIDS, tuberculosis, and malaria (Federal Democratic Republic of Ethiopia 2010). Following PASDEP, the government developed the Growth and Transformation Plans I and II from 2010–2015 and from 2016–2020, respectively. This ten-year growth and transformation plan was used as a road map for the country's vision to achieve lower-middle-income country status by 2025. Growth and Transformation Plans built on the lessons learned from the implementation of PASDEP (Federal Democratic Republic of Ethiopia 2010).

Health System Reform in 2003 and the Launch of the Health Extension Program

An evaluation of the HSDP II in 2003 showed that health services and higher-level health professionals were not reaching people at the grassroots level (Sebhatu 2008). In order to address this problem, the government launched a new health care strategy, known as the accelerated expansion of PHC coverage, a truly community-based approach (Sebhatu 2008). To achieve universal PHC coverage that reaches low-income, rural households, the government of Ethiopia launched the HEP in 2003 during the HSDP II implementation period. The aim of HEP was to enable the government to achieve PASDEP's strategic objectives and extend health coverage to rural villages, or *kebeles* (Federal Democratic Republic of Ethiopia 2010).

Before 1993, Ethiopia had a six-tier health care delivery system with a principal focus on urban-centered curative health care (World Health Organization 2012). The national health policy of 1993 tried to reorganize and decentralize the health care delivery system so that it could make a stronger contribution to the socioeconomic development of the country (Federal Democratic Republic of Ethiopia 2002; Wamai 2009).

In line with decentralization and expansion of the PHC system, the reorganization of the health system transferred administrative and operational power to its eleven regional governments (including two cities), with the Federal Ministry of Health mainly playing a coordinating and policy-making role (World Health Organization 2012). Through this decentralized structure, respective regional health bureaus, zonal health departments (subdivisions of regions), and *woreda*/district health offices took the responsibility of supervising health facilities and managing the delivery of health services. Community-level health committees participated in identifying major health problems, budgeting, planning, implementing, monitoring, and evaluating health services (Kloos 1998b).

Currently, Ethiopia's health service is structured into a three-tier system: primary, secondary, and tertiary levels of care (Ministry of Health, n.d.), as depicted in figure 8.2. PHC services are rendered at the primary tier, which is comprised of one health post for five thousand people, a health center for a twenty-five thousand to forty thousand, and a primary hospital for sixty thousand to one hundred thousand people. The health posts are staffed by two salaried health extension workers (HEWs). A health center and five health posts jointly form a primary health care unit (PHCU). Health center construction expanded enormously under the HEP, though the goal of increased numbers of health facilities has not yet been reached.

The Community Health Platform of Ethiopia

The community health service of Ethiopia is mainly implemented by the HEWs and supported by communities; HEP is a pioneering community-centered strategy. Its primary purpose is to deliver disease prevention, health promotion, and selected high-impact curative interventions at the health post, schools, community, and household levels. The program bridges community engagement through awareness creation, behavioral change, community organization, and mobilization.

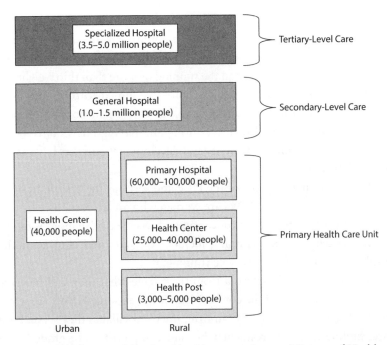

Figure 8.2. The Ethiopian three-tiered health system. Source: Ministry of Health, n.d.

The first experience with extension programs in Ethiopia was actually in the agricultural sector (Ghebreyesus 2013). Under that program, the agricultural extension workers taught farmers best practices in agronomy. The government adapted this program to form the HEP. The HEP's focus on community-level provision of essential health care services promoted the principle that the transfer of appropriate knowledge and skills to households would lead to communities producing and maintaining their own health.

HEWs also capture health-related data in their community. They continuously update the data and use this information for action. They send reports weekly, monthly, quarterly, and annually to their supervising health center. Health centers compile a PHCU report (for the health center and five about health posts combined) and submit it to the woreda/district office.

During the early stages of the implementation of the HEP, key stakeholders, partners, donors, health professionals, and communities were not in agreement on its PHC focus (Ghebreyesus 2013). However, after the government set a target that "every village needed to have a health post staffed with a minimum of two HEWs" and demonstrated its commitment to the program by funding its implementation, stakeholders took notice of this firm, high-level commitment and supported the program (Ghebreyesus 2013).

The community platform was designed as part of the national health system and has received sustained political commitment throughout its implementation. This commitment has resulted in the construction of more than sixteen thousand health posts and the training of more than thirty-eight thousand HEWs over the past years. The initiative aimed to train and deploy two HEWs per health post, with an average catchment population of five thousand. Costs associated with recruiting and paying HEWs have been financed by the government, while several development partners have assisted with HEW training.

HEWs are the main agents of the HEP and serve as the first point of contact with the PHC system. HEWs are women who are at least 18 years of age and have at least a tenth grade education and receive twelve months of training prior to deployment. Training includes didactic and clinical modules and substantial practical in-service training.

HEWs are preferably selected from the villages that they will be serving and speak the language of the community. However, some HEWs are selected from the district towns rather than from the rural villages they serve. For instance, finding a female resident who had completed tenth grade has not been possible in some places (Kitaw et al. 2007). HEWs are recruited through active community participation that involves committees made up of elected representatives from the community and local administration (Perry et al. 2017). Following their training, HEWs commence their activities by preparing maps of their assigned villages and identifying the main health priorities in their catchment area. HEWs are public sector employees and salaried civil servants with a monthly compensation of about US$84 as of 2014 (Perry et al. 2017). Health center staff make regular visits to health posts to supervise HEWs, and HEWs also attend monthly meetings at health centers (Perry et al. 2017).

The creation of the cadre of HEWs has greatly expanded access to a range of basic but also potentially lifesaving interventions. The design of HEP packages was based on analysis of major health problems and the disease burden of the population. Initially, sixteen health packages were organized into four principal categories: (1) family health, (2) disease prevention and control, (3) personal hygiene and environmental health, and (4) health education and promotion.

In addition to the provision of services at the health post, HEWs also provide free, door-to-door health services under these four main categories. Since each health post has two HEWs, the routine is for each HEW to spend half of her time in the community and half at the health post. Usually, the HEWs rotate so that one day one HEW is in the community while the other is at the health post, and the next day they reverse their locations.

Recently the scope of services has increased, particularly for children and women, so that it now includes integrated community-based case management of common childhood illnesses (e.g., childhood pneumonia, malaria, diarrhea, measles, and malnutrition), community-based newborn care, and provision of long-acting family planning methods (injectable contraceptives and contraceptives implanted subcutaneously in the forearm). The health services rendered by HEWs both at the health post and in the community are free of charge. HEP packages are mainly implemented at health posts and in homes but also at schools and youth centers.

Communities fully participate through WDA, often also referred to as the Health Development Army. The WDA is a networking and organizing mechanism for neighboring households. It meets regularly to discuss health issues and design local strategies for addressing challenges they encounter. The community becomes involved in health activities and implements the HEP with the support of the WDA. In addition to health promotion, the WDA also participates in other development activities, such as saving, agriculture, education, and environmental protection. Different sectors, such as Women, Child, Youth Affairs, agriculture, and education support the WDA structures at the grassroots level. Leaders at the national, regional, and district levels are linked with women's groups in every village across the country. There are steering committees at all levels, which brings all these sectors together. These sectors are expected to jointly plan, review, and monitor WDA activities. In addition, development partners and other stakeholders are encouraged to contribute to the implementation of the program by providing health materials and supplies as well as training and monitoring (Banteyerga 2011). The HEP relies on locally available technologies, knowledge, skills, and the wisdom of communities. The program is tailored to the local context and lifestyle of the community, so HEP packages differ across agrarian, pastoral, and urban settings.

This evolution occurred in steps. Following the successful implementation of the agrarian HEP launched in 2003, the HEP expanded to pastoral and urban areas in 2007 and 2010, respectively. The HEP packages and implementation modalities were revised and contextualized with the input of the pastoral and urban communities and according to their needs. In order to address challenges in recruiting qualified individuals in pastoralist and semipastoralist areas, the rules were revised to allow men and those with a sixth to eighth grade education (rather than a tenth grade education) to serve as HEWs. Urban HEWs are nurses with an additional three months of training on the community health program. Between 2003 and 2013, Ethiopia recruited, trained, and deployed more than thirty-eight thousand HEWs (Perry et al. 2017).

HEWs see patients at the health post and also make home visits. This arrangement is meant to improve access to health services. The HEP is serving as a platform to link the community with health facilities for early and better health care and for referrals for more complicated cases when required. HEWs receive support and supplies from health centers and, when necessary, from the woreda/district health offices. Primary hospitals serve as the referral and training hubs for the PHC units. The HEP designed and implemented the WDA Initiative in 2011 to further strengthen the program.

Formation of the Women's Development Army

HEWs were initially supported by community volunteers. Ethiopia has a long history of different types of volunteer community health programs. Community health volunteers with different names, such as community health agents, trained traditional birth attendants, volunteer health promoters, and others have played an important role in the provision of health care services, including health promotion. These community volunteers were members of the community and were early adopters of health actions; they volunteered to practice "doable" health actions and volunteered to show these to their neighbors and relatives. They were trained by HEWs and district health staff.

The HEP applied the social diffusion theory, which states that when introducing a new idea or innovation in a society, a select group of people are more apt to first adapt the introduced change, leading to a process whereby the change will eventually diffuse to others in the social system. To this effect, HEWs and then, later, community health workers identified and trained "model families"—households that actively participated in the different HEP health practices and implemented HEP packages. By giving these households social recognition and credibility, the program aimed to encourage others to follow their lead and adopt the desired health behaviors and practices. This brought about impressive health outcomes. However, there was a gap in quality and comprehensiveness. Hence, the WDA was initiated in 2011 to engage everyone in the community in an organized and inclusive manner, particularly disadvantaged and underserved groups (Damtew et al. 2018).

The WDA is a broad-based community engagement platform and a networking and organizing mechanism for households. Around thirty households in a neighborhood are organized into a group called a women's development team. The women's development team is divided into five smaller groups, with six households each, commonly referred as a one-to-five network. Once the households are networked, they elect a leader (called a WDA leader) for each network based on merit: good performance in the implementation of HEP packages, volunteerism to serve others, and other personal attributes.

WDA leaders spearhead the community through participatory learning and action meetings. The WDA has facilitated identification of local bottlenecks and come up with locally accepted strategies and feasible solutions to overcome them. HEWs mentor and build the capacity of WDA leaders. Because HEWs live where they work, they have context-specific knowledge of their communities. They learn by doing and build on the indigenous knowledge in the community with knowledge they have received from their trainings (Kanjo 2012; Damtew 2013). Hence, the close collaboration and rapport among HEWs and WDA leaders promote community ownership that in turn facilitates scaling up of best practices in a well-structured and near-to-community manner. WDA leaders are volunteers from the community, so they do not receive any salary or financial incentives, but they do receive certificates and recognition from their communities as well as from the HEWs with whom they work.

Many PHC centers constructed maternity waiting homes with the help of communities, and communities also made financial contributions to cover the cost of purchasing and operating ambulances. WDA leaders often facilitated this community engagement. This has led to improved health outcomes such as reduced maternal mortality in the northern part of Ethiopia (Godefay et al. 2015). The focus of the WDA, as their name implies, is not only on health but on other aspects of women's role on development activities such as education, agriculture, environmental protection, and savings and loan groups.

Expansion of the Primary Health Care Infrastructure

To address the staffing shortages and improve the coverage of PHC services, the government started to focus on the training of community-level and mid-level health workers. For instance, the training and scale-up of HEWs began in 2003. Over the next decade, the government trained thirty-eight thousand HEWs, giving them twelve months of formal training and a full-time government salary of approximately US$80 per month, providing one HEW for every twenty-five hundred people. The government also launched the accelerated health officer training program in 2005 in five universities and twenty hospitals to provide health resources for the PHC centers, which each served twenty-five thousand to forty thousand people. In addition, to address the human resource requirements for comprehensive obstetric care and emergency surgery at the PHC level, a master's degree program in emergency surgery was developed at five universities. In 2009, the government launched an accelerated midwifery training program for nurses in fifteen regional health science colleges. In the subsequent three years, thirty-two hundred nurses graduated from the midwifery training program and were deployed nationwide (UNFPA Ethiopia, 2014).

The number of health posts increased from 2,899 in 2004 to 16,480 in 2016, and the number of health centers increased from 519 in 2004 to 3,727 in 2016 (Assefa et al. 2018). In a similar way, to address the critical shortage and misdistribution of doctors, new medical schools have been established with a new integrated curriculum that enhances both the clinical skills and the social accountability of medical doctors (Ministry of Health, n.d.). Overall, between 2006 and 2013, Ethiopia was able to increase its human resources for health density (number of doctors, nurses, and midwives per one thousand population) from 0.25 to 1.3 (Assefa et al. 2018)—still quite low but nonetheless showing quite significant progress.

Impact Achieved through Primary Health Care in Ethiopia

As shown in table 8.1, Ethiopia made impressive gains in coverage of high-priority interventions between 2005 and 2015. Usage of family planning more than doubled, antenatal care coverage more than doubled, delivery by a skilled provider increased more than fourfold, immunization coverage doubled, and notable gains were achieved in prevalence of exclusive breastfeeding among infants younger than six months of age and in care seeking for children with symptoms of pneumonia. In 2015, Ethiopia achieved all the MDGs for health except for maternal health, which it almost achieved. Compared to baselines for 1990, there was a 67% decline in under-5 mortality, a 71% decline in maternal mortality (while the goal was a 75% decline), a 90% decline in new HIV infections, a decrease in malaria-related mortality by 73%, and a more than 50% decline in mortality from tuberculosis (Assefa et al. 2018). Despite these achievements, the gains were not equitable, with substantial differences remaining among regions and between urban and rural areas (Assefa et al. 2018).

Table 8.1. Coverage of high-priority interventions before and after full implementation of the Health Extension Program

Indicators	2005	2016
Coverage of use of any modern family planning method among married women (%)	14	35
Under-5 mortality/1,000 live births	123	67
Coverage of antenatal care (%) provided by skilled provider	28	62
Coverage of delivery assisted by skilled provider (%)	6	28
Percentage of children (12–23 months) who received all basic vaccinations	20	39
Percentage of infants younger than 6 months who are exclusively breastfed	49	58
Percentage of children with symptoms of pneumonia taken to an appropriate provider	19	30

Sources: Ethiopia Demographic and Health Survey, 2005 and 2016.

It is difficult to determine how much to attribute these health improvements to the PHC system: HEP versus other interventions that were implemented during the same time period in Ethiopia. However, there are indications that HEP's contribution has been important. The effectiveness of HEP emanates from its service provision approach, which involves services close to the community, including house-to-house visits, school-based activities, youth-centered programming, and workplace- and community-level advocacy and engagement.

Several studies have shown the impact and cost-effectiveness of HEP on specific health programs. For instance, a study conducted on cost-effectiveness of tuberculosis treatment by HEWs showed that community-based treatment by HEWs cost only 39% of what treatment by other health professionals at the health facilities cost, and the results are just as good as those obtained by higher-level workers (Datiko and Lindtjørn 2010). Involving HEWs in tuberculosis treatment is a cost-effective alternative (Datiko and Lindtjørn 2010). A cross-sectional survey conducted between December 2008 and December 2010 from a representative sample of 117 kebeles estimated the prevalence of high-quality maternal and newborn care practices, and a program intensity score revealed that for every unit increase in the score the odds of receiving antenatal care increased by 13% and the odds of birth preparedness increased by 31%. The odds of receiving postnatal care increased by 60% and the odds of initiating breastfeeding immediately after birth increased by 10% (Karim et al. 2013).

Ethiopia has made remarkable progress in improving access to PHC over the past two decades through massive expansion of health centers and health posts as well as deployment of frontline and mid-level health care providers (Ministry of Health, n.d.). A recent study showed that the HEP has increased access to health workers and health facilities, particularly for the lower-income quintiles of the population. However, significant inequities in maternal and child health outcomes persist (when comparing outcomes for those in the lower-income quintiles with those in the higher-income quintiles) despite overall population gains in health status (Memirie et al. 2016.

The commitment and effort of the government to PHC, to focused and pro-poor health policies and strategies, coupled with the country's overall gains in socioeconomic development and improvements in infrastructure have had a synergistic effect on improving health outcomes since the 1990s. Nonetheless, abundant challenges remain, not the least of which involve further strengthening of the HEW program by addressing their high workloads, low salaries, lack of career advancement opportunities that had been promised, and needs for infrastructure improvements and logistical support at health posts (Assefa et al. 2019).

Improving Essential Health Services through the Second-Generation Health Extension Program

As the literacy level and the socioeconomic status of the population improve, the demand for quality and comprehensive health services also increases. Changing demographic trends, epidemiology, and urbanization also require more comprehensive services covering a wide range of quality health services close to the community. To respond to the rapidly changing situations, the government is revisiting and calibrating the HEP (Damtew et al. 2018). The second-generation HEP includes upgrading the credentials of all HEWs from level III (certificate) to level IV (diploma). There are also now efforts to improve the capacity of health posts to provide services through expansions and renovations as well as improvements in equipment and supplies. The sixteen HEP packages have been revised and expanded into eighteen packages by incorporating some important new topics including noncommunicable diseases, mental health, neglected tropical diseases, and institutional hygiene, which includes hygiene of institutions in rural areas, such as schools and religious and other service-rendering institutes.

Multisectoral Approach and Integrated Systems

HEWs are considered to be "a critical asset for effective delivery of health services" in Ethiopia and have been given a range of responsibilities and roles that span health and also span multiple sectors at local, regional, and national levels (Perry et al. 2016). At the local level, HEWs and WDA leaders are engaged with helping communities overcome barriers to accessing health services. At the national level, multiple ministries, including the Federal Ministries of Health, Education, Labor, Finance, and Public Service and Human Development, are all involved in supporting community health programs. High-level political leadership from the prime minister's office and from leaders of the Federal Ministry of Health have been key to the rapid and successful scale-up of the program (Perry et al. 2016).

HEWs and the WDA interconnect with the rest of the health system in several ways. HEWs work closely with other sectors (e.g., education and agriculture) at their kebele/village and its administration. They jointly discuss their monthly performance reports and find local solutions for problems encountered. They also work with other community-based institutions and other influential people in their locality, such as religious leaders and clan leaders, to tackle community health problems.

LINKAGES WITH THE HEALTH SYSTEM

HEWs are generally well integrated into the health system and its governance, financing, and training functions. HEWs are now full-time, public sector, formal health workers. According to one recent systematic review of the literature on the topic of community health programs, Ethiopia is among "the most strongly integrated CHW programs in the world" (Perry et al. 2017). HEWs get close technical and logistical support from the PHC center they report to.

HEWs are the first point of contact for community members who need to access higher levels in the health system. An inclusive, organized, and participatory implementation of community-led PHC is the bedrock of basic health services. The country has gradually expanded access to a spectrum of services and essential medicine (Admasu et al. 2016). Ethiopia has established the International Institute for Primary Health Care-Ethiopia, which contributes to achieving health for all through PHC by maintaining Ethiopia's primary health programs as a role model for the rest of the world. The institute contributes to the national effort to meet the growing needs of the population by assessing current policies and programs and by suggesting alternative policies and programs that can further improve community health. IIPHC-E fosters joint learning about health systems that can respond better to the changing health needs of Ethiopia and beyond.

COMMUNITY HEALTH INFORMATION SYSTEM

HEWs use a family health folders system for placing health-related information about all the members of a family. Each folder is kept at the health post according to the name of the community and the number of the house as shown on the outside of the house and on the map established for the village. This folder is the basic unit of the community-based health information system designed according to the principles of standardization, integration, and simplification to provide information for decision-making (Federal Ministry of Health 2008). This record-keeping system enables HEWs to keep track of their catchment area: who is in their catchment area and who needs services. There is a plan to computerize the community health information system, and pilot testing is now underway.

HEWs use information from the system to guide home visits, giving priority to family members who need services. They also record information in the family health folder as services are provided, whether at the health post or in the community. The HEW takes these folders with her when she visits the community. Each HEW then summarizes her activities in a monthly report submitted to her supervising health center. Subsequently, the health center compiles the report of the PHCU and submits a report for the district health office, which then summarizes and compiles all the PHCU reports within the district and similarly passes them on to the zonal health departments, the regional health bureaus, and then the central Federal Ministry of Health through the automated Health Management Information System. The staff members of the PHCU meet monthly to evaluate their performance and set priority actions for the following month.

Bottom-Up, Community-Engaged Planning, Organization, and Control

Ethiopia's health care delivery system is undergoing a reform into a more decentralized and cost-effective system as part of the government's a strategy to improve the overall socioeconomic status of the country (Federal Ministry of Health 2008). The primary objectives of the political, administrative, and economic decentralization policy are to increase local participation aimed at increasing ownership in the planning and management of government health services, to expand efficiency in resource allocation, and to improve accountability of the government's health services to the population.

The Federal Ministry of Health is the central coordinator of the health care system of Ethiopia. The main responsibility of the ministry is formulating policy, developing national strategies, mobilizing resources, and providing support and capacity-building to the regional health bureaus, who then disseminate these trainings in a cascaded fashion. Health services are managed in accordance with the decentralized structures of the country. Hence, responsibility for the management of health service delivery falls to the respective regional health bureaus, zonal health departments, and woreda/district health offices. As a result, management of health facilities, personnel, and health training institutions within the region is undertaken by the regional health bureaus with the support of zonal health departments and woreda/district health offices.

Health Care Financing

Ethiopia's priority in terms of scaling up PHC is for all Ethiopians to be able to provide a complete package of needed, priority health services through an effective, equitable, and efficient health care system (Ministry of Health, n.d.). Hence, the country is also scaling up a community-based health insurance program for the informal sector to provide protection against catastrophic health expenditures. The Health Sector Transformation Plan calls for mobilizing funding by designing different financial schemes, ensuring efficient budget utilization, and facilitating alignment and harmonization of stakeholders. This minimizes duplication of efforts and misuse of resources, which in turn facilitates the development of sustainable financing for the health sector (Ministry of Health, n.d.).

Conclusion

The Ethiopia experience since 2003 demonstrates how, with strong national leadership, a national PHC can be transformed in only a decade. The rapid scale-up over a ten-year period in a vast country of more than one hundred million people of a national program of CHWs that provides access to PHC services that previously were not available is a major achievement. A strengthened PHC system has made important contributions to the notable health improvements of the Ethiopian population. In the past decade, the country has witnessed a major expansion in immunization coverage, marked reductions in child and maternal mortality, and notable reductions in morbidity and mortality from communicable diseases.

The government's HEP has brought community participation into the PHC system through awareness creation, behavioral change communication, and community mobilization. The WDA strategy of using a network of neighboring households through an inclusive and organized movement in the community increases the reach of HEWs into the community. The successful rapid scale-up of PHC services over the period of a decade in one of Africa's most populous countries has been studied and admired by many, though challenges remain. As the demand from the community for quality health service is increasing, HEWs have been given an increasing number of responsibilities and tasks. Maintaining the effectiveness of the national PHC system will require addressing pressing issues related to workload, remuneration and career advancement for HEWs, and improvements in health post infrastructure, equipment, and supplies.

In sum, the Ethiopian innovative approach of building a strong community health platform has great potential, not only for the Ethiopian health sector but also as an example of a best practice for other countries that are seeking to improve their PHC systems. The establishment of the International Institute for Primary Health Care-Ethiopia facilitates knowledge management and knowledge about PHC that can be shared with other countries. Ethiopia is committed to continual improvements in its PHC system, revising the essential health service package, improving the effectiveness of its management structure, strengthening the referral system, using appropriate technology, engaging the community, and providing protection against catastrophic health expenditures.

REFERENCES

Admasu, K., T. Balcha, and T. Ghebreyesus. 2016. "Pro-poor pathway towards universal health coverage: Lessons from Ethiopia." *J Glob Health* 6 (1): 010305.
Assefa, Y., D. Tesfaye, W. van Damme, and P. S. Hill. 2018. "Effectiveness and sustainability of a diagonal investment approach to strengthen the primary health-care system in Ethiopia." *Lancet* 392:1473–1481.
Assefa, Y., Y. A. Gelaw, P. S. Hill, B. W. Taye, and W. van Damme. 2019. "Community health extension program of Ethiopia, 2003–2018: Successes and challenges towards universal coverage for primary healthcare services." *Glob Health* 15 (24): https://globalizationandhealth.biomedcentral.com/articles/10.1186/s12992-019-0470-1.
Balabanova, D. 2013. "Good health at low cost 25 years on: Lessons for the future of health systems strengthening." *Lancet* 381 (9883): 2118–2133.
Banteyerga, H. 2011. "Ethiopia's health extension program: Improving health through community involvement." *MEDICC Rev* 13 (3): 46–49.

Damtew, Z. 2013. "Harnessing community knowledge for health: Case studies from the community health services and information systems in Ethiopia." PhD diss., University of Oslo. http://heim.ifi.uio.no/~jensj/Damtew2013HarnessingCommunityKnowle dgeForHealth.pdf.

Damtew, Z. A., A. M. Karim, C. T. Chekagn, N. Fesseha Zemichael, B. Yihun, B. A. Willey, and W. Betemariam. 2018. "Correlates of the Women's Development Army strategy implementation strength with household reproductive, maternal, newborn and child healthcare practices: A cross-sectional study in four regions of Ethiopia." *BMC Pregnancy Childbirth* 18 (Suppl. 1): 373.

Datiko, D. G., and B. Lindtjørn. 2010. "Cost and cost-effectiveness of smear-positive tuberculosis treatment by health extension workers in Southern Ethiopia: A community randomized trial." *PLoS One* 5 (2): e9158.

UNDP Ethiopia. 2014. *Ethiopia MDG report*. https://www.et.undp.org/content/ethiopia /en/home/library/mdg/EthiopiaMDG2014.html.

Federal Democratic Republic of Ethiopia. 2002. *Sustainable development and poverty reduction program*. https://www.imf.org/external/np/prsp/2002/eth/01/073102.pdf.

———. 2010. *Growth and transformation plan 2010/11-2014/15*. Addis Ababa. http://www.ethiopians.com/Ethiopia_GTP_2015.pdf.

Federal Ministry of Health. 2008. Health Management Information System (HMIS) Monitoring and Evaluation (M&E): Strategic Plan for Ethiopian Health Sector. Addis Ababa, Ethiopia. https://www.hfgproject.org/wp-content/uploads/2015/02 /Health-Facility-Governance-in-the-Ethiopian-Health-System.pdf.

Ghebreyesus, T. 2013. *Transforming health care in Ethiopia*. https://www.bcgperspectives .com/content/interviews/public_health_health_care_payers_providers_adhanom _ghebreyesus_transforming_health_care_ethiopia/.

Godefay, H., P. Byass, W. J. Graham, J. Kinsman, and A. Mulugeta. 2015. "Risk factors for maternal mortality in rural Tigray, Northern Ethiopia: A case-control study." *PLoS One* https://journals.plos.org/plosone/article?id=10.1371/journal.pone.0144975.

Kanjo, C. 2012. "In search of the missing data: The case of maternal and child health data in Malawi." https://pdfs.semanticscholar.org/baf6/384777210f50161ba99245ea 9e69232816b3.pdf?_ga=2.13858359.1293930127.1568147588-1993406079 .1568036952.

Karim, A. M., K. Admassu, J. Schellenberg, H. Alemu, N. Getachew, A. Ameha, L. Tadesse, and W. Betemariam. 2013. "Effect of Ethiopia's Health Extension Program on maternal and newborn health care practices in 101 rural districts: A dose-response study." *PLoS One* 8 (6): e65160.

Kitaw, Y., Y. Ye-Ebiyo, A. Said, H. Desta, and A. Teklehaimano. 2007. "Assessment of the training of the first intake of health extension workers." *Ethiop J Health Dev* 21 (3): 232–239.

Kloos, H. 1998a. "Primary health care in Ethiopia under three political systems: Community participation in a war-torn society." *Soc Sci Med* 46 (4–5): 505–522.

Kloos, H. 1998b. "Primary health care in Ethiopia: From Haile Selassie to Meles Zenawi." *Northeast Afr Stud* 5 (1): 83–113.

Memirie, S. T., S. Verguet, O. F. Norheim, C. Levin, and K. A. Johansson. 2016. "Inequalities in utilization of maternal and child health services in Ethiopia: The role of primary health care." *BMC Health Serv Res* 16 (1). https://bmchealthservres .biomedcentral.com/articles/10.1186/s12913-016-1296-7.

Ministry of Health. n.d. Ethiopia health system transformation plan, 2010–2015. Addis Ababa, Ethiopia: Government of Ethiopia. https://phe-ethiopia.org/admin/uploads/attachment-721-HSDP%20IV%20Final%20Draft%2011Octoberr%202010.pdf.

Perry, H., L. Akin-Olugbade, A. Lailari, and Y. Son. 2016. *A comprehensive description of the three national community health worker programs and contributions to maternal and child health and primary health care: Case studies from America (Brazil), Africa (Ethiopia) and Asia (Nepal).* https://www.chwcentral.org/sites/default/files/Perry-CHW%20Programs%20in%20Brazil%2C%20Ethiopia%20and%20Nepal-2016.pdf.

Perry, H., R. Zulliger, K. Scott, D. Javadi, J. Gergen, K. Shelley, L. Crigler, I. Aitken, S. H. Arwal, N. Afdhila, Y. Worku, J. Rohde, Z. Chowdhury, and R. Strodel. 2017. *Case studies of large-scale community health worker programs: Examples from Afghanistan, Bangladesh, Brazil, Ethiopia, Niger, India, Indonesia, Iran, Nepal, Pakistan, Rwanda, Zambia, Zimbabwe.* https://www.mcsprogram.org/resource/case-studies-large-scale-community-health-worker-programs-2/.

Sebhatu, A. 2008. *The implementation of Ethiopia's Health Extension Program: An overview.* http://www.ppdafrica.org/docs/ethiopiahep.pdf.

UNFPA Ethiopia. 2014. "Investing in midwives: Stories from Ethiopia." https://ethiopia.unfpa.org/en/publications/investing-midwives-stories-ethiopia.

Wamai, R. G. 2009. "Reviewing Ethiopia's health system development." *JMAJ* 52 (4): 279–286.

World Health Organization. 1978. "Declaration of Alma-Ata." http://www.euro.who.int/__data/assets/pdf_file/0009/113877/E93944.pdf.

World Health Organization. 2015. "Improving health system efficiency: Ethiopia human resources for health reforms." Health System Governance and Financing. https://apps.who.int/iris/bitstream/handle/10665/187240/WHO_HIS_HGF_CaseStudy_15.6_eng.pdf?sequence=1&isAllowed=y.

———. 2012. "Ethiopia: Health system outcomes." http://www.aho.afro.who.int/profiles_information/index.php/Ethiopia:Health_system_outcomes.

CHAPTER NINE

Health Improvement through the Primary Health Care Approach

Case of Nepal

KEDAR PRASAD BARAL, NADIA DIAMOND-SMITH, AND RITA THAPA

Nepal is one of the signatories of the 1978 Alma-Ata Declaration on primary health care (PHC). Forty years later, Nepal still endorses and continues to practice the core values and principles of PHC as fundamental approaches in policy formulation and program implementation. Furthermore, Nepal has made rapid progress on health indicators compared to other countries with a similar level of benchmark indicators (see chapter 2). This chapter reflects on Nepal's successes as lessons for future implementation of the PHC goals outlined in the Astana Declaration. Nepal's delivery of the promise of PHC in its policies and programs has evolved over the past forty years across changing landscapes of political, economic, and epidemiological contexts.

Nepal is a landlocked country bordered by India in the east, west, and south, and China in the north. It occupies 147,181 square kilometers, rising from as low as 59 meters at the tropical Terai (the northern rim of the Indo-Gangetic Plain) up to Earth's highest summit (Mount Everest) at 8,848 meters. Nepal has three distinct ecological belts—namely, the mountainous, hilly, and Terai—occupying areas of 51,817, 61,345, and 34,019 square kilometers, respectively (Central Bureau of Statistics 2015). Most mountainous areas are uninhabitable and are therefore sparsely populated. The population density varies across the regions, with a population density of 34 people per square kilometer in the mountains, 186 in the hills, and 392 in the Terai (Central Bureau of Statistics 2015). The first national census of Nepal, conducted in 1952–1954, estimated Nepal's population to be around eight million (Pant 1955), and as of 2017 the population stands at roughly twenty-eight million.

Nepal's feudal history and a complex social fabric with deep-rooted traditions and culture, endowed with natural resources along with diverse ethnic identities, challenging terrain, and frequent natural disasters, make it a challenging place to provide health care. The 1951 revolution broke the 104-year rule of the autocratic Rana family, opening the country to development and legalizing girls' formal schooling. Over the subsequent period, there were two popular movements and a protracted ten-year spell of violent civil conflict, and Nepal has undergone a tremendous social transformation, from feudal monarchy to a secular republic. The 1990 People's Movement brought in a multiparty political system while transforming the king into a constitutional monarch. Following the violent 1996 Maoist People's Movement, which ended in 2006 with a peace accord, the Constitution of Nepal institutionalized a Federal Democratic Republic of Nepal. The Constitution of 2015 guarantees an inclusive society, multiparty democracy, equitable social and economic development, the rule of law, and human rights. Basic health services, safe motherhood, women's reproductive health, and children's health were also enshrined in the constitution as fundamental rights, for the first time in the history of Nepal.

Despite decades of political instability, frequent natural disasters, poor infrastructure, challenging terrain, and lackluster economic growth, Nepal's health indicators have shown amazing progress over the past forty years (table 9.1). However, inequalities in absolute and relative terms persist for women, ethnicity, and rural areas, despite two decades of programmatic priorities directed to address the gap.

Background and Contextual History

For most of the twentieth century, Nepal was a subsistence economy, overwhelmingly dependent on agriculture and primarily controlled by landowners. Nepal's near-total lack of physical infrastructure, including roads, telecommunications, hospitals, and schools, further contributed to poor development and health outcomes before 1950. Rugged topography, lack of statistics, and an apathetic central government would have made it impossible to realize development needs.

In the 1950s, only 2% of Nepali people were literate, and there were only three hundred college graduates in the country. An estimated one in four individuals in the Terai region suffered from malaria before the malaria program was started in 1956. Unattended home delivery was universal, and the maternal mortality ratio was estimated at above fifteen hundred per one hundred thou-

Table 9.1. Nepal's health and development indicators over time

Indicators	1981	1991	1996	2001	2006	2011	2016
GNI per capita	160[1a]	210[1a]	210[1a]	240[1a]	340[1a]	600[1a]	730[1a]
Total fertility	6.3[2b]	5.6[2b]	4.64[1b]	4.1[2b]	3.1[2b]	2.6[2b]	2.3[1b]
IMR	117[2a]	97[2a]	73.74[2a]	64[2a]	48[2a]	46[2a]	32[2a]
Youth female literacy		17.38[3]	24.86[2]	34.88[3]		48.83[3]	64[2c]
Literacy rate							
Total	23.3[2c]	39.6[2c]		54[2c]		65.9[2c]	
Female	12[2c]	25[2c]		42.8[2c]		57.4[2c]	
MMR		750[1]	539[4]	415[4]	281[4]	250[4]	258[1]
Life expectancy							
Total	47.25[6]	55.13[6]	59.34[6]	63.08[6]	66.07[6]	68.33[6]	70.25[6]
Female	47.61[6]	55.75[6]	60.21[6]	64.17[7]	67.36[6]	69.83[6]	71.88[6]
Water supply coverage			69.8[8]	84.5[8]	81.8[8]	86.5[8]	87.0[8]
Sanitation coverage			22[8]	43[8]	41[8]	59[8]	87.3[8]
Gender development Index			0.75[9*]	0.77[9**]	0.832[9***]	0.885[9]	0.921[9]

Note: GNI, gross national income; IMR, infant mortality rate; MMR, maternal mortality ratio.
*Denotes the data from the nearest date: *1997**2002***2007.

[1] https://www.indexmundi.com/facts/nepal/mortality-rate

[1a] https://www.indexmundi.com/facts/nepal/gni-per-capita.

[1b] https://www.indexmundi.com/nepal/total_fertility_rate.html.

[2a] https://nepalindata.com/data/?request&secid=20,subsecid=118,indid=900&infant-mortality-rate-imr.

[2b] https://nepalindata.com/data/?request&secid=20,subsecid=118,indid=899,chart=table,year=2011&total-fertility-rate-tfr.

[2c] https://nepalindata.com/data/?request&secid=20,subsecid=39,indid=510,chart=table,year=2018&literacy-rate.

[3] https://data.worldbank.org/indicator/SE.ADT.LITR.FE.ZS?end=2018&locations=NP&start=1981&type=points&view=chart.

[4] https://dhsprogram.com/pubs/pdf/TR5/TR5.pdf.

[5] https://www.healthynewbornnetwork.org/resource/nepal-demographic-health-survey-2016-key-indicators/.

[6] https://countryeconomy.com/demography/life-expectancy/nepal.

[8] http://www.ess.gov.np/uploads/ck/a__1512380405_WASH%20SSR%202016%20-%20sent%20to%20printing%202017%20May%2017.pdf.

[9] United Nations Development Program, Human Development Reports, 1990–2015, http://hdr.undp.org/en/data#.

sand live births. The under-5 mortality rate was more than three hundred to four hundred per one thousand live births (Worth and Shah 1969), and the percentage of married women using modern contraceptives was at zero (Nepal Family Planning 1976). Life expectancy was around 28 years (Boch-Isaacson et al. 2001) overall, and it remained lower for women than men until the 2000s.

The 104-year-old Rana regime came to an end in 1951, and there was a brief beginning of a democratic system under a monarchy. However, in 1960

King Mahendra dissolved parliament, outlawed all political parties, and established a party-less panchayat political system consisting of five tiers of governance, from local to central. The absolute power remained with the king. The party-less panchayat system would rule Nepal for thirty years, until 1990.

In 1956, Nepal entered into a centralized planning system, with the first five-year plan covering 1956 to 1962 (Nepal National Planning Commission 1956). This was the beginning of national-scale public health programs, starting with the malaria eradication project in 1956, followed by smallpox eradication in 1962, family planning and maternal child health (FP-MCH) (Taylor and Thapa 1972) in 1965, as well as tuberculosis (Das 1996) and leprosy control (Mali 1996) in 1965.

Between the late 1970s and the 1990s, Nepal experienced an awakening of consciousness. Political leaders emphasized helping the common people realize their rights. They focused on developing skills, enabling the common people to join local issues of interest and establish a link to national issues. Particular emphasis was given to political freedom, rights, and social justice. During the 1980s, tension could be felt across careers and professions as a result of the political awakening of the common man and woman. Many left their jobs to contribute to political movements. Many promising professionals and students left their urban positions to go back to their villages and volunteer their time and skills to the political parties. The popular ways of mass consciousness-building were through youth, student, schoolteacher, professional, and village informal leaders. Therefore, human investments have had an extremely important bearing on Nepal's social development and transformation, including health. In 1990, political parties formed an alliance of all parties and organized a people's movement, which compelled the king to establish parliamentary democracy with a constitutional monarch. Since 1991, parliamentary democracy started and continues to date.

During the1990s, people's expectations reached an aspirational high, and leaders committed themselves to delivering services. Nepal liberalized its economy by entering into the open market system. Gradually, profit and nonprofit private organizations brought their initiatives into Nepal for development purposes. The new generation of leaders opened doors to new ideas and encouraged risk-taking in policy decisions. Nepal adopted innovative local initiatives and global best practices from within and outside in all sectors, including health.

In 1991, a multiparty democracy saw the promulgation of a new constitution and new leadership in the country. This era emphasized and further strengthened periodic plans. The overall delivery structure was continued, but the direction for development shifted drastically toward reaching rural people. In 1991, the first National Health Policy (Nepal Ministry of Health 1991) was enacted and enshrined PHC as the foundation. This was a watershed moment in the development of Nepal's public health system and is credited for providing much-needed momentum to PHC initiated earlier as the Integrated Community Health Service Development Project (ICHDP) in achieving the health developments Nepal has achieved today.

Unfortunately, during the 1990s, the nation found itself in the middle of another tumultuous period. The multiparty democracy could not live up to the people's expectations, and the economy especially failed to address the concerns of unemployed youth. The country was once again thrown into conflict, with a section of leaders organizing the Maoist People's Movement for violent conflict. The Maoists' goal was to establish a socialist system, including a constitutional assembly election.

Women's Status in Nepal

Nepal has long struggled with issues related to gender equality. Culturally, Nepal is a patriarchal society, and men have been the dominant decision-makers and actors in households and communities. Nepal used to score very low on measures of gender equality and women's empowerment, even compared to other South Asian countries (Smith et al. 2003). Son preference exists in Nepal, leading to a gender gap in education and health care–seeking behavior (Pokhrel et al. 2005). In adulthood, gender discrimination leads to high levels of domestic violence and unequal distribution of food within households (Atteraya et al. 2015). Qualitative research of women found that they felt that they and their communities had become more empowered through the 1990s and 2000s, aligning with large efforts to improve gender equality and women's status in Nepal (Leve 2007). An interesting study by Lauren Leve (2007) explored the meaning behind the large role that women had in the Maoist insurgency in Nepal, including women holding many high-level positions. In the past fifteen to twenty years, Nepal has made impressive progress, as shown in the growth of the Gender Development Index in table 9.1. Evidence exists about women's empowerment groups providing critical disaster relief and emergency response in their communities (Dhungel and Ojha 2012). As another example, women's groups that were part of the Nepal health development project identified a need for clean cookstoves in their communities, gained the skills to build these stoves, and then helped their own community members build them and taught their communities how to use them (Purdey et al. 1994). There are numerous examples of women-led community development projects, and these are only a few. Ultimately, extensive experience with multipronged, multisectoral development interventions led to a wide acceptance that women's rights are indispensable to realizing all human rights. From this foundation, the seventh constitution of Nepal extended and protected many fundamental women's rights in 2015.

Gender parity, an idea that once held little meaning within the sociolegal composition of Nepal, today is discussed with significant gravitas. This transformation in national consciousness gained momentum through education and was supported by political movements including the Maoists' activist actions. Over the years, Nepal's activists have crusaded against gender disparities to address obstacles faced by women. Recognition of women's needs and challenges struggled against a culture in which traditional values were laced with male superiority. It gradually was accepted that women face barriers that men may not deal with. Coordinated efforts across sectors were launched for education and consciousness-building among the female population as part of political movements in Nepal. This gave new impetus to Nepal's women's movement. The Local Self Governance Act of 1999 made special provisions for women, economically and socially disadvantaged ethnic groups, and indigenous groups to be represented in the village- and ward-level development committees. It also gave operational and management responsibility of health services to village-level committees. Social auditing was used to devolve authority and improve accountability to communities served, especially the poor and marginalized (World Health Organization 2018). What was in the beginning a movement to redress private inequalities gained widespread momentum to affect the public sphere, ensuring women's participation in various sectors including the parliament and the judiciary and executive branches. Although there is still much to be desired, the recognition of women's rights as a fundamental right under the latest constitution of Nepal is definitely a step in the right direction.

Nepal's Health Achievements: What Has Worked?

Policy, Structure, and Program Evolution: From Past to Present

Nepal is known to be one of the few countries that has managed to achieve the Millennium Development Goals, despite geographical and economic barriers, and it continues to improve life expectancy even after decades of political instability. This section narrates the changes to the health development sector over time in Nepal and highlights factors that contributed to health system improvement and improved health outcomes.

Nepal's Department of Health Services and the Civil Medical School were established in 1933. In 1956, Nepal started a centralized periodic planning system for the development of all sectors, including health, with the first five-year plan (Nepal National Planning Commission 1956). Subsequently, regional development plans and administrative mechanisms were also advanced. Credit is due to academics and development experts of that time for providing technical input into the development plans, especially plans concerning regional development. In addition to the periodic five-year plans, the first long-term health plan spanned the fifteen-year period of 1975–1990 and introduced basic minimum need goals.

In 1972, the Institute of Medicine was established at Tribhuvan University, and all mid-level health training was brought under it. It also started an innovative community-oriented bachelor of medicine and bachelor of surgery program in 1978, a groundbreaking step that helped motivate most medical graduates to work in rural areas. Until the mid-1970s, the focus of health policy was a rather concentrated approach for controlling endemic communicable diseases. These were vertical target projects managed semiautonomously and financed primarily with foreign aid. These were envisioned as short-term, temporary projects, wrapping up as soon as their purpose was achieved. There were efforts to improve public health administration, develop long-range national plans, and ultimately integrate all the vertical projects into the public health system in the 1970s. Subsequently, in 1975, the ICHDP was established under the Department of Health Services and started an agenda of comprehensive PHC. The integration process was piloted in six districts and gradually scaled up. All vertical projects and programs were reorganized under one overall umbrella of the Department of Health Services by 1993.

The aim of the ICHDP was to integrate services provided by vertical projects into district health systems. The system includes district hospitals and district public health offices, under which all peripheral-level health facilities (PHC center, health post, subhealth post) and outreach activities are linked and supported by community-based, salaried village health workers (VHWs) and unsalaried female community health volunteers (FCHVs) to provide an integrated package of PHC services. The ICHDP subsequently institutionalized community participation in health planning within village development committees (VDCs) with the implementation of the Local Self Governance Act of 1999. The district public health offices were responsible for the delivery of public health services through health post and outreach activities working together with community-based health workers such as VHWs and FCHVs. By 1985, there were 745 health posts. In the mid-1980s, responsibility for Nepal's basic minimum needs goal was brought under the National Planning Commission, which was managed by the prime minister's office. The reason was to bring all the ministries together for coordinated intersectoral actions.

During the 1980s, a concept was introduced where at least nine *ilika* (subdistrict) health posts (Dixit 1995) in each of the seventy-five districts were to organize PHC through a team headed by a health assistant, who oversaw auxiliary health workers (AHWs), auxiliary nurse midwives (ANMs), and a VHW for each VDC area. A VDC divided into nine small geographical localities called wards. One FCHV was trained in each ward. VHWs are responsible for outreach activities through home visits and by organizing outreach clinics. At the VDC (then panchayat) level, an integrated service delivery package was envisioned to be delivered by FP-MCH health aids, malaria field workers, and vaccinators during early phases of the integration process.

Although Nepal established a Department of Health Services and its Civil Medical School as early as 1933, the seeds of PHC were sown in the late 1950s, well before the Alma-Ata Declaration. It started with the training of mid-level health workers such as male AHWs and female ANMs. These cadres of health workers, though limited, were responsible for providing the first level of care in rural heath posts. Earlier, the five vertical public health projects started training their respective community-based workers as frontline workers to deliver basic and proven packages of PHC services at the population level from the late 1950s onward.

Vertical projects had a parallel system of service delivery and were managed outside the Department of Health Services. The focus on PHC allowed the Department of Health Services to maintain its identity and merge available resources to establish the ICHDP in 1975 under the Department of Health Services. Nepal's malaria eradication project, using almost 50% of the total national health budget, had reached its targeted maintenance level by 1972, but there was no basic health service infrastructure to maintain this gain. The external donors were pulling out their previously agreed-upon support. This is when the government changed its policy from a "vertical approach" to an "integrated approach," establishing the ICHDP. This was a mega-project, born out of an imminent need of maintaining malaria eradication efforts while creating an integrated basic health infrastructure that could deliver PHC services at doorsteps in rural areas.

It was a prescient, pro-poor public health decision. Had this not been done, one or more vertical projects would have dominated the public health delivery system of Nepal, without having any basic structures to deliver PHC services to rural communities. The ICHDP allowed space for all vertical projects to gradually come under one structure.

Evolution of Female Community Health Volunteers

Community mobilization was part of Nepal's public health program. From early on, different projects deployed salaried community health workers under different names. In the FP-MCH program, they were called health aides. They were called malaria home visitors in the malaria program and smallpox vaccinators in the smallpox program. These three categories of community-based, salaried health workers were unified as VHWs under the ICHDP. FCHVs evolved as an important missing link that ensured PHC services reached households. The ICHDP realized quite early that it was not possible for one VHW to deliver outreach services to all nine wards of a village development area. Thus evolved the idea of piloting the training of one FCHV from each ward of the respective village panchayat (later VDC). FCHVs are ward-based volunteers recruited for training with the support of local mothers' groups. The FCHV idea was pilot tested based on a twenty-day staggered training module at respective health posts in 1977 (Thapa et al. 1973). FCHV candidates are chosen by local mothers' groups, and this enhances their acceptability to the people they serve. The ICHDP had piloted the concept of training nonsalaried FCHVs in the late 1970s. In 1988, based on the demonstrated effectiveness of FCHVs, the health minister made the Female Community Health Volunteer Program a national program of the Ministry of Health (Nepal Ministry of Health 1988). The program was subsequently rolled out throughout the country, reaching every ward. The FCHV program's thirty years of success has made a remarkable contribution to PHC in Nepal.

FCHVs are an interesting example of women (potentially) gaining more status in their communities (Perry et al. 2013) and obtaining a role in which they have the opportunity to impact community health. We might expect FCHVs to be more empowered in their communities because of their role in providing critical health information and services based on the additional knowledge acquired through training and experience. Furthermore, one might expect them to be empowered in their households because of their added income (through limited incentives) and their ability to improve the

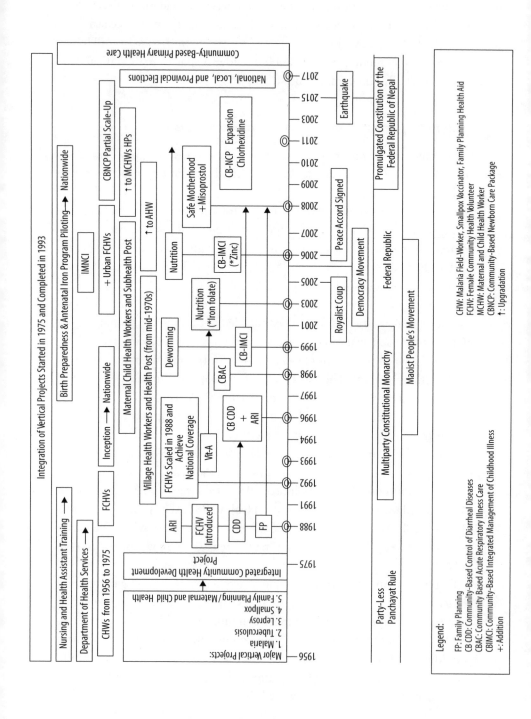

health of their households based on the knowledge they have gained. Past qualitative research with FCHVs found that the main reason they worked on this mostly volunteer basis was a sense of obligation to their community and to earn religious merit (dharma) (Glenton et al. 2010; Swechhya and Kamaraj 2014). Previous studies have found that FCHVs valued the recognition from their communities, suggesting that the status component is important (Glenton et al. 2010). Some qualitative research has suggested that FCHVs do feel that their role has empowered them. Specifically some have stated that being a FCHV has given them knowledge to improve the health of their own families (Swechhya and Kamaraj 2014). Because they are self-employed volunteers, they often achieve more respect and power than salaried, community-based health workers such as VHWs. The structure of the FCHV program also potentially provides the opportunity for other women in the community to have a voice and impact because local mothers' groups and the Village Development Committee are involved in the selection and oversight of FCHVs (Perry et al. 2013). Apart from the government, FCHVs are highly sought after by NGOs intending to promote PHC in communities. In this way, FCHVs are self-employed and empowered women. However, there is still inadequate evidence about whether being a FCHV actually changes a woman's level of empowerment, either in her household or community, and more definitive work is necessary.

Community-based systems and FCHVs improve access for disadvantaged populations in rural and remote areas and have been effective at carrying out increasing activities over time despite their low educational level and skills at the time of recruitment. FCHVs are selected from the mothers' groups within each community, and the basic requirement is that she must belong to the catchment area, should be married, and should display interest and willingness to serve as a volunteer for her community. As shown in figure 9.1, the responsibilities of FCHVs have increased over time. FCHV attrition is low—4% of FCHVs leave their posts annually. According to a national survey conducted in 2014, FCHVs had an average of 13.9 years of experience, with 46% of FCHVs having served for sixteen years or more (Family Health Division 2014). In addition to receiving government incentives, FCHVs became a valued resource sought after by several NGOs/INGOs to engage with them in community-level work, which provides additional training and various incentives. These incentives provide direct and indirect benefits that contribute to a supportive environment and recognize the importance of

Figure 9.1. Evolution of primary health care in Nepal.

FCHVs' work. Nationally, FCHVs are recognized, and Nepal celebrates FCHV day on December 5 nationwide. A dress allowance (blue saris designed with the FCHV logo accompanied by an official name badge) gives FCHVs recognition in the community. The government provided well-designed, meaningful wallboards that are strategically placed to identify each FCHV's house. Work by FCHVs has been nationally recognized, and good practices are endorsed through the national FCHV day.

Over time, the demographic profile of FCHVs has changed. As of 2007–2008, they were younger, with a median age of 38 and only 4% older than 60, unlike before that time. They are more educated, with 62% of all FCHVs literate (New Era 2008). FCHVs' current work portfolio includes services related to family planning, HIV/AIDS, maternal and newborn care, community-based pneumonia treatment, diarrhea care, vitamin A and deworming, and immunization. They have remained frontline workers of Nepal's PHC system to this day (figure 9.2).

Nepal's community health system has slowly expanded to include a comprehensive package of MCH services delivered by the village teams. The FCHVs are strategically placed as an interface between the formal and community system. Regular contact with local citizens enables them to be cognizant of the problems and concerns of the community. As part of the communities, FCHVs enjoy the advantages of being included in the community-based solving of health problems. Their familiarity with local context gives them communication advantages as compared to outsiders. FCHVs often have personally acquired the ability to identify with pain and suffering, as well as the sociocultural constraints of women in the community. They have come to understand the essentials of a rural woman's life. Their cultural competence allows other women to share their problems, giving FCHVs a chance to be supportive and search for solutions together. Bonds between FCHVs and women strengthen over time, which in turn helps to build confidence and self-esteem in their fellow mothers. FCHVs' communication is not limited to mothers' group meetings. Outreach activities happen during work; while walking to fetch water, firewood, and fodder; in the forest or the field; or in other forums organized for other activities.

Developing a community program on a nationwide scale is a gradual process, as shown in figure 9.3. It is important to recognize that Nepal's public health leaders have made choices that were locally as well as socioculturally appropriate. Interventions were very strategically rolled out over time and were responsive to emerging common health needs of the population. The stewardship and harmonization of community-level service provision has

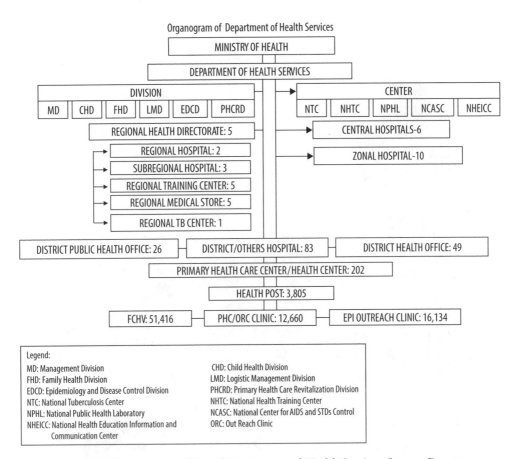

Organogram of Department of Health Services

| MINISTRY OF HEALTH |
| DEPARTMENT OF HEALTH SERVICES |

| DIVISION | CENTER |

MD | CHD | FHD | LMD | EDCD | PHCRD

NTC | NHTC | NPHL | NCASC | NHEICC

REGIONAL HEALTH DIRECTORATE: 5

CENTRAL HOSPITALS-6

REGIONAL HOSPITAL: 2
SUBREGIONAL HOSPITAL: 3
REGIONAL TRAINING CENTER: 5
REGIONAL MEDICAL STORE: 5
REGIONAL TB CENTER: 1

ZONAL HOSPITAL-10

DISTRICT PUBLIC HEALTH OFFICE: 26 | DISTRICT/OTHERS HOSPITAL: 83 | DISTRICT HEALTH OFFICE: 49

PRIMARY HEALTH CARE CENTER/HEALTH CENTER: 202

HEALTH POST: 3,805

FCHV: 51,416 | PHC/ORC CLINIC: 12,660 | EPI OUTREACH CLINIC: 16,134

Legend:
MD: Management Division
FHD: Family Health Division
EDCD: Epidemiology and Disease Control Division
NTC: National Tuberculosis Center
NPHL: National Public Health Laboratory
NHEICC: National Health Education Information and
Communication Center

CHD: Child Health Division
LMD: Logistic Management Division
PHCRD: Primary Health Care Revitalization Division
NHTC: National Health Training Center
NCASC: National Center for AIDS and STDs Control
ORC: Out Reach Clinic

Figure 9.2. Organogram of Nepal Department of Health Services. Source: Department of Health Services, *Annual Report* 2016/17

been critical. In contrast to workers offering services in a clinic, FCHVs are present in their communities at all times. There is no facility to be absent from and no clinic that can be closed or offer inconvenient hours. The most important dimension of the community is building trust, bonding, and strengthening the traditional cohesiveness around the topic of shared health concerns. Until now, most of the villages in remote parts of Nepal were in a subsistence economy. Relationships with neighbors and relatives are based on shared values and resources. Helping and respecting each other is part of day-to-day life. Elders and mothers are the most respected people. Public health professionals are observant that resolving issues during community meetings along with delivering service strengthens members' confidence, self-esteem, and

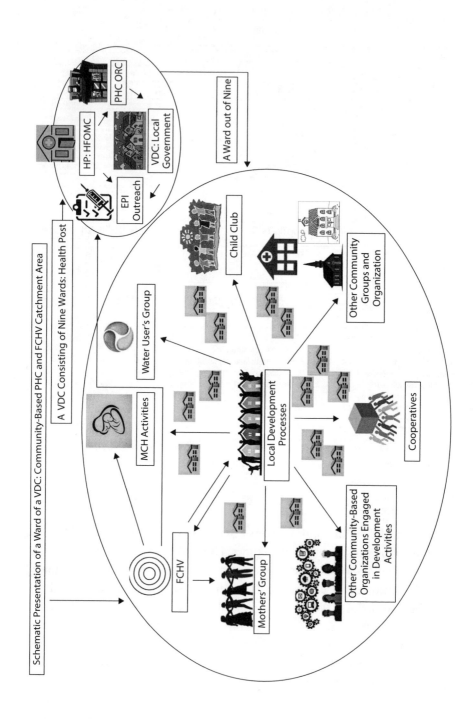

Schematic Presentation of a Ward of a VDC: Community-Based PHC and FCHV Catchment Area

A VDC Consisting of Nine Wards: Health Post

A Ward out of Nine

PHC ORC

HP: HFOMC

VDC: Local Government

EPI Outreach

Water User's Group

Child Club

Other Community Groups and Organization

MCH Activities

Local Development Processes

Cooperatives

FCHV

Mothers' Group

Other Community-Based Organizations Engaged in Development Activities skills, and increases the likelihood of contact with other persons, including health workers and visitors.

Gradually, the communities have started recognizing FCHVs as their leaders, going so far as to endorse them as informal community leaders. Now, a FCHV's role transcends just health since they are key stakeholders in local development programs. Over time, FCHV representation has also been mandated by guidelines. A pertinent example is their inclusion on operation and management committees for local health facilities. FCHVs served as election educators in the last election, a decision accepted by all at the national to village level because of the trusted and neutral role they play in communities. For the past several years, FCHVs have increased their representation in women cooperatives, water user groups, and other village development initiatives. In the last election, a sizeable number of FCHVs campaigned for leadership, and many of them have been elected to serve in their local government.

The Era of Democratic Government: Beyond 1990

Nepal's political transition from the traditional, party-less panchayat system to a multiparty democracy opened new doors of opportunity for expanding health and development interventions. In 1991, the health minister for the interim government formulated the first National Health Policy (Nepal Ministry of Health 1991). The new democratic government's National Health Policy in 1991 identified the reasons behind the poor improvement in health. It was attributed to weakness in implementation of preventive, promotive, and curative health programs at the grassroots level (Nepal Ministry of Health 1991). The statement set out a goal to expand services to peripheral levels. The focus concentrated on reducing child and maternal mortality, reducing fertility, and increasing life expectancy. The 1991 first National Health Policy prioritized resource investment to further scaling of the PHC services by establishing subhealth posts along with increased human resources. These new investments promoted health research, community participation, better monitoring, better supervision, and better mobilization of resources. A new organogram developed to realize the objectives as policy evolved.

The 1991 National Health Policy further prioritized and revitalized health care service delivery at the community level and made services accessible to

Figure 9.3. Village development committee and female community health volunteer catchment area.

Table 9.2. Nepal Health and Related Policy Milestone and Events

Events	Dates
Department of Health Service Established	1933
End of Rana Regime	1951
Insect Borne Disease Control Bureau	1952
Nepal General Election-Parliament	1959
King Mahendra Dissolved Cabinet	1960
Constitution-Established Party-less Panchayat System	1962
The Food Act	1966
First Long-Term Health Plan	1975
Expanded Program on Immunization	1977
National Immunization Program	1979
Control of Diarrheal Diseases	1983
Solid Waste Act; Control of Acute Respiratory Infection Program	1987
Higher Secondary Education Act; Nepal Drinking Water Corporation Act	1989
Nepal Health Research Council Act; Nepal Agriculture Research Council Act; National Health Policy; Pesticides Act; Birth, Death and Other Person or Private Incident Act	1991
National Blood Policy; Council for Technical Education and Vocational Training Act; Primary Health Care Outreach Strategy	1993
National Drug Policy; National Mental Health Policy; National HIV and AIDS Policy	1995
Human Rights Commission Act; Nepal Health Professional Council Act; Nepal Health Service Act; Second Long-Term Health Plan 1997–2017	1997
Iodized Salt (Production, Sale, and Distribution) ACT; Human Body Organ Transplantation (Regulation and Prohibition) Act; Nepal Veterinary Council Act; Slaughter House and Meat Checking Act; Local Self-Governance Act; Local Self-Governance Regulations; Community-Based Integrated Management of Childhood Illness (CBIMCI) Program	1999
National Plan of Action (Education) 2001–2015; National Ethical Guidelines for Health Research in Nepal	2001
Poverty Alleviation Ordinance; National Safe Abortion Policy; National Health Research Policy of Nepal; Strategic Plan for Human Resources for Health; Nepal Health Sector Strategy; National Guidelines for Counseling, Testing, and Referral	2003
Drinking Water Management Board Ordinance; Drinking Water Tariff Charge Fixation Commission Ordinance; Human Rights Commission Ordinance; Information Technology Academy Ordinance; Poverty Alleviation Fund Ordinance; Safe Delivery Incentive Program	2005
Right to Information; Human Trafficking and Transportation (Control) Act; Three-Year Interim Plan Approach Paper; Nepal Interim Constitution; Free Health Care Policy; Policy on Quality Assurance in Health Care Services; National Medicines Policy; Implementation Guide on Adolescent Sexual and Reproductive Health; National Work Force Policy	2007
Nepal Human Rights Action Plan; Nepal Health Sector Program Implementation Plan-II (NHSP-IP2); Guideline for Below Poverty Level Medical Treatment Support Program; Operational Guidelines for DDCs and VDCs; National Youth Policy; Drug Control Policy	2010
Social Service Unit Establishment and Operational Guidelines; National FCHV Program revised Strategy; Multi-Sector Nutrition Plan for Accelerating the Reduction of Maternal and Child Under-Nutrition in Nepal 2013–2017; National Guidelines for Minimum Services Packages for Children Affected by AIDS (CABA); National Plan of Action for Children	2012
Organized Crime Prevention Act; Mutual Legal Assistance Act	2014

Dates	Events
1934	Civil Medical School Established
1952	Total Hospital Beds 600
1956	Nepal Malaria Eradication Organization; Five-Year Periodic Plan Started, First Nursing Training Started
1960	Established National Planning Commission
1961	Banned Political Party
1964	Nepal Citizenship Act; Small Pox Control Act; Infectious Disease Act; Nepal Medical Council Act
1971	National Education Committee Act; Education Act
1976	Birth, Death, and Other Personal Event Registration Act; Narcotics Drugs (Control) Act
1978	Drug Act; Under-graduated Medical Program Started
1982	Natural Calamity (Relief) Act; Disabled Persons Protection and Welfare Act; Disaster Management Policies in Nepal
1986	Trafficking in Human beings (Control) Act
1988	Ayurveda Medical Council Act; Female Community Health Volunteer (FCHV)
1990	Municipality Act; District Development Community Act; Village Development Community Act; Communication-Related Act
1992	National Dairy Development Board Act; Children's Act; Water Resources Act and Regulation; Mothers Milk Substitute (Control of Sale and Distribution) Act
1994	Nepal National Policy on Sanitation
1996	Nepal Nursing Council Act; Policy on the Participation of Non-Government Organization in Water Supply and Sanitation Program
1998	Drinking Water Regulation; Safe Motherhood Policy; FCHV Strategy
2000	Child Labour (Prohibition and Regulation) Act; Nepal Pharmacy Council Act; National Adolescent Health and Development Strategy; National Reproductive Health Research Strategy
2002	National Academy for Upliftment of Aboriginal and Ethnic Group Act; Prevention of Corruption Act; National Academy of Medical Sciences Ordinance; National Safe Motherhood Plan (2002–2017); Nepal National HIV/AIDS Strategy; Abortion Legalized
2004	Education (Eight Amendment) Ordinance; National Nutrition Policy and Strategy; Rural Water Supply and Sanitation; National Policy and Strategy; Health Sector Strategy; An Agenda for Reform; Nepal Health Sector Program-Implementation Plan (NHSP-IP); SWAP Adopted; National Neonatal Health Strategy; Nepal Red Cross Society Health Policy
2006	Nepal Water Management Board Act; National Policy on Skilled Birth Attendant; Health Sector Information System National Strategy; Mental Health (Treatment and Protection) Act; Health Care Technology Policy; Environmental Impact Assessment of Nepal Health Sector Program-Implementation Plan 2004–2009; Health Care Waste Management in Nepal Assessment of Present State and Establishment of a Framework Strategy and Action Plan for Improvement; Vulnerable Community Development Plan for NHSP-IP; National Safe Motherhood and Newborn Health Long-Term Plan; Labor and Employment Policy
2009	Domestic Violence Act; Aama Program; Community-Based Newborn Care Package; Five-Year Operational Plan for In-Service Training of Skilled Birth Attendants; Health Sector Gender Equality and Social Inclusion Strategy; National ART Gridlines
2011	National HIV/AIDS Strategy 2011–2016; National Guidelines on Prevention of Mother to Child Transmission (PMTCT) of HIV in Nepal; National Plan of Action on Human Trafficking
2013	National Oral Health Policy; The National Anti-tobacco Communication Campaign Strategy for Nepal; Integrated Noncommunicable Diseases (NCDs) Prevention and Control Policy of Nepal; Guidelines for Community Health Insurance; Local Health Governance Strengthening in Nepal; A Collaborative Framework
2016	Human Organ Transplant Act; National Strategy for Reaching the Unreached; Directive for Treatment of Ultra Poor (Bipanna) Fund; Nepal Health Sector Strategy; Implementation Plan

Note: The first Constitution Assembly Election of the Federal Democratic Republic of Nepal was held in 2008, but the assembly failed to finalize the constitution and the second election was held in 2013. The assembly promulgated the constitution of the Democratic Republic of Nepal in September 2015. The constitution established three levels of government, and the election for all levels was held in 2017; since then, all the levels of government are in place.

even the remotest communities. It considered sociocultural context and viability, and therefore trained health workers to have expertise and sensitivity to these factors. It was designed to have adequate supervision of the system and to be suitable to reach the rural, underserved, and disadvantaged populations. Over a period of several years, the public health system decentralized, and specific policies, protocols, and guidelines on health service delivery, human resources, health information systems, and the cost of services guided the health delivery mechanism. The policy milestones shown in table 9.2 illustrate that Nepal's health policy environment was progressively evolving over the decades since the 1960s. Policy changes had been initiated based on the application of established international best practices and informed by the results from local pilot and feasibility studies. One of the best examples for research translated into program policy was the vitamin A supplementation program among children aged 6–59 months (Gottlieb 2007).

Nepal was able to attract foreign assistance and received substantial resources to support government efforts for scaling up evidence-based interventions, and government investment in public health priority sectors increased after 1991. This was primarily due to advocacy by health professionals and civil society along with responsive leadership. Since the adoption of a sector-wide approach in 2004, fragmentation and duplication have been greatly reduced. Subsequent joint annual work plans and a review process undertaken together with stakeholders assisted in maintaining a less fragmented approach to program planning and implementation, and has created more ownership, joint accountability, and strong government stewardship. There was strong national ownership and stewardship of the health strategy especially after the initiation of the Nepal Health Sector Strategy Implementation Plan, which was first started in 2004 (Nepal Ministry of Health 2004). Currently, Nepal is implementing the third plan (2016–2021), along the lines of the second long-term Health Plan and National Health Policy 2014.

The primary orientation toward providing essential health care services for free has been sustained through changes in the political system. The Nepalese health system utilizes a mix of public and private service delivery. There is a degree of coordination and support from nonprofit and for-profit sectors for selected public health interventions or selected areas. Notable examples are FP-MCH services. The Ministry of Health is the sole guarantor of publicly funded health services for rural, disadvantaged, and underserved populations. The health policy is developed, standardized, and governed at the central level by the Ministry of Health.

Health services are delivered from the central level to the community level, as shown in figure 9.3. The community level includes the VDC and the ward. PHC services at the VDC are delivered through health posts, which are staffed by salaried employees of the Ministry of Health: health assistants, AHWs, and ANMs. The nonsalaried FCHVs provide PHC at their respective ward with technical backup support of the health post for their VDC catchment area. The PHC services are provided below the VDC in two modes:

1. *At the community level,* there are regular periodic outreach activities that are organized from the health post and coordinated and supported by the FCHVs. The outreach packages, including health promotion, are provided by teams consisting of an AHW, an ANM, VHWs, and a FCHV, who sensitize the community well before each of the outreach events. The outreach teams offer almost the full range of outreach services as those provided by the health post.

2. *At the ward level,* routine services are provided in the community by FCHVs. This cadre of service providers delivers a basic, routine essential services package that has expanded over time. These services include elements of essential maternal and newborn care, child health services, family planning, antenatal care, immunization, and nutrition, as well as distribution of vitamin A and iron tablets to pregnant women, awareness of HIV/AIDS, the importance of using condoms for safe sex, and avoiding reuse of used syringes. These PHC services provided by FCHVs are linked with formal referral services at health posts, district hospitals/district health offices, and zonal hospitals. The establishment of health facilities in each VDC, with its regular monthly outreach clinics delivering scientifically proven and operationally feasible interventions at the community level, was the most significant contribution for achieving high coverage with equity accruing good health outcomes.

Nepal's health system introduced reforms in the comprehensive sense of Alma-Ata, and the platform of delivery and community participation also upheld this vision. Community health workers such as VHWs and FCHVs are the backbone of public health in Nepal to date. They are conveniently located in communities to address health across multiple sectors, and they provide scientifically tested, nationally prioritized packages of health interventions at the defined platforms of the community.

Modern Drivers and Movers of Health Development in Nepal

The Constitution of Nepal 2015 guarantees that "every citizen shall have the right to free basic health care services from the state, and no one shall be deprived of emergency services." These results have not been an overnight success. Progress began more than fifty years ago, with the intensity of the efforts increasing in the 1980s. The struggle was for the recognition of fundamental rights, especially freedom of organization, speech, and association.

As one of the signatory countries, the government of Nepal endorsed and committed to implementing the Alma-Ata Declaration. The principles of the Alma-Ata Declaration were woven into the country's integrated community-based health service system as appropriate.

Despite political instability, social consciousness has steadily increased. People have harnessed their rich cultural traditions that encourage cohesiveness and community kinship. People have used traditional norms of solidarity to find their unique path in maintaining functional local communities even during the country's weakest moments. Although the Panchayat era severely restricted the growth of civil society and community group initiatives, it established several community-based public health programs, including FCHVs, which have become the foundation for PHC. The tide began changing in 1991, with the growth of civil society and community groups. Since then, nongovernmental organizations, community groups, and users' groups have started to directly involve themselves in the local development process, and they have become development partners in government efforts. More importantly, they have taken a place as free voices in a democratic society.

For a long time, political instability had been a part of Nepal's political sphere. Nepal has made steady progress toward stable government and basic law enforcement but very slow progress controlling corruption. At the community level, different mechanisms evolved including social auditing and users' groups for village-level development projects (e.g., water user and forest user groups). In the health sector, establishment of the mothers' groups in each ward of the VDC and organization of health facility operation and management committees are examples of institutions with limited roles but that offer points of entry for people to express their voices. These also served as watchdogs for service accountability, alongside NGOs and community-based organizations and users' groups.

For the past twenty-five years, Nepal, with its low gross national income, has been contributing a minimum of 3% to a maximum of 7% of the national government budget to the health sector. Since the sector-wide approach has started, Nepal has also succeeded in garnering donors' support in a progressive manner. For the first time in 1995–1996, the central government started providing 300,000 rupees (about $US2,700) as a development grant directly to all the VDCs. This paved the way for local bodies to prioritize local needs. Until then, only centrally itemized budgets went to the VDC level; thus, the opportunities for development of local needs were infrequent. The guideline of the village development fund mandated that its 5% had to be invested in social sectors, including health. The amount increased as time went by, and it served as a catalyst for cascading locally prioritized development activities that facilitated its local ownership among four thousand VDCs then in the country. This decision has a historic bearing for the grassroots movement and has had a tremendous impact in the health sector.

Maintenance of Health Systems Despite Political Conflict

While there were negative consequences of the Maoist People's Movement, there were some collateral benefits that came from it. The Maoist People's Movement led to a social awakening of the people, especially regarding fundamental human rights. Although the movement was violent, participants characteristically refrained from hostile acts toward health facilities and activities. Even during the first national measles vaccination campaign, conducted during a time when the western districts of Nepal were ravaged by conflict, the Maoists allowed access to the program. During intense periods of conflict, during which the government was absent at VDCs and subdistricts, community members had to devise their own strategies to ensure physical access. Some health services were continuing during the conflict in rural and remote areas. Wherever the Maoist Party was, all government activities were under surveillance, and thus projects were made accountable and retention of health workers improved. Therefore, despite the conflict Nepal's public health indicators continued to progress during this period. Gender equality, abolishing the caste system, and inclusion of the rights of ethnic minorities were among the important social agenda items of the Maoists and are important issues in Nepal's context. The Maoists recruited women within their ranks and attempted to implement education and awareness programs in communities where they had a stronghold. This gave rise to an unseen but healthy competition between the government and the Maoists. Consequently, the government also increased participation of women in the Nepal Army and the Nepal Police, as well as in other sectors. Ultimately, through a peace accord both sides came into agreement and continued to pursue a progressive agenda together. Finally, the 2015 Constitution of Nepal mandated a one-third female composition in parliament and also other ethnicities' and castes' representation in different positions.

Conclusion and Lessons

Nepal's achievements were not an accident but required conscious effort in policy formulation, implementation, and community mobilization by the health system over time, with review and lessons drawn periodically. A progressive policy environment, early piloting of community involvement, establishment and recognition of community volunteers, and initiation of interventions with clear objectives were important turning points for health in Nepal before the 1990s. Appropriate selection of interventions, utilization of global evidences, and local research for the development of a national system began as early as the 1970s. Placing mid-level health workers for service delivery together with VHWs and FCHVs at an interface between the national health system and the community in the public health delivery system was appropriate and successful. Careful introduction of interventions, empowerment of FCHVs for delivery of selected interventions, and development of a well-supported, community-based health system helped attain high coverage that was sustainable. More recently, civil society movements, improved literacy and women's status, and improved demand for services facilitated by better road access, communication, and media were linked to an improved supply of services. Progress in health development was possible because Nepal's public health leaders made a deliberate choice to identify and maintain strong community engagement in health facilitated by the FCHVs (see box on page 221).

Historically, Nepal faced the challenge of preventing appallingly high rates of maternal and child mortality, with a severe lack of materials, budget, and trained health workers. Universal home delivery of infants was the historical norm. In order to meet these challenges, Nepal took initiatives that have worked well.

Unlike in neighboring countries, the Family Planning Programme developed in Nepal as an integral component of MCH. The system created a new cadre of community-based health workers together with FCHVs in every village. Working together with local health posts and with a technical backstop of respective district health offices, they form the backbone of Nepal's health system today.

Case Study of one Female Community Health Volunteer: A Common Happening in Villages of Nepal

Maya Devi Thakuri is a 57-year-old female community health volunteer (FCHV) in the Dailekha district, a remote village in Nepal. She is also an active member of a cooperative and participates in the local community forestry group. She is a devoted crusader for the Water and Sanitation User's Group during the regular village drinking water and Sarsafai (cleanliness) Campaign.

It's time for Maya to resume her responsibility as the moderator in the forthcoming monthly mothers' group meeting. It is scheduled to begin tomorrow, and there are important items to be discussed along with regular updates and education. The proposed agenda items are the upcoming biannual vitamin A supplementation and deworming campaign, the campaign for measles supplemental immunization activities, and contribution to the declaration of open defecation free village, as well as regular updates. This morning Maya met with Rup Kumari, a 20-year-old Dalit woman who is from a more remote part of her village, to discuss health issues. Maya has specifically invited Rup to attend the upcoming meeting.

Compelled to drop out of school at age 12 to help support her family, Rup joins an adolescent life-skills program facilitated by FCHVs. There she is exposed to various issues pertaining to her sexual and reproductive health, and grows to understand the reason behind the death of her mother's firstborn son. Married at the age of 12, twenty-five years earlier, her mother suffered the loss of her first child at the age of 15. Learning from this, Rup chooses to marry Krishna, whom she has known for several years, but decides to wait until she is 21. They then adopted a temporary family planning method, which they receive from the FCHV regularly. Two years later, Rup and Krishna decide to have a child. In the previous mothers' group meeting, she was informed about the benefits of antenatal checkups as well as danger signs to look out for during pregnancy, delivery, and the postpartum period.

Subsequently, a pregnant Rup attends a health post primary health care outreach clinic, and the FCHV lends support by accompanying her there for the first time. She gains further information during antenatal care. Having already received two tetanus toxoid injections, she makes sure to take iron and folate regularly during her pregnancy. On her final visit, she is advised to go to a primary health care center (PHCC), where a skilled birth attendant is available.

Rup and Krishna put aside some rupees as suggested by the mothers' group, and Krishna discusses transport options with his neighbors for when she enters into labor. When Rup goes into labor, friends help carry her to the nearest PHCC. There, Rup is examined by Jhuma Limbu, an auxiliary nurse midwife and a skilled birth attendant. In a normal procedure, Rup gives birth to a healthy baby girl, whom Jhuma dries and wraps after washing her hands with soap and water. Jhuma waits for the umbilical cord to stop pulsating, then clamps and cuts it with a sterile blade and applies chlorhexidine to the cord stump. Rup immediately puts her new baby on her belly to keep her warm and commences breastfeeding. The baby also receives 200,000 IU of vitamin A.

Three days later, Rup and her daughter are visited by a FCHV, who confirms that her supplies of iron and folate are replenished. She discusses exclusive breastfeeding, family planning, vaccination of her baby in six weeks, and vitamin A supplementation, but only after her child reaches six months.

The FCHV counts her supplies and prepares her report, which will be submitted for review at the monthly FCHV meeting at her health post next week. There, all of the FCHVs will discuss their progress and the challenges of the past month and plan for the next.

Thousands of mothers across Nepal are receiving such care and support from FCHVs each day. Over the course of the past twenty to twenty-five years, FCHVs have changed the landscape of access to PHC services in Nepal.

Community-based health workers were responsible for delivering a set of safe and proven basic MCH-FP technologies. A few examples of these are health education and communication about basic hygiene, family planning, a homemade oral rehydration solution (Noon-Chini Aushadhi Paani) that cuts diarrhea mortality by half, immunization, the promotion of breastfeeding, infant and child nutrition, and the treatment and prevention of protein-calorie malnutrition with homemade and affordable foods such as sarbottam pitho. There are many other examples.

With the imminent risk of malaria reemergence in 1970s, the government changed its policy from a vertical to an integrated approach, creating an integrated community health services development project. This project focused mainly on delivering the basic health care provided earlier by five vertical projects through health assistants, community-based VHWs, and FCHVs.

Along with the integrated community health services development project came the establishment of the integrated district health offices, which pooled the district-level resources of the previously existing five vertical projects. For example, the resources of twenty-five FP-MCH district offices established by 1971 were reorganized under the integrated district health offices. By the end of the sixth five-year plan (1980–1985), an integrated health care delivery system was operational in forty-eight out of seventy-five districts. Over time, Nepal's national health system evolved into a community-based pyramid whose base was rooted at the community level.

An appropriately designed scale-up plan guided strategies to target the population through a suitable selection of delivery platforms together with meaningful community participation. Having national ownership and stewardship of the PHC approach was critical for Nepal's past health development. The country is now scaling up universal coverage through a strategy of health insurance. The lessons learned from Nepal's comprehensive and result-oriented PHC offer an excellent foundation for future health development.

REFERENCES

Atteraya, Madhu Sudhan, Shreejana Gnawali, and In Han Song. 2015. "Factors associated with intimate partner violence against married women in Nepal." *J Interpers Violence* 30 (7): 1226–1246.

Boch-Isaacson, Joel M., Christa Sherry, Kerry Moran, and Kay M. Kalavan. 2001. *Half-a-century of development: The history of US assistance to Nepal, 1951–2001.* Kathmandu, Nepal: Multi Graphics Press.

Central Bureau of Statistics. 2015. *Statistical year book 2015.* Ramshahpath, Kathmandu, Nepal: Government of Nepal National Planning Commission. https://cbs .gov.np/wp-content/upLoads/2019/02/Statistical-Year-Book-2015.pdf.

Das, G. S. L. 1996. "Tuberculosis in Nepal: Past, present and future." *J Nepal Med Assoc* 1966 (4): 8–15.

Dhungel, Rajesh, and Ram Nath Ojha. 2012. "Women's empowerment for disaster risk reduction and emergency response in Nepal." *Gender Dev* 20 (2): 309–321.

Dixit, Vishwa Deep. 1995. *The quest for health.* 1st ed. Mahakalthan, Kathmandu: Educational Enterprises.

Family Health Division. 2014. *Female community health volunteer national survey.* Teku, Kathmandu, Nepal: Department of Health Services, Ministry of Health and Population.

Glenton, Claire, Inger B. Scheel, Sabina Pradhan, Simon Lewin, Stephen Hodgins, and Vijaya Shrestha. 2010. "The female community health volunteer programme in Nepal: Decision makers' perceptions of volunteerism, payment and other incentives." *Soc Sci Med* 70 (12): 1920–1927.

Gottlieb, J. 2007. "Reducing child mortality with vitamin A in Nepal." In *Case studies in global health: Millions saved,* edited by Ruth Levine, 25–32. Burlington, MA: Jones and Bartlett.

Government of Nepal. 2015. "Constitution of Nepal." http://www.lawcommission.gov .np/en/wp-content/uploads/2018/09/10272.pdf.

Leve, Lauren. 2007. "'Failed development' and rural revolution in Nepal: Rethinking subaltern consciousness and women's empowerment." *Anthropol Q* 80 (1): 127–172.

Mali, I. B. 1996. "Leprosy services in Nepal." *J Nepal Med Assoc* 1966 (3): 225–229.

Nepal Family Planning. 1976. *Maternal Child Health Project, Nepal Fertility Survey.* His Majesty's Government of Nepal and World Fertility Survey.

Nepal Ministry of Health. 1988. Female Community Health Worker Program.

———. 1991. "National health policy." Ramshahpath, Kathmandu, Nepal: Government of Nepal. www.lawcommission.gov.np.

———. 2004. Nepal Health Sector Program: Implementation Plan. Ramshahpath, Kathmandu, Nepal.

Nepal National Planning Commission. 1956. "First plan." https://www.npc.gov.np /images/category/FirrstPlan_Eng.pdf.

New Era. 2008. *An analytical report on national survey of female community health volunteers of Nepal*. USAID. https://dhsprogram.com/pubs/pdf/FR181/FCHV _Nepal2007.pdf.

Pant, Y. P. 1955. "Nepal's first census." *Econ Weekly* 7 (31): 912–914.

Perry, Henry, Rose Zulliger, Kerry Scott, Dena Javadi, and Jess Gergen. 2013. "Case studies of large-scale community health worker programs: Examples from Bangladesh, Brazil, Ethiopia, India, Iran, Nepal, and Pakistan." *Afghanistan: Community-Based Health Care to the Ministry of Public Health*. Washington, DC: USAID/MCHIP. https://www.mcsprogram.org/resource/case-studies-large-scale-community-health -worker-programs-2/

Pokhrel, Subhash, Rachel Snow, Hengjin Dong, Budi Hidayat, Steffen Flessa, and Rainer Sauerborn. 2005. "Gender role and child health care utilization in Nepal." *Health Policy* 74 (1): 100–109.

Purdey, Alice F., Gyan Bahadur Adhikari, Sheila A. Robinson, and Philip W. Cox. 1994. "Participatory health development in rural Nepal: Clarifying the process of community empowerment." *Health Educ Q* 21 (3): 329–343.

Smith, Lisa C., Usha Ramakrishnan, Aida Ndiaye, Lawrence Haddad, and Reynaldo Martorell. 2003. *The importance of women's status for child nutrition in developing countries*. International Food Policy Research Institute. https://core.ac.uk /download/pdf/6289649.pdf.

Swechhya, Baskota, and R. Kamaraj. 2014. "Female community health volunteers program in Nepal: Perceptions, attitudes and experiences on volunteerism among female community health volunteers." *Int J Interdiscip Multidiscip Stud* 1 (5): 9–15.

Taylor, D., and R. Thapa. 1972. *Country profiles, Nepal*. New York: Population Council. https://files.eric.ed.gov/fulltext/ED063153.pdf.

Thapa, R, Y. N. Sharma, and K. B. Singh. 1973. "Manpower development for Maternal-Child Health and Family Planning program—A Nepalese case study." *J Nepal Med Assoc* 11 (4): 109–126.

World Health Organization. 2018. "Global Health Expenditure Database." Geneva. http://apps.who.int/nha/database/Home/Index/en/.

Worth, Robert M., and Narayan K. Shah. 1969. *Nepal health survey, 1965–1966*. Honolulu: University of Hawaii Press.

CHAPTER TEN

Four Decades of Community-Based Primary Health Care Development in Ghana

James F. Phillips, Fred N. Binka, John Koku Awoonor-Williams, and Ayaga A. Bawah

Introduction

When Ghana signed the World Health Organization's Alma-Ata Declaration in 1978, it embraced a vision of a health system that prioritized those in greatest need (World Health Organization 1978; Ministry of Health Republic of Ghana 1995; Saleh 2012). Yet, by the early 1990s, services remained inaccessible to the rural poor (Nyonator and Kutzin 1999). In search of practical means of achieving Health for All, the Ministry of Health convened an advisory panel in 1991 to define a new course for community health care programming. A program of implementation research and action was launched that has contributed to community-based primary health care (PHC) development ever since. Experience gained illustrates a strategy for moving beyond a pilot trial to national programming while also tailoring change to local cultural conditions and capabilities of relevant administrative units. This chapter presents a country case study of ways to leverage health system reforms developed in one location by spreading implementation capacity throughout a country.

Ghana's history of evidence-driven program development is portrayed in figure 10.1. Questions concerning what should be done in response to evidence of continuing high fertility and high mortality remained the subject of policy debate in the 1990s. The provision of PHC remained remote from the population in need or dispersed to poorly supervised and inadequately trained volunteer health workers whose services often did more harm than good (Skeet 1985; Peter, Davidson, and Burger 1987; Walt, Perera, and

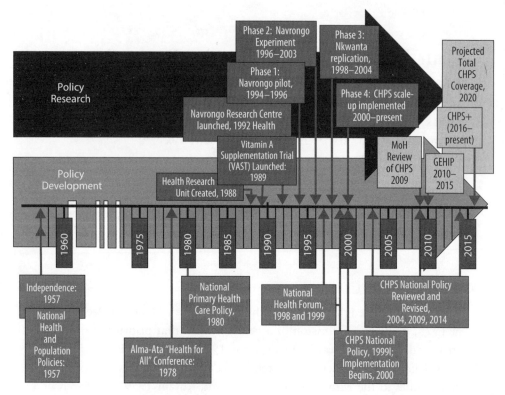

Figure 10.1. The process of community-based primary health care development in Ghana, 1978–2018.

Heggenhougen 1989). Despite international consensus that community-based PHC could save lives, the appropriate strategic responses to this consensus were unresolved in the 1990s and are still evolving three decades later (Perry et al. 1999; Freeman et al. 2012; Singh and Sachs 2013). This chapter presents a country case study of ways to guide the process of PHC development with a phased program of research, evidence-based policy reform, and organized spread of implementation capacity throughout a country.*

Ghana's 1980 Primary Health Care Policy aimed to develop the organizational structure that is shown in figure 10.2. Although Level A was

*Preparation of this chapter was supported by grants of the Doris Duke Charitable Foundation's (DDCF) African Health Initiative to the Mailman School of Public Health, Columbia University. The authors gratefully acknowledge advisory support of members of the DDCF African Health Advisory Council and guidance of the CHPS+ Strategic Advisory Committee chaired by Dr. Anthony Nsiah-Asare, director general, Ghana Health Service.

planned to comprise primary service points that would function as the main community-based care point, budget constraints had prevented essential health post construction that the Level A agenda required. Subdistrict care had been established in clinics, termed Level B, with each clinic serving a population ranging from ten thousand to twenty-five thousand in a given subdistrict. Each of these subdistrict health centers was staffed by medical assistants, "enrolled nurses," and midwives with the goal of providing access to basic ambulatory health care. Level C consisted of a hospital led by at least one physician who was supported by a team of paramedics. Each district in Ghana was provided with a district health management team (DHMT) convened with administrative authority over the system shown in figure 10.2. By 1990, each of the ten regions of Ghana was equipped with a referral hospital and a regional health administration to coordinate the activities of each DHMT. In 1996, an act of parliament consigned the policy and political functions of the health sector to the Ministry of Health; implementation functions of the health care system, as shown in figure 10.2, were consigned to the newly constituted Ghana Health Service (GHS).

By the early 1990s, a cadre of community health nurses (CHNs) had been created and nearly two thousand had been hired, trained for eighteen months, and deployed to districts throughout Ghana. Each CHN was mandated to provide immunizations, care for childhood illness, dispense family planning methods, and deliver other PHC services (table 10.1). However, the absence of revenue for constructing Level A community facilities, purchasing essential equipment, and providing logistics support, prevented CHN community deployment. Instead, CHNs were assigned to already fully staffed Level B subdistrict health centers and Level C district hospitals, where their redundant services amounted to one episode of care per worker per day. Thus, despite the creation of the CHN cadre, more than half of all households were located nine kilometers or more from the nearest Level C hospital or Level B clinic. It was apparent to program planners in Accra that Level A in the system shown in figure 10.2 existed in name only.

To provide evidence that could guide the development of policy to address the need for accessible PHC, the Ministry of Health established a health research unit of the Policy, Planning, Monitoring and Evaluation Division in Accra with a mandate to establish health research centers in each of the three ecological zones of Ghana (Agyepong and Adjei 2008).

By 1992, the northern ecological zone version of these centers was established in the Kassena-Nankana District of the Upper East Region (UER) from institutional capabilities that had been generated by research on vitamin A

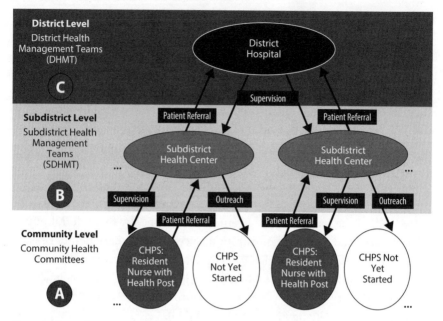

Figure 10.2. The organizational structure of primary health care services in Ghana at the community (A), subdistrict (B), and district hospital (C) levels.

supplementation (VAST Study Team 1993). The Navrongo Health Research Centre, based in Navrongo, was accorded a mandate to convert an existing cohort research system into a population research platform for the demographic evaluation of community-based PHC (Binka et al. 1999). The UER was Ghana's most impoverished region. The core mandate of the Navrongo Health Research Centre was to research means of addressing the challenging health development problems of Sahelian northern Ghana (Binka et al. 1995; Adongo et al. 1998; Ngom et al. 1999; Doctor 2007). UER mortality rates were well above national levels, and cultural traditions were known to sustain high fertility (Adongo et al. 1997) and constrain health development (Ngom et al. 2003). The study area economy was dominated by subsistence agriculture, literacy was low—particularly among women—and traditions of marriage, kinship, and family-building emphasized the economic and security value of large families. Parental health-seeking behavior was governed more by tradition than by the pursuit of modern health care (Ngom et al. 2003).

Table 10.1. Primary health care modalities and services provided at the community level.

Category	Health Intervention Provided by Community-Based Health Planning and Services (CHPS) as of January 2018
General population	
Malaria prevention	• Cost-free insecticide-treated bed net distribution • Residual spraying, environmental management • Training for improved malaria case management and referral
Childhood preventive and curative care	
Expanded program in immunization	• Comprehensive immunization care with Bacille Calmette-Guerin, Diphtheria-pertussis-tetanus, Haemophilus influenza, Hep (B-1, 2, and 3), oral polio vaccine (1, 2, and 3), Rotavirus vaccine, Pneumoccocal vaccine (1, 2, and 3), measles • Vitamin A supplementation
Integrated management of childhood illness	• Training and deployment of all community health officers in diagnosis, care, and referral of febrile illnesses—for example, antibiotics for pneumonia and acute ear infections, malaria treatment (artesunate/amodiaquine), and referral of febrile diarrheal disease cases for clinical care • Care and referral for watery diarrheal diseases via oral rehydration therapy
Reproductive health: prepregnancy and pregnancy	
Community-based family planning	• Provision of oral contraceptives, injectables, condoms, information services, referral for side effects or provision of clinical methods; clinic-based provision of intrauterine device and subdermal methods
Clinical services	• Intrauterine device, subdermal contraception, tubectomy, oral contraceptives, and condoms • Care for side effects
Perinatal health	
Antenatal care	• Routine four visits, including checkup and referral • Tetanus toxoid, iron supplementation • Intermittent preventive treatment of malaria in pregnancy with Sulfadoxine pyrimethamine
Promotion of facility based care	• Promotion of facility-based delivery • Immediate postdelivery care

Source: World Health Organization 1997, 2005, 2009, 2012; Community Directed Interventions Study Group 2010; V. Patel and Andrews 2000.

Note: All modalities and modes of delivery employed by the Navrongo Project and subsequently by CHPS were approved in advance by the Ministry of Health and endorsed for community-based services by the World Health Organization.

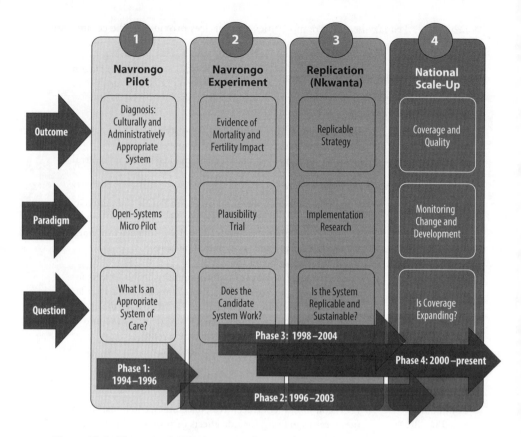

Figure 10.3. Phases in the application of research to community-based primary health care development in Ghana.

Developing Community-Based Primary Health Care

The Primary Health Care Steering Committee was chaired by the director of public health of the Ministry of Health, with participating members that included the director of maternal and child health, the director of the health research unit, and other research experts. Instead of risking public investment in a large-scale, unsuccessful program, the committee sponsored the creation of a four-phased learning process for guiding deliberations on policy.

Phase 1: Participatory Planning Research

Phase 1 was comprised of a three-village learning process that aimed to develop culturally appropriate strategies for providing PHC (Nazzar et al. 1995). Discussion groups comprised of community leaders, women's social

Lessons from Phase 1: The Navrongo Three Community Pilot

- Community-based primary health care is in great demand.
- When traditional leaders were consulted, they sponsored the creation of community health committees.
- With support from leaders, these committees organized the convening of consensus-building events termed *durbars*.
- Durbars fostered community commitment to constructing interim health posts.
- Community-engagement processes were critical to sustainable development of volunteerism and community support for the work of nurses.

networks, and frontline workers were convened to comment on service needs and strategies. Based on community advice, services were implemented and discussion was reconvened to gauge reactions. Traditional community gatherings, known as "durbars," were used to build consensus for relocating nurses from subdistrict and hospital clinics to community locations. The pilot also clarified strategies for recruiting, training, and deploying volunteers for supplementing nurse services with rudimentary syndromic care and referral for childhood illnesses (see box on this page). Attention was also directed to eliciting community contributions of labor and materials for constructing community health compounds, where nurses were to be posted for resident health service work.

Phase 2: The Navrongo Trial

To generate evidence on the possible impact of Phase 1 strategies, a Phase 2 plausibility trial was launched in four subdistricts, each corresponding to policy options for providing convenient, low-cost, and comprehensive service delivery operations. Cells of the trial corresponded to subdistricts where fully functioning clinics were available for medical assistants and nurses to provide the full regimen of PHC. One such subdistrict was set aside as a comparison area. The four subdistricts of Kassena-Nankana were randomly allocated to two operational dimensions.

The community health officer dimension of the project involved reorienting existing subdistrict health centers to community health care and deploying them to community locations that would improve efficiency and develop the quality and intensity of child health services. CHNs were retrained to function as village resident personnel, known as community health

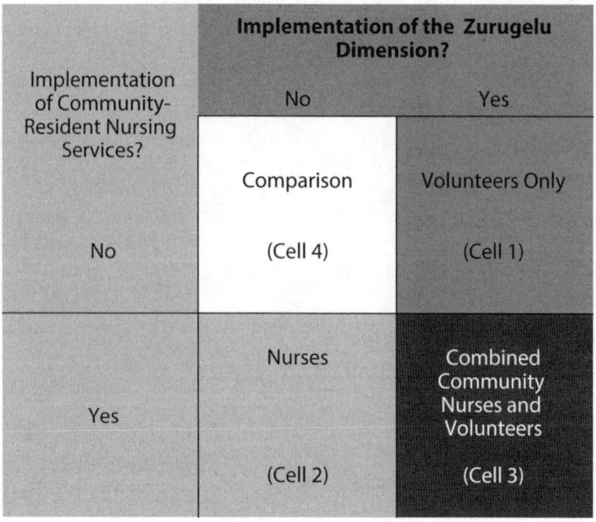

Implementation of Community-Resident Nursing Services?	Implementation of the Zurugelu Dimension?	
	No	Yes
No	Comparison (Cell 4)	Volunteers Only (Cell 1)
Yes	Nurses (Cell 2)	Combined Community Nurses and Volunteers (Cell 3)

Figure 10.4. Cells of the Navrongo Experiment design.

officers (CHOs), with training added to develop CHO skills in community engagement and doorstep service delivery.

The Zurugelu dimension mobilized cultural resources of chieftaincy, social networks, village gatherings, volunteerism, and community support. Volunteers were provided with six weeks of training in syndromic screening and referral. Volunteer deployment was posited to represent an affordable and feasible means of providing essential health services to the rural poor, premised on the observation that vibrant African social institutions could provide a platform for recruiting, supervising, and sustaining volunteer effort. Broad outlines of this volunteer-focused approach were advocated by the UNICEF-sponsored Bamako Initiative (Knippenberg et al. 1990). However, no systematic evidence had emerged showing that volunteers with limited syndromic treatment capabilities could save lives (Golden 1991; Lairumbi et al. 2011; Greenspan et al. 2013).

Since the Navrongo worker deployment dimensions could be configured independently, jointly, or not at all, a four-celled experiment was implied by the design (figure 10.4). The joint implementation cell tested the impact of relocating nurses as resident CHOs for ambulatory and preventive health services with backstopping and referral services provided by volunteers. Taken together, the two arms of the trial addressed key themes of policy debate about the effectiveness of volunteers and the sustainability of professional nursing (Binka et al. 1995). Experimentation was needed in the 1990s because

Lessons from Phase 2: The Navrongo Experiment

Cell 1: The Zurugelu Area with Primary Health Care Provided by Volunteers

- Volunteers could have been deployed and sustained with community support, but this strategy had no impact on child survival or fertility.

Cell 2: The Community Health Officer Deployment Area

- Nurse deployment saved lives.
- Impact was concentrated among post-infants (an integrated management of childhood illness effect).
- Nurses' deployment without volunteers had no impact on fertility. Family planning requires comprehensive social engagement that includes outreach to male networks and opinion leaders.

Cell 3: The Community Health Officer and Zurugelu Volunteers Backed Up by Community Engagement

- Cell 3 was adopted in 1999 as national PHC policy.
- Where volunteers were deployed together with nurses, both fertility and mortality declined.
  - Child survival effects were equivalent to Cell 2: MDG4 in seven years.
  - Fertility decline of 15% in five years, equivalent to one birth relative to Cells 1, 2, or 4.

Cell 4: The Comparison Area

- Where subdistrict clinic services functioned without community-based care, neither mortality nor fertility declined.
- Caseloads at subdistrict health center were very low: about one patient per worker per day.

there was no rigorous scientific evidence that supplying family planning services would work in a demand-constrained, rural African setting or that community-based PHC could significantly improve childhood survival (see box on this page).

This conclusion was corroborated by qualitative research showing that parents dealing with childhood illness tended to seek traditional healers as their first provider, owing to customs of trust and respect that permitted the healers to allow parents to defer payments with the expectation that they would eventually be compensated for their care. The trust between traditional providers and their clients represented a form of social insurance that ensured access to traditional health care that was otherwise unaffordable (Nyarko et al. 2002). By replicating this custom of social insurance for deferring payment, the CHO could provide modern health technologies that replaced traditional medicine, a substitution effect that immediately improved survival (Wells-Pence et al. 2007) and eventually achieved MDG4 within seven years

(Phillips et al. 2006; Binka et al. 2007). In addition, with training and supervision, their outreach to men focusing on family planning provided critical organizational capabilities for the project to achieve reproductive health impact (Debpuur et al. 2002). Therefore, the "combined cell" was adopted as the service model for the national health policy.

Phase 3: Replication-Related Implementation Research

In 1998, the Ministry of Health convened a conference of district and regional health officials to disseminate preliminary results and discuss implementation implications. Rather than accept results as a basis for moving forward, most participants in the meeting questioned the relevance of Navrongo research to their respective capabilities and needs elsewhere in the country. The remoteness of Navrongo, its research resource base, and unique administrative structure were cited as reasons to question the replicability and sustainability of the Navrongo model. However, the DHMT in Nkwanta District had already launched a process of replicating the Navrongo model. After discussing this initiative, conference participants resolved to reconvene deliberations within a year to review the experience of this replication and gauge the policy relevance of lessons Nkwanta provided as a basis for researching this implementation process, documenting its details, and demonstrating the process to visiting implementation teams.

Based on the Nkwanta experience, six steps were documented as national policy for implementing the program, which are phased in zone by zone over time wherever CHPS is implemented (figure 10.5).

1. *Preliminary planning.* Communities are comprised of contiguous clusters of extended households with a common lineal leader or chief and elders representing coresident lineage heads (Lyon 2003). Since household membership in a community is unambiguous, Nkwanta planning started with social mapping of the boundaries of chieftaincy domains and locations of the households of traditional leaders. Three to five communities were clustered into geographic "zones," defining nurse community health care service areas.
2. *Community entry.* Meetings, dialogue, and community diplomacy involving traditional leaders and elders was to build community ownership of the program and launch traditional public gatherings termed *durbars* for engaging community support (Tindana et al. 2011).

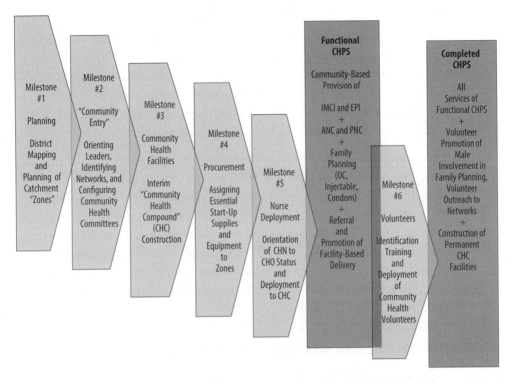

Figure 10.5. The Nkwanta milestones for launching community-based health policy services at the community level.

3. *Community health compound construction.* Community involvement enabled the Nkwanta team to organize volunteer construction of facilities that could act as service points for community-based health care. The process of constructing permanent facilities for public health programs involved procedural delay associated with acquiring revenue, awarding contracts, and completing the construction process. The Nkwanta process of soliciting community volunteer support for constructing traditional housing for CHPS operations uncoupled implementation with these construction formalities. Temporary community construction has been critical to accelerating CHPS operations wherever rapid scale-up has occurred.

4. *Essential equipment procurement.* Implementing CHPS required investment in equipment, supplies, and logistics arrangements.

5. *In-service training on community engagement.* Nurses were retrained in community organizational tasks that enable them to effectively liaise with community institutions.

6. *Volunteer training and deployment.* Community health volunteers were recruited and trained in community health mobilization, methods of promoting family planning and reproductive health among men, and procedures for backstopping nurses.

Phase 3 implementation research showed that the Nkwanta replication was feasible and effective (Awoonor-Williams et al. 2010) (see box on this page). Prior to CHPS implementation, family planning usage in Nkwanta District was estimated to be less than 4%. Within two years, prevalence had increased to 8.6%. The odds that infants were fully immunized was 2.4 times greater among children living in CHPS areas relative to areas not yet provided with CHPS. CHPS exposure was associated with odds ratios of 2.8 and 3.6 for completing the polio and DPT/Penta series, respectively (Awoonor-Williams et al. 2004).

Lessons from Phase 3: The Nkwanta Replication Trial

- The Navrongo service model is replicable, but local strategic adjustments are essential. Local pilots and phasing in can clarify the adjustment process.
- There are six critical milestones for implementing Community-Based Health Planning and Services (CHPS) in each nurse deployment zone:
  1. planning district implementation by mapping and assessing traditional leadership;
  2. engagement of community leaders for convening community health committees and launching community durbars;
  3. community team facility development by traditional construction or renovation of interim community health compounds, where nurses live and work;
  4. marshaling essential equipment, supplies, and furniture for a given community health compound;
  5. orienting nurses to community-engagement tasks and deploying nurses with community-engagement backing; and
  6. recruiting community health committee volunteers, training volunteers, and deploying them to backstop nurses.
- Nkwanta and Navrongo could serve as transfer of innovation localities for catalyzing national scale-up by providing practical demonstration of the six milestones.
- Replication was associated with greater impact than had been observed in Navrongo.
- District leadership workshops failed if training lacked practical field team demonstration of the implementation process.

While the Nkwanta six-milestone approach to community-based care was found to be too complex to describe in workshops, it proved to be relatively simple to demonstrate, particularly when demonstration involved teams of peer counterparts learning about the initiative by seeing their respective roles in action. Accordingly, thirty-two DHMTs were selected among the 126 districts by regional directors of health services to observe the Nkwanta implementation process with the goal of disseminating practical implementation experience to each of Ghana's ten regions. Each participating DHMT was requested to assemble teams of managers, subdistrict supervisors, and frontline CHOs to travel to Nkwanta, where they would be assigned to peer counterparts for witnessing milestone achievement, and plan for the transfer of this experience to their home districts.

This transfer process was catalyzed by small start-up grants to participating DHMTs, ranging between US$18,000 and $28,000, for financing an initial pilot CHPS zone in each participating district. These small grants were intended to catalyze CHPS start-up activities. While the GHS had made budget provisions for salaries, supplies, and equipment, there was no budget provision for start-up costs. To generate essential revenue, pilot zone activity was intended to generate grassroots political commitment for the allocation of development revenue for health post construction costs. This additional revenue could be marshaled by district assemblies if local political consensus was manifest. To build this political consensus, grassroots politicians from the district assembly were invited to participate in pilot zone communication and community consensus–building activities, a process that accorded opportunities for communities to demonstrate their support for CHPS and opportunities for politicians to garner popular support from voters by demonstrating their support of improving access to health care. Once started, this process of scaled-down, zone-by-zone spread of commitment to CHPS often catalyzed the diffusion of community commitment to implementation throughout participating districts. During the start-up period, from 2000 to 2008, nearly all CHPS implementation was concentrated in the thirty-two districts where implementers had visited Nkwanta and had experienced practical demonstration of the CHPS start-up process.

Phase 4: Scaling Up the CHPS Program

To achieve its national mandate of removing geographic barriers to health care, CHPS planners have always sought to enable district managers throughout Ghana to adapt approaches to community health care to local traditions

Lessons from Monitoring the Scaling-Up Process

- Initial scale-up was rapid in districts where teams had received on-site implementation orientation in Nkwanta.
- Workshops for district leaders without demonstration failed to have an impact on implementation unless district teams had also experienced on-site demonstration of the Community-Based Health Planning and Services (CHPS) implementation process.
- The absence of earmarked budget lines and start-up revenue delayed implementation.
- CHPS is sustainable with Ghana Health Service investments in staff, supplies, and logistics once start-up problems are resolved.

- CHPS scale-up is a process of guided diffusion within districts:
  - Demonstration: Within districts, scale-up progressed if pilot zones were established, funds were provided for financing a start-up community, and a process of community to community demonstration exchanges emerged.
  - Champions: Organizational change was accelerated if committed individuals were engaged in demonstrating the feasibility of CHPS implementation and its benefits to the community.
  - Political engagement: The popularity of CHPS catalyzed political support for development investment in start-up costs.

and sustain implementation with available resources. While the process for pursuing this goal was developed in Phase 1 in Navrongo, tested in Phase 2, and refined in Phase 3, an additional phase was required to provide lessons from monitoring the scaling-up process. Policy learning was embedded in CHPS replication and scale-up research (see box on this page).

Effective CHPS Implementation Requires Decentralized and Phased Implementation

Rather than transferring CHPS operations to entire districts, Nkwanta exchanges transferred the process of phased learning to participating trainee districts. Once equipped with this capability, DHMTs could convene a process of community exchanges within their district, catalyzing the spread of community commitment to CHPS implementation once pilot services were established in one or two demonstration zones—a process akin to the diffusion of innovation (Davis and Cherns 1975; Mintrom 1997; Muula et al. 2004; Mintrom and Norman 2009). Component activities of the CHPS program have been designed to foster the diffusion of operational innovation (Rogers 1962; Awoonor-Williams et al. 2010). Success on a small scale can catalyze the spread of innovation within districts.

Progress Is Enhanced by Guiding Diffusion with Consensus-Building Activities

In response to the observation that scaling up can be accelerated by diffusion of CHPS implementation, the CHPS Initiative has been organized more in the manner of a social movement than a bureaucratic program. Where district managers have directed resources and training to community exchanges, local CHPS implementation can proceed. However, diplomacy and outreach to the political community is important to resource mobilization and consensus-building.

The Importance of Champions

This diffusion process has been catalyzed by ideational leadership. The CHPS experience suggests that organizational change is highly effective when it is driven by committed individuals who demonstrate that change is not only feasible as a process but is associated with outcomes that are in the interest of the community at large (Standing and Chowdhury 2008).

Knowledge Management for Fostering Change

Developing a program that relies on "guided diffusion" requires strategic attention to mechanisms for communicating lessons about progress to stakeholders at all levels of the system (Godlee et al. 2004; Hyder et al. 2007; Travis et al. 2004; Chen et al. 2006; Shoo et al. 2012; Awoonor-Williams et al. 2013; Ghiron et al. 2014; Phillips et al. 2018). In the CHPS program, communication tools, such as a newsletter, were developed for the flow of "bottom-up" lessons learned. Ghana has also developed mechanisms for "top-down" communication: policy conferences, policy guidelines, monitoring and evaluation feedback, and other mechanisms for communicating to district managers national policy commitment to the CHPS agenda. These mechanisms, in turn, were supported by "lateral communication" comprised of peer-to-peer demonstration of implementation at the district level. Though incomplete in its current execution, this communication system has developed awareness throughout the GHS system of the importance of CHPS scale-up, the feasibility of its strategies, and progress throughout the country in achieving widespread access to health care. In this manner, the management of CHPS knowledge has been a systems approach grounded in the channels of communication and action that move the change process forward.

Credibility

While national health programs throughout Africa have adopted the sector-wide approach to integrated health planning and decentralization, districts provided with the mandate to plan their operations are often ill-equipped to do so (Berman and Bossert 2000; Dujardin 2009; Peters et al. 2009; Vaillan-court 2009; Peters et al. 2012). The diffusion of organizational change is most likely to occur if the proposed alternative represents a clear improvement over existing operations and if the required changes are perceived to be both reasonable and achievable. CHPS fosters district-to-district demonstration designed to focus implementers on developing a manageable operational change agenda.

Ownership

Studies of the diffusion of organizational change consistently indicate that changes that are perceived by stakeholders as being imposed from the outside are less acceptable than those that are perceived to be initiated internally (Kirigia et al. 2005; Sivhaga et al. 2012; Sherr et al. 2013). In health system development, researchers are thus often marginalized from decision-making processes (Godlee et al. 2004; Damschroder et al. 2009). The sense of joint management-researcher ownership of change that characterizes the CHPS program arises from collaborative exploration of alternative operations, teamwork in planning change, and consensus-building regarding the practical implications of findings.

Reforming CHPS

The evidence from Navrongo and Nkwanta showed that community health care could save lives if essential services were conveniently available and if workers were trained to provide the full range of essential PHC. But, the first decade of Phase 4 monitoring showed that CHPS was not living up to its full potential. The pace of scale-up was unacceptably slow in districts where leaders had not participated in Nkwanta exchanges. Moreover, CHPS was not adequately contributing to improvement in newborn survival (Binka et al. 2009; Atinga et al. 2018). A process of CHPS reform was instituted that revisited the logic of the framework shown in figure 10.3 with a renewed process of phased implementation research (figure 10.6).

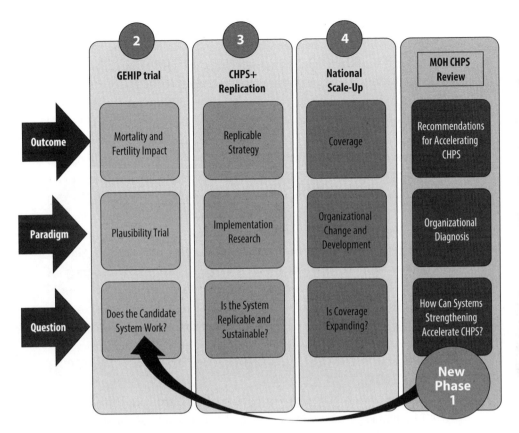

Figure 10.6. Guiding community-based health policy services reform with a renewed process of phased implementation research.

CHPS Reform Phase 1: The Changing Political Context and Diagnostic Appraisal
THE POLITICAL CONTEXT

From the onset of CHPS, evidence generated by research has had a political audience. The 2008 election launched a new era of CHPS political support for CHPS systems grounding. In that election, all political parties in Ghana supported CHPS implementation owing to the grassroots popularity of CHPS that was evident everywhere. Public concern about access to care emerged as a theme of political commentary, with the major parties promising that public demand for PHC could best be pursued by electing their candidates. The president of Ghana who was elected in this contest campaigned on a promise of making CHPS implementation a national priority.

The president had a personal understanding of research results related to the CHPS model. He had been the vice president of Ghana at the time of the 1999 National Health Forum for announcing the CHPS policy. Thus, in his capacity as the key convener of this conference, he presided over the rollout of CHPS as national policy. His advocacy of the initiative at that time was based on his personal understanding of the potential benefits of CHPS field operations.

To underscore his commitment to CHPS after the election, he sponsored a 2009 act of parliament that imposed a special tax on all government employees for financing CHPS implementation. The revenue generated by this action was inconsequential, but the symbolic value of this commitment was transformative for CHPS. Presidential speeches and political gatherings were focused on garnering support for CHPS implementation throughout Ghana. This national support, combined with a vibrant grassroots democracy in Ghana, provided political backing to act on the evidence generated by Navrongo and Nkwanta. The CHPS learning process that was intended to base PHC on Alma-Ata inspired a commitment that promoted a process of adapting strategy to the unique needs and capabilities of each participating district (Gilson et al. 1994; Gilson and Shalley 2004; Shalley and Gilson 2004; Gilson et al. 2005).

Political will was allied with resources to act. Petroleum-led economic growth of Ghana's economy in the late 2000s enabled financing for CHPS. Revenue sources for CHPS shifted from external aid for vertical programs to Government of Ghana investments in the CHPS system of community-based PHC. External support shifted from grants to lending agreements that shifted down programming to decentralized systems investment controlled by district assemblies. With the new national political leadership and expanded flexible revenue at the periphery, CHPS became the component of the health care system that commanded political attention and priority at all levels of government. After 2000, district and regional managers' performance indicators included criteria that were linked to be coverage of CHPS services. And these standards were not limited to the health sector. Development sector budget lines and resource allocations were revamped to provide opportunities to link health financing needs with district development resources. DHMTs became integrated political stakeholders in the district-level development system. With grassroots politicians in command of local budgets, community demand for CHPS had an audience that could respond by consigning small, but meaningful, resources to its start-up costs.

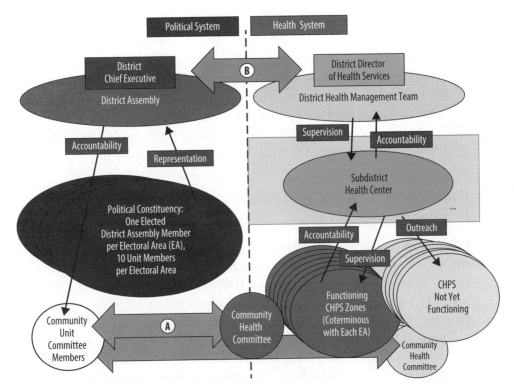

Figure 10.7. The emergence of a political and health system partnership for supporting community-based health policy services implementation and reform (2009–2019).

The dynamic that emerged is depicted in figure 10.7 as a modification of the bureaucratic design portrayed in figure 10.2: An existing consensus involving grassroots politicians and community health committees defined the climate of demand for PHC services well before the 2008 election (figure 10.7A). What changed, however, was the partnership that emerged when district assembly members cooperated with subdistrict supervisors and traditional leaders in the process of organizing support for CHPS milestone transitions (as in figure 10.6). What changed was the emergence of partnership of the district chief executive and district director of health services, who from 2009 onward were formally instructed to consign priority to CHPS implementation (figure 10.7B). A new implementation research sequence was mandated to guide action that the political system was keen to embrace.

The Phase 1 Qualitative CHPS Review

In 2009, the Ministry of Health responded to the challenge implied by Phase 4 monitoring results by commissioning a review of the CHPS implementation process with the goal of clarifying factors that explained why implementation was proceeding rapidly in some districts but not at all in others (Binka et al. 2009). The report identified a need to focus more on CHPS components that emphasize field observation, teamwork, and community engagement.

Phase 2 of CHPS Reform: The Ghana Essential Health Interventions Program

Policy lessons that emerged from the 2009 Ministry of Health review were assembled into a systems strengthening research project known as the Ghana Essential Health Interventions Program (GEHIP). GEHIP emphasized two goals: (1) systems strengthening and (2) service development to address gaps in the range and quality of care that CHPS was capable of providing (table 10.2).

Although much was learned in Navrongo and Nkwanta about making community health services work, less was learned about how to make district management systems capable of implementing these lessons at scale. GEHIP was therefore designed to shift the research and action agenda from testing delivery strategies to developing and testing means of making district leadership work.

Results of the 2009 appraisal showed that PHC budgets were so rigidly structured in all study districts that the allocation of flexible revenue to cover start-up costs was not administratively possible. Deliberations tended to focus on the district-wide costs of doing everything rather than the zone-by-zone capabilities of communities to take action. Some district managers would delay implementation until external revenue could be acquired to defray start-up costs for a comprehensive service package. In contrast, leaders in rapid implementation districts established practical means of surmounting budgetary constraints with a grassroots process of political mobilization to support the utilization of development revenue for CHPS together with cost reduction strategies such as marshaling volunteer labor for constructing health posts and using less costly construction methods and materials. Where leaders had acquired practical experience with the organizational requirements of launching CHPS, through observation and participatory learning, there was understanding of the process of community- and political-engagement strategies for supporting CHPS rollout. Pilot implementation

Table 10.2. GEHIP systems strengthening and service development interventions

Systems Strengthening "Pillar" for Improving . . .	Interventions Designed to Improve the Pace of Community-Based Health Planning and Services (CHPS) Scale-up and the System of Support for Primary Health Care
. . . access to care	• Reform of the process of developing health posts to emphasize community-engaged construction of interim facilities where CHPS services can be provided without delay (Awoonor-Williams, Sory, Nyonator, et al. 2013)
. . . expanding the range of services and the and improving worker skills	• Training all frontline workers in community newborn care interventions (Asuru et al. 2013) • Launch a community-engaged emergency referral system (Awoonor-Williams, Patel, et al. 2015) • Train community members and volunteers in danger-sign recognition and referral (Olokunde et al. 2015)
. . . information for decision-making	• Simplify the service information system to eliminate redundant procedures and enhance data use for decision-making (Awoonor-Williams, Stone, et al. 2016) • Develop mortality audit procedures and systems for clinical review and response
. . . essential drugs and equipment	• Provision of low-cost tricycle ambulances with cell phone systems, communication arrangements, and community outreach for essential emergency services (Adamtey et al. 2015; Furuya and Kamara 2011; Patel et al. 2016; Awoonor-Williams, Patel, et al. 2015, 2017)
. . . planning, budgeting, and finance	• Develop and test procedures for linking planning and budgeting to burden of disease profiles (Nyonator et al. 2015; Awoonor-Williams, Schmitt, et al. 2016) • Provide $0.85 per capital per year for three years in flexible financing (Awoonor-Williams et al. 2013)
. . . supervision, leadership, and governance	• Develop outreach procedures for facilitative supervision (Frimpong et al. 2011) • Implement observational and community-based participatory training as a component of leadership training (Nyonator et al. 2005) • Engage grassroots politicians in Ghana Essential Health Interventions Program field activities and community celebration of CHPS milestone achievement (Awoonor-Williams, Phillips, and Bawah 2016)

Continued

Table 10.2. continued

Systems Strengthening "Pillar" for Improving . . .	*Interventions Designed to Improve the Pace of Community-Based Health Planning and Services (CHPS) Scale-up and the System of Support for Primary Health Care:*

Interventions Designed to Expand the Range of CHPS Services (beyond table 10.1) to Include CNC

Postnatal care of mothers and newborns (Darmstadt et al. 2005; Lawn, Wilczynska-Ketende, and Cousens 2006; Bazzano et al. 2008; Bhutta et al. 2009; Kinney et al. 2010; World Health Organization 2013) via comprehensive CNC	• Training and equipping all frontline workers and paramedics to respond to asphyxia (Bang et al. 1999; Loidl et al. 2000; Bhutta and Soofi 2008; Singhal and Bhutta 2008; Wall et al. 2009; Engmann et al. 2012) • Birth monitoring and follow-up with care and referral, as needed (four postdelivery home follow-up visits)[115]–[116]. • Frontline worker trained in case management and identifying danger signs assess and classify the child's illness, and provide oral drugs as needed to ensure effective management of childhood illness and manage triage and referral (Aborigo et al. 2014; Mbalinda et al. 2014) • Community education and mobilization required for ensuring family identification of danger signs and recognition of the need to seek care or referral from a community health officer (Olokunde et al. 2015) • Observation of the neonate for twenty-four to forty-eight hours, including helping babies breathe, referral, exclusive breastfeeding, and cord care (Chan et al., n.d.; Zaidi et al. 2011) • Community volunteers trained to provide neonatal integrated management of childhood illness and IMCI at other ages differ due to the dosages of medicines used (Kruse and Høgh 2004)
Diagnosis and treatment of neonatal febrile illnesses	• Community treatment of pneumonia with amoxicillin and malaria with artesunate/amodiaquine • Promotion and provision of facility-based care for all neonatal illness
Care for low-birthweight newborns	• Supplementing existing hospital-based skin-to-skin contact via kangaroo mother care for thermal control for low birthweight infants (Lawn et al. 2010) with community-based KMC provided by all community workers and volunteers (Bhutta and Soofi 2008)
Improved delivery services and immediate postdelivery maternal and child care	• Upgrading CHO to midwife status (Speciale and Freytsis 2013; Sakeah et al. 2014) • Volunteers trained to report home births, visit newborns, and refer cases for facility-based care (Hommerich et al. 2007; Penfold et al. 2010, 2013) • CHO home-based care for neonates (Bang et al. 1999; Bhutta et al. 2005; Baqui et al. 2008; Darmstadt et al. 2005) • Incentives for volunteers to conduct CNC referrals of home births via mobile phones (Darmstadt et al. 2005; Baqui et al. 2009; Dawson et al. 2013) to report home deliveries to supervisors to enable prompt CNC by nurses

Source: Adapted from Awoonor-Williams et al. 2013.

could be used to generate public support and consensus for action that offset prevalent managerial concerns that starting CHPS operations would create unsustainable grassroots pressure for an unaffordable program.

In response to the Ministry of Health 2009 report, the GHS launched a new policy to strengthen CHPS implementation. A project was convened to test means of implementing this policy and refining its strategies for saving maternal and newborn lives. GEHIP shifted the focus of research from conducting community studies to investigating district managerial and political leadership of CHPS implementation.

GEHIP involved six activities:

1. Implementation zones were developed within each GEHIP district, and exchange activities allowed subdistrict implementation teams to observe all essential CHPS start-up activities to foster and spread CHPS implementation capacity.
2. District managers instituted community engagement for volunteer construction of temporary health post facilities.
3. Field implementation–based learning was integrated into the training process and focused on practical demonstration to supervisors on how to undertake community engagement and liaison with traditional leaders.
4. Leadership development began to involve political and development officials, including budgeting and planning modules designed to catalyze grassroots efforts to expand the resource base of CHPS and improve GEHIP impact.
5. Supplemental funding amounting to $0.85 per capita per year for three years was added to the health budget as "catalytic revenue" for district managers to use for activities aimed at building popular support for CHPS.
6. There was a new focus on emergency services in maternal and neonatal care (table 10.2) (Patel et al. 2016), with motorcycle ambulances and volunteer drivers trained in emergency transport. CHOs were trained in acute care triage and referral with attention directed to prehospital first aid. Community outreach was directed to ensuring appropriate use of the system.

The impact of GEHIP on CHPS coverage was immediate and pronounced (figure 10.8). HPS zones that were functioning in 2010 covered 20% of the population in the four GEHIP treatment districts. By 2015, all of the GEHIP target population was covered by CHPS services, a level of coverage that was

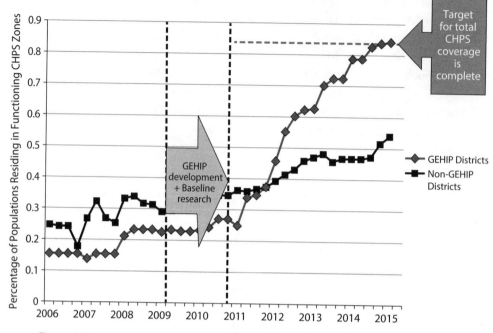

Figure 10.8. Percentage of Ghana Essential Health Intervention Program treatment district populations and comparison district populations residing in functioning community-based health policy services service zones by quarter, 2006–2015.

double the proportion reached in comparison areas (Awoonor-Williams, Phillips, et al. 2016). Childhood mortality declined markedly in the UER during GEHIP, with declines in neonatal mortality decline associated with GEHIP interventions (Bawah et al. 2019).

CHPS Reform Phase 3: The CHPS+ Initiative

There were deliberate efforts to build district leadership capacity. Going forward, the next phase, called CHPS+, has been designed to help leaders institutionalize systems learning for CHPS (Phillips et al. 2018). Initial CHPS+ activities focused on creating four systems learning districts (SLDs) where GEHIP functionality could be demonstrated to visiting implementation teams from other districts in two participating regions. Participating management team members who visit could then return to their districts to replicate the process of CHPS implementation (Phillips et al. 2018). This process of demonstration and counterpart support is accompanied with the provision of catalytic financing to support the creation of pilot communities in each participating district, where learning by doing can commence in ways that cascade CHPS reform through each district as community leaders replicate what has been demonstrated in SLDs. To evaluate the project, a stepped wedge design accompanies the pace of implementation, together with monitoring tools, a cluster sample survey, and mixed method implementation research. The CHPS+ implementation process is designed to provide continuous learning and knowledge management, and to develop national capacity to scale-up CHPS programming.

Conclusion

It is common for health research projects to end without impacting large-scale operations (Binswanger and Aiyar 2003; Cummings et al. 2007), in part because scaling up tends to terminate research rather than sustain the process of evidence-based organizational change (Simmons and Shiffman 2007). Ghana's experience with sequential implementation research has addressed this problem. This learning process was not confined to the periphery. A continuous process of applying sequential implementation science to catalyzing the scale-up of community health service innovations has institutionalized evidence-based decision-making. At each level of the system, the process of learning by doing has been nationally commissioned, coordinated, and implemented at the regional and district levels. Peer learning combined with a system of demonstration that involves communities, districts, and regions of excellence can function as a catalytic process of spreading implementation learning to other regions, districts, and communities. In keeping with the community-guided diffusion concept, each SLD can function as a learning locality for spreading understanding of the community-based, scaling-down "learning by doing" activity for institutionalizing implementation innovation in participating districts.

Ghana's CHPS research paradigm has emerged as a capability for evidence-driven systems development that will be a resource for guiding health systems development in the future. No health care system is perfect. Implementation science is showing that the key components of Ghana's UHC agenda are not fully functioning as planned. For example, the National Health Insurance Scheme was launched with the goal of making health care affordable to all Ghanaians (Abiiro and McIntyre 2012; Mills et al. 2012). Yet, despite its important achievements, the National Health Insurance Scheme must address challenging implementation problems if it is to successfully ensure financial access to health care (Akazili 2010; Akazili et al. 2014; Awoonor-

Williams, Tindana, et al. 2016; Kanmiki et al. 2018). Similarly, while CHPS represents a pillar of UHC policy by facilitating essential care accessibility, CHPS implementation is often associated with quality of care lapses and organizational challenges (Frimpong et al. 2011, 2014; Atinga et al. 2018). Reforms that will be essential to achieving UHC will benefit from the institutional capacity of the GHS to conduct pilots, trials, replication studies, and scaling-up procedures that CHPS has pioneered.

The Future of Primary Health Care in Ghana

The Ghana experience enabled senior managers to introduce research-based innovations that simultaneously required people-centered action at the periphery. With qualitative and quantitative research providing evidence on the content, coverage, and pace of change, the implementation of community-based PHC could be consistent with national evidence and yet adapted to local realities, needs, and resources.

Monitoring data for the 2009–2018 period suggest that the past decade has been transformative, generating national-, regional-, and district-level political commitment to CHPS implementation. By 2010, the pace of CHPS scale-up accelerated. National monitoring provides evidence of a marked upward disjuncture in the pace of CHPS implementation that was associated with policy change in 2009. Ghana's phased implementation paradigm could have an impact on CHPS scaling-up capacity at each level of health systems functioning, from communities to districts. Lead districts serving as points of innovation, implementation research, and training are transforming regional capacity to manage scale-up. National dissemination programs are being utilized to communicate knowledge about the health impact of community-based care and the feasibility of scaling up CHPS operations through the scaling-down paradigm. At the current pace of CHPS coverage expansion, Ghana will achieve CHPS for All by the year 2022.

REFERENCES

Abiiro, Gilbert Abotisem, and Di McIntyre. 2012. "Achieving universal health care coverage: Current debates in Ghana on covering those outside the formal sector." *BMC Int Health Hum Right* 12 (25). https://doi.org/10.1186/1472-698X-12-25.
Aborigo, R. A., Cheryl A. Moyer, M. Gupta, Philip B. Adongo, John Williams, Abraham R. Hodgson, P. Allote, and C. M. Engmann. 2014. "Obstetric danger signs and factors affecting health seeking behaviour among the Kassena-Nankani of Northern Ghana: A qualitative study." *Afr J Reprod Health* 18:78–86.

Adamtey, R., Josephine Frimpong, Romanus D. Dinye, and T. Čater. 2015. "An analysis of emergency healthcare delivery in Ghana: Lessons from ambulance and emergency services in Bibiani Anhwiaso Bekwai District." *Ghana J Dev Stud* 12 (1–2): 71–87.

Adongo, Philip B., James F. Phillips, and Fred N. Binka. 1998. "The influence of traditional religion on fertility regulation among the Kassena-Nankana of northern Ghana." *Stud Fam Plan* 29 (1): 23–40.

Adongo, Philip B., James F. Phillips, Beverly Kajihara, Clara Fayorsey, Cornelius Debpuur, and Fred N. Binka. 1997. "Cultural factors constraining the introduction of family planning among the Kassena-Nankana of northern Ghana." *Soc Sci Med* 45 (12): 1789–1804.

Agyepong, Irene Akua, and Sam Adjei. 2008. "Public social policy development and implementation: A case study of the Ghana National Health Insurance Scheme." *Health Policy Plan* 23 (2): 150–160.

Akazili, James. 2010. "Equity in health care financing in Ghana." PhD dissertation, University of Cape Town, South Africa.

Akazili, James, Paul Welaga, Ayaga Bawah, Fabian S. Achana, Abraham Oduro, John Koku Awoonor-Williams, John E. Williams, Moses Aikins, and James F. Phillips. 2014. "Is Ghana's pro-poor health insurance scheme really for the poor? Evidence from northern Ghana." *BMC Health Serv Res* 14 (1): https://doi.org/10.1186/s12913-014-0637-7.

Atinga, Roger A., Irene Akua Agyepong, and Reuben K. Esena. 2018. "Ghana's community-based primary health care: Why women and children are 'disadvantaged' by its implementation." *Soc Sci Med* 201 (March): 27–34.

Awoonor-Williams, John Koku, Patricia E. Bailey, Francis Yeji, A. E. Adongo, P. Baffoe, A. Williams, and S. Mercer. 2015. "Conducting an audit to improve the facilitation of emergency maternal and newborn referral in northern Ghana." *Glob Public Health* 10 (9): 1118–1133.

Awoonor-Williams, John Koku, Ayaga A. Bawah, Frank K. Nyonator, Rofina Asuru, Abraham Oduro, Anthony Ofosu, and James F. Phillips. 2013. "The Ghana Essential Health Interventions Program: A plausibility trial of the impact of health systems strengthening on maternal and child survival." *BMC Health Serv Res* 13 (Suppl. 2). https://doi.org/10.1186/1472-6963-13-S2-S3.

Awoonor-Williams, John Koku, E. S. Feinglass, R. Tobey, et al. 2004. "Bridging the gap between evidence-based innovation and national health-sector reform in Ghana." *Stud Fam Plan* 35 (3): 161–177.

Awoonor-Williams, John Koku, James F. Phillips, and Ayaga A. Bawah. 2016. "Catalyzing the scale-up of community-based primary healthcare in a rural impoverished region of northern Ghana." *Int J Health Plan Manage* 31 (4): e273–e289.

Awoonor-Williams, John Koku, Margaret L. Schmitt, Janet Tiah, Joyce Ndago, Rofina Asuru, Ayaga A. Bawah, and James F. Phillips. 2016. "A qualitative appraisal of stakeholder reactions to a tool for burden of disease–based health system budgeting in Ghana." *Glob Health Action* 9 (1): 30448.

Awoonor-Williams, John Koku, Paulina Tindana, Philip A. Dalinjong, Harry Nartey, and James Akazili. 2016. "Does the operations of the National Health Insurance Scheme (NHIS) in Ghana align with the goals of primary health care? Perspectives of key stakeholders in northern Ghana." *BMC Int Health Hum Rights* 2:1–16.

Awoonor-Williams, John Koku, Maya Vaughan-Smith, and James F. Phillips. 2010. "Scaling-up health system innovations at the community level: A case study of the

Ghana experience." In *Social determinants of sexual and reproductive health: Informing future research and program implementation Geneva*, edited by Shawn Malarcher, 51–70. Geneva: World Health Organization.

Bang, A. T., R. A. Bang, S. B. Baitule, M. H. Reddy, and M. D. Deshmukh. 1999. "Effect of home-based neonatal care and management of sepsis on neonatal mortality: Field trial in rural India." *Lancet* 354 (9194): 1955–61.

Baqui, Abdullah H, Shams El-Arifeen, Gary L Darmstadt, Saifuddin Ahmed, Emma K Williams, Habibur R Seraji, Ishtiaq Mannan, et al. 2008. "Effect of community-based newborn-care intervention package implemented through two service-delivery strategies in Sylhet District, Bangladesh: A cluster-randomised controlled trial." *Lancet* 371 (9628): 1936–1944. https://doi.org/10.1016/S0140 -6736(08)60835-1.

Bawah, Ayaga A., John Koku Awoonor-Williams, Patrick O. Asuming, Elizabeth F. Jackson, Christopher B. Boyer, Sebastian F. Achana, James Akazili, and James F. Phillips. 2019. "The child survival impact of the Ghana Essential Health Interventions Program: A regional health systems strengthening initiative in northern Ghana." *PLoS One* 14 (6): e0218025.

Bazzano, Alessandra N., Betty R. Kirkwood, Charlotte Tawiah-Agyemang, Seth Owusu-Agyei, and Philip Baba Adongo. 2008. "Beyond symptom recognition: Care-seeking for ill newborns in rural Ghana." *Trop Med Int* 13 (1): 123–128.

Berman, Peter A., and Thomas J. Bossert. 2000. "A decade of health sector reform in developing countries: What have we learned?" In *DDM Proceedings of a symposium on appraising a decade of health sector reform in developing countries*. Data for Decision Making Project, USAID.

Bhutta, Zulfiqar A., and Sajid Soofi. 2008. "Community-based newborn care: Are we there yet?" *Lancet* 372:1124–1126.

Bhutta, Zulfiqar A., Anita K. M. Zaidi, Durrane Thaver, Quratulain Humayun, Samana Ali, and Gary L. Darmstadt. 2009. "Management of newborn infections in primary care settings." *Pediatr Infect Dis J* 28 (Suppl.): S22–S30.

Binka, Fred N., Moses Aikins, Samuel O. Sackey, Richmond Aryeetey, Mawuli Dzodzomenyo, Reuben Esena, Philip B. Adongo, Patricia Akweongo, and Kwabena Opoku-Mensah. 2009. *In-depth review of the Community-Based Health Planning Services (CHPS) programme: A report of the Annual Health Sector Review, 2009*. Accra, Ghana: Ministry of Health. http://www.moh.gov.gh/wp-content/uploads/2016/02 /Review-of-Ghana-Health-Sector-2009.pdf.

Binka, Fred N., Ayaga A. Bawah, James F. Phillips, Abraham Hodgson, Martin Adjuik, and Bruce B. Macleod. 2007. "Rapid achievement of the child survival Millennium Development Goal: Evidence from the Navrongo Experiment in northern Ghana." *Trop Med Int Health* 12 (5): 578–583.

Binka, Fred N., Alex Nazzar, and James F. Phillips. 1995. "The Navrongo Community Health and Family Planning Project." *Stud Fam Plan* 26 (3): 121–139.

Binka, Fred N., Pierre Ngom, James F. Phillips, Kubaje Adazu, and Bruce B. MacLeod. 1999. "Assessing population dynamics in a rural African society: The Navrongo Demographic Surveillance System." *J Biosoc Sci* 31 (3): 373–391.

Binswanger, Hans P., and Swaminathan S. Aiyar. 2003. "Scaling up community driven development: Theoretical underpinnings and program design implications." https:// pdfs.semanticscholar.org/3d69/d96ae9386fba487d0a489908b004836b8b7a.pdf.

Chen, Lincoln, David Evans, Timothy Evans, Ritu Sadana, Barbara Stilwell, Phyllida Travis, Wim V. Lerberghe, and Pascal Zurn. 2006. *Working together for health: The World Health Report 2006.* Geneva, Switzerland: World Health Organization.

Community Directed Interventions Study Group. 2010. "Community-directed interventions for priority health problems in Africa: Results of a multi-country study." *Bull World Health Organ* 88 (7): 509–518.

Cummings, Greta G., Carole A. Estabrooks, William K. Midodzi, Lars Wallin, and Leslie Hayduk. 2007. "Influence of organizational characteristics and context on research utilization." *Nurs Res* 56 (Suppl. 4): S24–S39.

Damschroder, Laura J., David C. Aron, Rosalind E. Keith, Susan R. Kirsh, Jeffery A. Alexander, and Julie C. Lowery. 2009. "Fostering implementation of health services research findings into practice: A consolidated framework for advancing implementation science." *Implement Sci* 4 (1): 50.

Darmstadt, Gary L., Zulfiqar A. Bhutta, Simon Cousens, Taghreed Adam, Neff Walker, Luc De Bernis, Lancet Neonatal, Survival Steering, and Luc De Bernis. 2005. "Evidence-based, cost-effective interventions: How many newborn babies can we save?" *Lancet* 365 (9463): 977–988.

Davis, Louis E., and Albert Cherns. 1975. *The quality of working life.* New York: Free Press.

Debpuur, Cornelius, James F. Phillips, Elizabeth F. Jackson, Alex K. Nazzar, Pierre Ngom, and Fred N. Binka. 2002. "The impact of the Navrongo Project on contraceptive knowledge and use, reproductive preferences, and fertility." *Stud Fam Plan* 33 (2): 141–164.

Doctor, H. V. 2007. "Has the Navrongo Project in northern Ghana been successful in altering fertility preferences?" *Etude Popul Afr* 22:87–106.

Dujardin, B. 2009. "Sector-wide approach and health policy reforms: SWAP is the answer, but what is the question." *Trop Med Int Health* 14:17–18.

Freeman, Paul, Henry B. Perry, S. K. Gupta, and B. Rassekh. 2012. "Accelerating progress in achieving the Millennium Development Goal for children through community-based approaches." *Glob Public Health* 7 (4): 400–419.

Frimpong, Jemima A., Stéphane Helleringer, John Koku Awoonor-Williams, Thomas Aguilar, James F. Phillips, and Franics Yeji. 2014. "The complex association of health insurance and maternal health services in the context of a premium exemption for pregnant women: A case study in northern Ghana." *Health Policy Plan* 29 (8): 1043–1053.

Frimpong, Jemima A., Stéphane Helleringer, John Koku Awoonor-Williams, Francis Yeji, and James F. Phillips. 2011. "Does supervision improve health worker productivity? Evidence from the Upper East Region of Ghana." *Trop Med Int Health* 16 (10): https://doi.org/10.1111/j.1365-3156.2011.02824.x.

Ghiron, Laura, Lucy Shillingi, Charles Kabiswa, Godfrey Ogonda, Antony Omimo, Alexis Ntabona, Ruth Simmons, and Peter Fajans. 2014. "Beginning with sustainable scale up in mind: Initial results from a population, health and environment project in East Africa." *Reprod Health Matters* 22 (43): 84–92.

Gilson, Lucy, Martin Alilio, and Kris Heggenhougen. 1994. "Community satisfaction with primary health care services: An evaluation undertaken in the Morogoro Region of Tanzania." *Soc Sci Med* 39 (6): 767–780.

Gilson, Lucy, Natasha Palmer, and Helen Schneider. 2005. "Trust and Health worker performance: Exploring a conceptual framework using South African evidence." *Soc Sci Med* 61:1418–1429.

Gilson, Lucy, and Christina E. Shalley. 2004. "A little creativity goes a long way: An examination of teams' engagement in creative processes." *J Manage* 30:453–470.

Godlee, Fiona, Neil Pakenham-Walsh, Dan Ncayiyana, Barbara Cohen, and Abel Packer. 2004. "Can we achieve health information for all by 2015?" *Lancet* 364 (9430): 295–300.

Golden, G. K. 1991. "Volunteer counselors: An innovative, economic response to mental health service gaps." *Soc Work* 36:230–232.

Greenspan, Jesse A., Shannon A. McMahon, Joy J. Chebet, Maurus Mpunga, David P. Urassa, and Peter J. Winch. 2013. "Sources of community health worker motivation: A qualitative study in Morogoro Region, Tanzania." *Hum Resourc Health* 11:52.

Hommerich, Lena, Christa von Oertzen, George Bedu-Addo, Ville Holmberg, Patrick A. Acquah, Teunis A. Eggelte, Ulrich Bienzle, and Frank P. Mockenhaupt. 2007. "Decline of placental malaria in southern Ghana after the implementation of intermittent preventive treatment in pregnancy." *Malar J* 6 (1). https://doi.org/10.1186/1475-2875-6-144.

Hyder, Adnan A., Gerald Bloom, Melissa Leach, Shamsuzzoha B. Syed, David H. Peters, and Future Health Systems: Innovations for Equity. 2007. "Exploring health systems research and its influence on policy processes in low income countries." *BMC Public Health* 7 (January): 309.

Kanmiki, Edmund W., Ayaga A. Bawah, James Akazili, John Koku Awoonor-Williams, and Kassem Kassak. 2018. "Moving towards universal health coverage: An assessment of unawareness of health insurance coverage status among reproductive-age women in rural northern Ghana." *Lancet* (March): S32.

Kirigia, J., L. Sambo, B. Nganda, G. Mwabu, R. Chatora, and T. Mwase. 2005. "Determinants of health insurance ownership among South African women." *BMC Health Serv Res* 5 (1): 1–17.

Knippenberg, Rudolf, Daniel Levy-Bruhl, Raimi Osseni, Kandjoura Drame, Agnes Soucat, and Christophe Debeugny. 1990. "The Bamako Initiative: Primary health care experience." *Children in the Tropics* 184/185:94.

Kruse, Alexandra Y., and Birthe Høgh. 2004. "International child health." *Arch Dis Child* 21:32–33.

Lairumbi, Geoffrey M., Parker Michael, Raymond Fitzpatrick, and Michael C. English. 2011. "Ethics in practice: The state of the debate on promoting the social value of global health research in resource poor settings particularly Africa." *BMC Med Ethics* 12 (January): 22.

Lawn, Joy E., Judith Mwansa-Kambafwile, Bernardo L. Horta, Fernando C. Barros, and Simon Cousens. 2010. "'Kangaroo Mother Care' to prevent neonatal deaths due to preterm birth complications." *Int J Epidemiol* 39 (Suppl. 1): 144–154.

Lyon, Fergus. 2003. "Community groups and livelihoods in remote rural areas of Ghana: How small-scale farmers sustain collective action." *Community Dev J* 38 (4): 323–331.

Mills, Anne, Mariam Ally, Jane Goudge, John Gyapong, and Gemini Mtei. 2012. "Progress towards universal coverage: The health systems of Ghana, South Africa and Tanzania." *Health Policy Plan* 27 (Suppl 1): i4–i12.

Ministry of Health Republic of Ghana. 1995. *Medium Term Health Strategy*. Accra: Republic of Ghana.

Mintrom, Michael. 1997. "Policy entrepreneurs and the diffusion of innovation." *Am J Pol Sci* 41 (3): 738–770.

Mintrom, Michael, and Phillipa Norman. 2009. "Policy entrepreneurship and policy change." *Policy Stud J* 37 (4): 649–667.

Mutale, Wilbroad, N. Chintu, C. Amoroso, John Koku Awoonor-Williams, James F. Phillips, Colin D. Baynes, Cathy Michel, A. Taylor, and Kenneth Sherr. 2013. "Improving health information systems for decision making across five sub-Saharan African countries: Implementation strategies from the African Health Initiative." *BMC Health Serv Res* 13 (Suppl. 2): https://doi.org/10.1186/1472-6963-13-S2-S9.

Muula, Adamson S., Humphreys Misiri, Yamikani Chimalizeni, Davis Mpando, Chimota Phiri, and Amos Nyaka. 2004. "Access to continued professional education among health workers in Blantyre, Malawi." *Afr Health Sci* 4 (3): 182–184.

Nazzar, Alex K., Philip B. Adongo, Fred N. Binka, James F. Phillips, and C. Debpuur. 1995. "Developing a culturally appropriate family planning program for the Navrongo experiment." *Stud Fam Plann* 26 (6): 307–324.

Ngom, Pierre, Patricia Akweongo, Philip Adongo, Ayaga Agula Bawah, and Fred Binka. 1999. "Maternal mortality among the Kassena-Nankana of northern Ghana." *Stud Fam Plan* 30 (2): 142–147.

Ngom, Pierre, Cornelius Debpuur, Patricia Akweongo, Philip Adongo, and Fred N. Binka. 2003. "Gate-keeping and women's health seeking behaviour in Navrongo, northern Ghana." *Afr J Reprod Health* 7:17–26.

Nyarko, Philomena Efua, Brian Pence, and Philip Baba Adongo. 2002. "Child morbidity and health-seeking behaviour of primary caretakers in the Kassena-Nankana District of northern Ghana." Unpublished report of the Health Research Unit, Policy Planning Monitoring and Evaluation Division, Ghana Health Service, Republic of Ghana, Accra, Ghana.

Nyonator, Frank K., and J. Kutzin. 1999. "Health for some? The effects of user fees in the Volta Region of Ghana." *Health Policy Plan* 14 (4): 329–341.

Olokunde, Tioluwa L., John Koku Awoonor-Williams, Janet A. Y. Tiah, Robert Alirigia, Rofina Asuru, Sneha Patel, Margaret L. Schmitt, and James F. Phillips. 2015. "Qualitative assessment of community education needs: A guide for an educational program that promotes emergency referral service utilization in Ghana." *J Com Med Health Educ* 5 (4). https://doi.org/10.4172/2161-0711.1000363.

Patel, Sneha, John Koku Awoonor-Williams, Rofina Asuru, Christopher Boyer, Janet Awopole Yepakeh Tiah, Mallory C. Sheff, Margaret L. Schmitt, Robert Alirigia, Elizabeth F. Jackson, and James F. Phillips. 2016. "Benefits and limitations of a community-engaged emergency referral system in a remote, impoverished setting of northern Ghana." *Glob Health Sci Pract* 4 (4): 552–567.

Penfold, Suzanne, Barbara A. Willey, and Joanna Schellenberg. 2013. "Newborn care behaviours and neonatal survival: Evidence from sub-Saharan Africa." *Trop Med Int Health* 18 (11): 1294–1316.

Perry, Henry, Nathan Robison, Dardo Chavez, Orlando Taja, Carolina Hilari, David Shanklin, and John Wyon. 1999. "Attaining Health for All through community partnerships: Principles of the census-based, impact-oriented (CBIO) approach to primary health care developed in Bolivia, South America." *Soc Sci Med* 48 (8): 1053–1067.

Peter, Berman A., Gwatkin R. Davidson, and Burger E. Susan. 1987. "Community-based health workers: Head start or false start towards Health for All?" *Soc Sci Med* 25 (5): 443–459.

Peters, David H., Sameh El-Saharty, Banafsheh Siadat, Katja Janovsky, Marko Vujicic, and A. von Haeseler. 2009. *Improving health service delivery in developing countries: From evidence to action.* Washington, DC: World Bank.

Peters, David H., Ligia Paina, and Finn Schleimann. 2012. "Sector-wide approaches (SWAps) in health: What have we learned?" *Health Policy Plan* 28 (8): 884–890.

Phillips, James F., Ayaga A. Bawah, and Fred N. Binka. 2006. "Accelerating reproductive and child health programme impact with community-based services: The Navrongo Experiment in Ghana." *Bull World Health Organ* 84 (12): 949–955.

Phillips, James F., John Koku Awoonor-Williams, Ayaga A. Bawah, Belinda Afriyie Nimako, Nicholas S. Kanlisi, Mallory C. Sheff, Patrick O. Asuming, Pearl E. Kyei, Adriana Biney, and Elizabeth F. Jackson. 2018. "What do you do with success? The science of scaling up a health systems strengthening intervention in Ghana." *BMC Health Serv Res* 18 (484): https://doi.org/10.1186/s12913-018-3250-3.

Rogers, Everett M. 1962. *Diffusion of innovations.* New York: Free Press.

Sakeah, E., H. V. Doctor, L. McCloskey, J. Bernstein, K. Yeboah-Antwi, and S. Mills. 2014. "Using the community-based health planning and services program to promote skilled delivery in rural Ghana: Socio-demographic factors that influence women utilization of skilled attendants at birth in northern Ghana." *BMC Public Health* 14 (344): 1–9.

Saleh, K. 2012. *World Bank study: A health sector in transition to universal coverage in Ghana.* Washington, DC: World Bank.

Shalley, Christina E., and Lucy L. Gilson. 2004. "What leaders need to know: A review of social and contextual factors that can foster or hinder creativity." *Leadership Q* 15 (1): 33–53.

Sherr, Kenneth, Jennifer Harris Requejo, and Paulin Basinga. 2013. "Implementation research to catalyze advances in health systems strengthening in sub-Saharan Africa: The African Health Initiative." *BMC Health Serv Res* 13 (Suppl. 2): S1.

Shoo, Rumishael, Willy Matuku, Jane Ireri, Josephat Nyagero, and Patrick Gatonga. 2012. "The place of knowledge management in influencing lasting health change in Africa: An analysis of AMREF's progress." *Pan Afr Med J* 13 (Suppl. 1): 3.

Simmons, Ruth, and Jeremy Shiffman. 2007. "Scaling-up reproductive health service innovations: A conceptual framework." In *Scaling up health service delivery: From pilot innovations to policies and programmes,* edited by Ruth Simmons, Peter Fajans, and Laura Ghiron, 1–30. Geneva: World Health Organization.

Singh, Prabhjot, and Jeffrey D. Sachs. 2013. "1 million community health workers in sub-Saharan Africa by 2015." *Lancet* 382 (9889): 363–365.

Singhal, Nalini, and Zulfiqar Ahmed Bhutta. 2008. "Newborn resuscitation in resource-limited settings." *Semin Fetal Neonatal Med* 13:432–439.

Sivhaga, Kennedy, Boniface Hlabano, and Penina Ochola Odhiambo. 2012. "Using partnership approach to reduce mortality and morbidity among children under five in Limpopo Province, South Africa." *Pan Afr Med J* 13 (Suppl. 1): 14.

Skeet, M. 1985. "Community health workers: Promoters or inhibitors of primary health care?" *Int Nurs Rev* 32 (2): 55–58.

Speciale, Anna Maria, and Maria Freytsis. 2013. "MHealth for midwives: A call to action." *J Midwifery Women's Health* 58 (1): 76–82.

Standing, H., and A. Mushtaque R. Chowdhury. 2008. "Producing effective knowledge agents in a pluralistic environment: What future for community health workers?" *Soc Sci Med* 66 (10): 2096–2107.

Tindana, Paulina O., Linda Rozmovits, Renaud F. Boulanger, Sunita V. S. Bandewar, Raymond A. Aborigo, Abraham V. O. Hodgson, Pamela Kolopack, and James V. Lavery. 2011. "Aligning community engagement with traditional authority structures in global health research: A case study from northern Ghana." *Am J Public Health* 101 (10): 1857–1867.

Travis, Phyllida, Sara Bennett, Andy Haines, Tikki Pang, Zulfiqar Bhutta, Adnan A Hyder, Nancy R. Pielemeier, Anne Mills, and Timothy Evans. 2004. "Overcoming health-systems constraints to achieve the Millennium Development Goals." *Lancet* 364 (9437): 900–906.

Vaillancourt, Denise. 2009. "Do sector-wide approaches achieve results? Emerging evidence and lessons from six countries." World Bank Independent Evaluation Group. http://siteresources.worldbank.org/EXTWBASSHEANUTPOP/Resources/wp4.pdf.

VAST Study Team. 1993. "Vitamin A supplementation in northern Ghana: Effects on clinic attendances, hospital admissions, and child mortality." *Lancet* 342 (8862): 7–12.

Walt, Gill, Myrtle Perera, and Kris Heggenhougen. 1989. "Are large-scale volunteer community health worker programmes feasible? The case of Sri Lanka." *Soc Sci Med* 29 (5): 599–608.

Wells-Pence, Brian, Philomena Nyarko, James F. Phillips, and Cornelius Debpuur. 2007. "The effect of community nurses and health volunteers on child mortality: The Navrongo Community Health and Family Planning Project." *Scand J Public Health* 35 (6): 599–608.

World Health Organization. 1978. "Primary health care: Alma-Ata." In *World health assembly*. Geneva, Switzerland: World Health Organization.

———. 1997. *The use of essential drugs*. Geneva, Switzerland: World Health Organization.

———. 2005. *Handbook IMCI: Integrated management of childhood illness*. Geneva, Switzerland: World Health Organization.

———. 2007. *Everybody's business: Strengthening health systems to improve health outcomes WHO's framework for action*. Geneva, Switzerland: World Health Organization.

———. 2009. *Expanded Programme on Immunization (EPI)*. Jakarta, Indonesia: World Health Organization Regional Office for South East Asia.

———. 2012. *Guidelines on neonatal resuscitation*. Geneva, Switzerland: World Health Organization.

———. 2013. *WHO recommendations on postnatal care of the mother and newborn 2013*. Geneva, Switzerland: World Health Organization.

Zaidi, Anita K. M., Hammad A. Ganatra, Sana Syed, Simon Cousens, Anne C. C. Lee, Robert Black, Zulfiqar A. Bhutta, and Joy E. Lawn. 2011. "Effect of case management on neonatal mortality due to sepsis and pneumonia." *BMC Public Health* 11 (Suppl. 3): S13. https://doi.org/10.1186/1471-2458-11-S3-S13.

Sri Lanka's Health Improvements as an Example of the Implementation of the Alma-Ata Declaration

Vinya Ariyaratne

Sri Lanka, an island nation located in the Indian Ocean at the southern tip of India, has demonstrated remarkable gains in population health despite a low per capita income. Sri Lanka's success story has been studied extensively (Halstead 1985; Caldwell 1986). Past scholarship has emphasized uniquely Sri Lankan advantages underlying these gains, based on geography, religion, and culture. However, the health achievements of Sri Lanka were not inevitable blessings of its history—a series of deliberate choices were made that others can learn from. Unlike other former British colonies that struggled to build operational public health systems, Sri Lanka embraced a system of local public health departments that have proven themselves as well as invested in making primary clinical services accessible to all residents.

Sri Lanka gained independence in 1948 with few macroeconomic advantages. Following independence, its political system underwent regular turmoil. Nevertheless, it was able to transform its communities' health by turning to a legacy of cultural traditions and a commitment to principles of multisectoral comprehensive community participation that are enshrined in the Alma-Ata Declaration. The institutions built in Sri Lanka were sorely tested by a long civil war, but they showed resilience despite this challenge. Being able to isolate design principles underlying that resilience will be of value for readers who are eager to build comprehensive primary health care (PHC) systems that can function and thrive under the challenges of political instability and economic resource scarcity.

The lessons of Sri Lanka are partly inseparable from its context but partly universal. In describing the Sri Lankan health success, I attempt to demarcate the uniquely Sri Lankan features, including the geographical, epidemiological, and political backdrop of the country. In subsequent sections, I narrate the series of policy choices that built the functional governmental and nongovernmental institutions that constitute the current systems contributing to the health of the Sri Lankan people. The chapter teases out those universal principles that readers can learn and apply in other contexts. This narrative cannot be confined to the health sector and health services. People's health is inextricably connected to and determined by social, economic, and political factors more than ever in history. This analysis and commentary is based on a public health practitioner's point of view and reflects a broad perspective on the major determinants of health.

Recent Trends in Health Status

Sri Lanka has a land area of 62,705 square kilometers and a population of 21.2 million. The country's key health indicators have shown steady improvement since the early decades of the twentieth century, particularly during the decades following independence from the British colonial rule.

Maternal and child mortality have decreased dramatically. As of 2013, the maternal mortality ratio stands at 26.8 per 100,000 live births, and the infant mortality rate is 8.3 per 1,000 live births (Ministry of Health 2016). Life expectancy, too, has risen steadily, to 76 for females and 72 for males (Ministry of Health 2016). The total fertility rate had declined to a below replacement level of 1.9 by 2006, though it increased to 2.3 in 2016 (DHS 2016). Still, challenges remain in child nutrition and health disparities based on region and gender. According to data from the Sri Lanka Demographic and Health Survey of 2016, the proportion of children with low birth weight stands at 15.7%. The proportions of children with stunting (17.3%), wasting (15.1%), and underweight (20.5%) have not fallen much compared to prior decades. There are also wide regional disparities in health indicators. For example, while the national level of low-birth-weight babies is recorded at 11.4 per 100 live births, it is recorded at a higher level of 17.8 for Nuwara Eliya District (Ministry of Health 2015). Similar disparities are seen in the lagging progress of health and nutrition among women of Sri Lanka (DHS 2016). This is evident especially among estate sector women. Nuwara Eliya District, which accounts for a large number of estate sector women, has one of the highest maternal mortality ratios of the country: while the national level indicates 32 deaths per 100,000 live births, it is reported at 62.7 in the Nuwara Eliya District (Ministry of Health 2015) (table 11.1).

Table 11.1. Annexure 1: demographic and health indicators, 1917–2018

	1917	1948	1958	1968	1978	1988	1998	2008	2018
Population	4,497,900[1]	6,657,300[1]	9,389,000[2]	11,992,000[2]	14,190,000[2]	16,586,000[2]	18,784,000[4]	20,217,000[5]	21,444,000[5]
Population above 65 years				443,842[3]	611,624[3]	883,716[3]	1,146,758[3]	1,873,000[6]	1,684,000[8]
Infant mortality rate				50.3[2]	37.1[2]	19.4[2]	14.3[7]	9.0[9]	8.5[8]
Under-5 mortality rate				75.3[3]	57.0[3]	22.4[3]	17.9[7]	11.1[9]	9.4[10]
Maternal Mortality ratio							27.0[7]	33.4[11]	33.8[11]
Crude death rate		13.0[1]	9.7[6]	7.9[2]	6.6[2]	5.8[2]	6.0[7]	5.9[7]	6.5[8]
Crude birth rate		38.9[1]	35.8[12]	32.0[13]	28.5[13]	20.7[13]	17.2[13]	18.5[13]	15.2[8]
Life expectancy at birth		42.8[1]	61.7[1]	63.144[3]	67.308[3]	69.209[3]	69.744[3]	74.207[3]	75.0[8]
Literacy rate (male, %)	56.3	75.9[1]	85.8[1]	85.6[1]	91.1[12]		92.6[4]	92.8[14]	94.1[5]
Literacy rate (female, %)	21.2	53.6[1]	67.5[1]	70.9[1]	83.2[12]		89.7[4]	90.0[14]	92.2[5]

Note: Sri Lanka has a land area of 62,705 square kilometers and a population of 21.2 million (Department of Census and Statistics 2016).
[1] Census of Population and Housing 1981.
[2] Food and Nutrition Statistics 1950–1990.
[3] World Bank 2019.
[4] Census of Population and Housing 2001.
[5] Economic and Social Statistics of Sri Lanka 2009/Central Bank of Sri Lanka.
[6] Statistical Abstract 2009.
[7] Bulletin of Vital Statistics 2010.
[8] CBSL Annual Report 2017.
[9] Statistical Abstract 2014.
[10] World Bank 2016.
[11] National Maternal Death Reviews, Family Health Bureau.
[12] Statistical Abstract 1994.
[13] Statistical Abstract 2016.
[14] Central Bank of Sri Lanka Annual Report 2009.

Health Infrastructure

Today in Sri Lanka, a health care facility can be found on average not farther than 1.4 kilometers from most homes, and free government health care services are available within 4.8 kilometers of most homes. Other physical infrastructure has also improved significantly over the past two decades, leading to greater ease of accessing these widely distributed facilities (Marga Institute 2006).

Historical Context

Sri Lanka has twenty-five hundred years of recorded history. The country was ruled by monarchies up until the start of British rule in 1815. The country was first occupied by the Portuguese (1505), followed by the Dutch (1656), and then by the British (1796). However, the Portuguese and the Dutch could only occupy the coastal areas of Sri Lanka, and it was solely the British who could conquer the entire island.

Buddhism was introduced to Sri Lanka in the fifth century B.C. Buddhism, practiced by a majority of people in Sri Lanka, has had a strong influence over health and well-being for more than two millennia. People's health was a primary concern of all kings who ruled the country, as Buddhism recognized care of the sick as a highly meritorious deed. Sri Lanka's archeological ruins include what may have been the first hospital ever built in the world. Ancient Sri Lankans also constructed sanitation works, leaving behind the remains of privies, urinals, and baths (Uragoda 1987).

Traditional practices and systems of medicine existed in Sri Lanka as well. Western, Ayurvedic, Unani, Siddha, acupuncture, and homeopathy systems of medicine are all practiced in Sri Lanka. However, the dominant system of medicine in Sri Lanka today, the Western allopathic system, was introduced to the country by the colonial powers. The Portuguese first brought the country into contact with Western medicine, but their influence on local medical practice was marginal (Uragoda 1987). The Dutch, toward the latter part of their rule, built hospitals in different parts of the island and managed them with their physicians and surgeons, primarily to serve the colonial expatriate workforce and secondarily to care for the local population.

During British rule (from 1796 to 1948), Western medicine took deep roots and transformed medical practice in the country. It is observed that, unlike the Portuguese and the Dutch, the British, from the very inception of their rule, were very concerned about the health of the local population. The

British could be credited for the establishment and expansion of preventive and curative Western health care.

During the British rule in the late nineteenth century, coffee, tea, and rubber plantations were introduced to Sri Lanka. As the local population was not willing to work as wage laborers on these plantations, the British planters brought down south Indian Tamil laborers to work on their estates in Sri Lanka. The British colonial government made the plantation owners responsible for the health of their workers. As these workers came from extremely poor communities in South India, living in unhealthy and unhygienic conditions, they were subjected to many infectious diseases. The plantation workers later became citizens of Sri Lanka as a distinct ethnic community known as "Tamils of Indian origin" (to distinguish them from "Sri Lankan Tamils," who inhabited the island long before the era of colonial rule in Sri Lanka). The health status of this estate population in Sri Lanka continued to lag behind compared to other ethnic communities living in the country.

Role of Education in Health Improvements

Traditionally, the people of Sri Lanka, irrespective of their ethnic and religious background, have always treated education as a virtue. They have seen its practical value as a means of upward social mobility. Long before the British introduced the formal, Western-modeled education system in the country, Sri Lanka had a temple-based (*pirivena*) education system. This societal demand for education for both sexes paved the way toward building a highly literate population, which in return provided a firm foundation on which public health could also be built. This does not mean that traditional beliefs and practices were not playing a role in the Sri Lankan population. Rather, Sri Lankan society has an interesting health-related belief system that is deeply, culturally rooted and coexists within a predominantly Western, modern medical care system. Especially when it comes to mental health issues, communities in rural areas of the country still resort to traditional rituals (*Yaaga*) for healing. In addition, communicable diseases such as chickenpox and measles are considered to be caused by supernatural forces.

Health Behavior

Given the importance assigned to people's health by the ancient rulers of Sri Lanka and the health care systems introduced during colonial rule, it is observed that the people of Sri Lanka have been, by and large, a "health conscious" population. Positive health behaviors and values have been transmitted across generations for several centuries and played a decisive role in creating receptivity to the public health initiatives of the health units in Sri Lanka. To illustrate, Pieris (1999) wrote:

It might be assumed that the traditional health beliefs would be weaker among an educated population, however, the study found the situation in Sri Lanka more complex. The treatments for illness have changed drastically without a concomitant change in health beliefs. Indeed, although most Sri Lankans hold traditional beliefs concerning illness causation and appropriate treatment, this does not prevent them from using modern medicine in preference to traditional medicine.

Sri Lankans believe, and have long believed, that illness can be cured through treatment and do[es] not have to be left [to] fate. For instance, the illnesses that people suffer [from] today as a result of changes in lifestyle, such as heart attacks and cancer, are regarded as being a result of bad *karma* (fate). Nevertheless, Sri Lankans recognize that these diseases can be treated, and, on occasion, cured through modern treatment.

While Ayurvedic treatment is most used for a few specific diseases, in a less obvious way it is used for other diseases, too. Many people, for example, use Ayurvedic medicine as a follow-up treatment to restore the equilibrium of the bodily fluids after modern medicine has quickly cured the symptoms of the disease.

The mortality decline in Sri Lanka is not entirely explained by the implementation of modern health care. Though the modern health system was an essential prerequisite for mortality decline, it would not have been effective had the people not willingly accepted and experimented with [a] new type of treatment. Sri Lankans were willing to accept the new health system since they saw sickness primarily as a physical problem, rather than, as is often the case elsewhere in South Asia, as a divine punishment. This attitude may be largely due to the influence of religious teaching, particularly of Buddhism. Sri Lanka's Buddhist heritage, encourages men and women to think of themselves and to make decisions independently. (239–240)

Governance and Politics

A strong demand for participatory governance is part of Sri Lankan political culture despite a history of monarchic and colonial rule. Prior to the British colonial rule, there existed a Gram Sabha (village council) system in Sri Lanka (Fernando 2010). It is widely accepted that this system was established during the Anuradhapura Kingdom and lasted until 1833, when the Gram Sabha system was formally abolished according to the recommendations of the Colebrook Commission. According to Professor Laksiri Fernando of the University of Colombo, inscriptions of the tenth century indicate that those Gram Sabhas were instrumental in making decisions related to law and order, water management, dispute resolution, and agricultural land allocation.

The citizens of Ceylon (as Sri Lanka was known at the time of the British colonial rule) had been agitating for their representation in administration since the early part of the twentieth century. As a result, the British Government introduced far-reaching political reforms, including limited representation of locals in the Legislative Council in 1910 and universal adult franchise of all men and women in 1931 (Election Commission of Sri Lanka, n.d.). Sri Lanka was the second country, after New Zealand, to enjoy universal franchise in the Asian and Australian region. The evolving competitive political system under the new constitution provided new capacity for elected representatives to articulate the urgent needs of their electorates on the Executive (the British Government) for larger allocation of resources for social services for their constituencies. At the same time, the citizens also found, through franchise, a powerful new tool to demand services to fulfill their basic needs by electing representatives who they believed could deliver those services. This especially emanates from the pre-1977 political system of the country, in which there was a single elected Member of Parliament responsible and accountable for an electoral constituency. Therefore, the constituents could hold their MP accountable for the effective delivery of public services in the area.

Hence, policies for essential social services such as health, education, and food subsidy started to evolve and develop well before the country gained independence (in 1948). Officials found that they could achieve electoral success through expansion of facilities for provision of state-supported health services and education in all parts of the country. Despite regular turnover of elected governments within the multiparty system, the state's commitment toward universal free health care did not change. As R. Rannan-Eliya and L. Sikurajapathy (2009) observed: "Once democracy had served to establish a widely dispersed government health infrastructure, accessible by all, it then acted to ensure its survival under often difficult, fiscal conditions. Subsequently, successful market-oriented and reform-minded governments in Sri

Lanka have generally understood that the cost of adequate public sector health services accessible to the poor was a small fiscal price to pay for the political support that they engender to enable other more important economic reforms." The political logic supporting and maintaining provision of fully state-supported health services and wide health coverage was the result of broader historical and social factors (Gunatilleke 1985, 1).

Establishment of the Health Unit System

One of the most important elements of the health system introduced during the British period was the health unit system. A health unit is a well-defined geographic area that is under the purview of a medical officer of health (MOH). An MOH is assisted by a team consisting of public health inspectors (PHIs), who are responsible for environmental health and control of communicable diseases, and public health nurses and midwives, who are responsible for maternal and child health (MCH). The network of health units paralleled the domestic system of district health offices that the British Parliament legislated for themselves in the Public Health Acts of 1848 and 1875 (Szreter 1988). In Sri Lanka, the government norm is for each MOH unit to cover a population of eighty thousand to one hundred thousand. Today, there are about three hundred MOH units delivering public health services. The MCH staff typically includes one to two public health nursing sisters, one to three supervising public health midwives, and a team of public health midwives. The PHI team is much smaller, typically consisting of one supervising PHI and a small team of PHIs. The government norm is for PHIs to cover a population of about ten thousand, while public health midwives cover about three thousand. The MOH supervises the work of both the MCH staff and the PHIs.

Sri Lanka's Health Unit Program has been cited as a model of "selective" PHC (Hewa 2011). However, I would argue that this view fails to recognize the longer history and much more extensive formal institutionalization of the health unit system in Sri Lanka. The MOH health unit system was not at all a model to deliver a few selective PHC interventions. Conversely, it was staffed with career public health professionals who were assessing and addressing a multitude of pertinent health issues. The staff in Sri Lankan health units were gauging community health issues and assuring local solutions just like their counterpart district health officers were back in England. For epidemiological reasons, Sri Lankan health units logically focused on

MCH, environmental health, and food hygiene. They certainly made use of selective interventions as appropriate, but their approach was far broader. Because Sri Lankan health units had built channels of surveillance, communication, and problem-solving they became natural platforms to contribute to the success of a host of "vertical" disease control programs, such as malaria, leprosy, and filariasis programs, all of which used the MOH health unit system in their preventive interventions (Ellepola and Dayaratne 2016). With a strong horizontal platform in place, each vertical program did not have to recreate the public health infrastructure it would need to succeed. Therefore, the health unit system should be seen as a model that provided a solid platform on which a range of public health services could be provided in a coordinated manner. This is the very definition of comprehensive PHC as opposed to selective PHC.

Alma-Ata Declaration

It is within this longer historical context of a progressive and equity-oriented public health system that the Alma-Ata Declaration became an important touchstone in the evolution of the health care sector in Sri Lanka. The Alma-Ata Declaration gave a tremendous boost and legitimacy to further build on core elements of Sri Lanka's health unit system. As can be clearly seen from the forgoing analysis, the basic elements of the PHC approach endorsed by the Alma-Ata Declaration were already an integral part of the Sri Lankan health system in 1978. Sri Lanka became an active promoter and subsequently a signatory to the Alma-Ata Declaration. Decades of experience with the Sri Lankan model were promoted at a Bellagio conference on PHC in 1985 and held up for emulation (Halstead 1985; Hewa 2011).

Community Participation in Primary Health Care in Sri Lanka

Sri Lanka has a rich tradition of community participation in various aspects related to fulfilling people's basic needs. Because of its agricultural economy, people's direct participation in managing and maintaining community resources including irrigation systems, as well as jointly preparing land for cultivation, harvesting, and marketing, has been a routine practice since precolonial times.

Historically, mobilizing public participation for health was triggered by the threat of infectious diseases. During the malaria epidemic of 1934–1935, more than a million people were affected, and there were more than 125,000 deaths. Arising from this devastating event, the Suriya Mal Movement mobilized a large number of volunteers to combat the epidemic among the poor and to address root causes in nutrition and housing. Various voluntary development organizations have facilitated community participation in addressing health and nutritional issues in rural villages, focusing on linking remote and inaccessible rural communities with government health services (Halstead 1985).

In the late 1970s, the emphasis was on building awareness and raising public consciousness regarding available services. Health volunteers became the link between the community and government health services, particularly in promoting MCH services. The communities had been passive recipients of services delivered by nongovernmental organizations (NGOs) and transitioned to a more "empowerment"-oriented approach. The concepts of PHC emerging from Alma-Ata gave new inspiration and legitimacy to community participation promoted by the NGOs. There emerged active engagement of communities in preventive health work including nutrition, water supply and sanitation, and early child education—areas directly connected to community health but not part of mainstream government health services.

In the late 1980s, community participation focused on combatting specific communicable diseases, such as malaria. For example, community groups deployed trained volunteers to detect cases of malaria. Starting in the early 1990s, community participation began to include control of sexually transmitted diseases and human immunodeficiency virus/acquired immunodeficiency syndrome (HIV/AIDS). The nongovernment sector was also important in building community collective action for health, as is illustrated by the Sarvodaya Shramadana Movement (see box on page 268).

In 2018, an extensive consultative and review process was carried out by the Ministry of Health, Nutrition and Indigenous Medicine in the reorganization of PHC in Sri Lanka. The subcommittee appointed to study the current status of beneficiary engagement, gender, and citizens' voice concluded that the current status of citizen engagement was unsatisfactory (Ministry of Health, Nutrition and Indigenous Medicine 2017). It was the unanimous opinion of the committee that "the health system must increase patient empowerment and engagement in their health," and it offered a series of recommendations that included establishing a formal mechanism for citizen engagement and a grievance redressal mechanism (Ministry of Health, Nutrition and Indigenous Medicine Sri Lanka 2017, 33). Coming years should see a reemphasis of this traditional feature of public health in Sri Lanka.

The Sarvodaya Shramadana Movement of Sri Lanka

The Sarvodaya Shramadana Movement is by far the largest grassroots nongovernmental development organization in the country. Founded in 1958, members of the Sarvodaya Shramadana Movement have worked with underprivileged and poverty-stricken communities in Sri Lanka to uplift their living standards through a unique, holistic, integrated, and participatory approach.

Main strategies of the organization in development or awakening of a village community is divided in to five stages, and they are concentrated on each dimension of empowerment (i.e., spiritual and ethical, cultural, social, economic, and political.

- Stage 1: Psychological infrastructure development
  Spiritual and ethical empowerment
- Stage 2: Social infrastructure development and training
  Cultural empowerment
- Stage 3: Satisfaction of basic human needs and institutional development
  Social empowerment
- Stage 4: Income and employment generation and self-financing
  Economic empowerment
- Stage 5: Sharing with neighboring villages and good governance
  Political empowerment

The lowest level of the Sarvodaya organization is at the village level. To initiate these activities at the village level, a group called the Sarvodaya Village Shramadana Samithiya is convened. Initial activities revolve around organizing Shramadana campaigns. These campaigns form a variety of groups such as women's groups, youth groups, children groups, farmers' groups, and so forth, and identify their own unique needs as the village-level organization is progressing. Sarvodaya provide initial leadership and skills training, and subsequently they often develop a Children's Services Center. They also try to solve the issues related to the provision of ten basic needs within the village, and the main Sarvodaya organization assists with these initial activities. The organization is expected to be progressing through the five strategic stages listed previously to ultimately reach the "Gram Swaraj" village status.

At each level, village communities are assisted by various units of the Sarvodaya Shramadana Movement. For example, the village organization is registered under the Societies Ordinance at Stage 3, and the legal unit of the main branch assists in the process. At Stage 4, the SEEDS (Sarvodaya Economic Enterprises Development Services) unit assists the village community to develop a micro-financial organization.

Sarvodaya has an outreach of fifteen thousand villages over a period of six decades, with fifty-four hundred villages having been formed as independent village organizations as described earlier. In the 1960s and 1970s, Sarvodaya's work in community health, such as early childhood development and nutrition, was regarded as a novel experiment in promoting people's health. Sri Lankan experiences helped inform the buildup to the Alma-Ata Conference in 1978 (United Nations Childrens' Fund, 1977).

The Sarvodaya Shramadana Movement, which covered the entire country with its community development programs, played a critical role in the satisfaction of basic needs in a large number of rural villages in Sri

Lanka. The ten basic needs approach adopted by Sarvodaya addressed the determinants of ill-health through participatory and voluntary action. For over five decades, Sarvodaya has evolved innovative programs to address emerging health challenges while continuing to address key social and economic determinants of health. As disease control activities had to be carried out during the height of armed conflict in Sri Lanka, Sarvodaya, being a neutral party involved in both humanitarian and development activities in war-affected areas, was able to deliver the services to the "last mile."

In addition to working at the community level and in close collaboration and coordination with the Ministry of Health and other key stakeholders working in the health sector, the Sarvodaya Shramadana Movement also works at the national level to influence policies related to health. Because of their organizational experience and credibility, Sarvodaya's leaders serve in national-level policy-making bodies such as the Nutrition Steering Committee on Noncommunicable Diseases, the National Committee on Mental Health, the Technical Advisory Committee on Health of Young Persons, and others. Sarvodaya is a founding member of the People's Health Movement, and since its inception in 2000, it has served as the national coordinator bringing together more than sixty organizations working in the health

sector, including a few key trade unions. The People's Health Movement in Sri Lanka has carried out extensive advocacy programs on national drug policy and the rights of sex workers and the LGBTQ community, and most importantly it has led in a nationwide campaign to include health as a fundamental right in the constitution of Sri Lanka.

The village level and the organization of communities create the foundations and the building blocks of Sarvodaya's work, where ownership of sustainable development lies with the communities themselves. The Sarvodaya Shramadana Movement has three related objectives: (1) the consciousness objective of transforming human consciousness through spiritual, moral, and cultural awakening, and deepening the societal commitment for nonviolence; (2) the economic objective of transforming the society through the creation of a fully engaged economic system that creates sustainable village economies, which meets the basic needs of all Sri Lankans through social, economic, and technological empowerment; and (3) the power objective of transforming the present political system to establish community self-governance, participatory democracy, and good governance through political and legal reforms. Empowerment would need to go a long way to create the socioeconomic and political order that serves justice and awakening to all.

The Civil War and the Impact on Health

Sri Lanka was engulfed in a violent internal armed conflict from 1983 to 2009. A separatist campaign by the Liberation Tigers of Tamil Eelam against the government resulted in hundreds of thousands of lost lives, largely those of civilians. There was widespread damage to livelihoods and property. The northern and eastern parts of the country were directly affected by the war, while the rest of the country also suffered due to attacks on civilians and as a result of the negative effects on the economy. Nearly a million people were internally displaced during the period of the war. The war came to an end in May 2009 with a comprehensive military victory by the government over the Liberation Tigers of Tamil Eelam. However, the war that had lasted for twenty-six years left a devastating impact on the population exposed to the war.

A country that had had a reputation of maintaining good vital statistics for more than a century found itself unable to collect, collate, and report the vital statistics for more than twenty years for the northern and eastern districts affected by the war. Hence, it was difficult to objectively evaluate trends of morbidity and mortality during the period of the war. It is still challenging to fully assess the health impact of the war on the population in Sri Lanka, and thus there is a paucity of epidemiological evidence (Siriwardhana and Wickramage 2014). However, based on findings of the few studies that are available, it could be concluded that there has been a significantly negative impact on the health status of people living in the conflict zones (Family Health Bureau 2010). A large number of people also suffer from psychological effects of the war, including post-traumatic stress disorder (de Jong et al. 2002). The war negatively affected overall public health and development across the nation. S. Johnson (2017) wrote: "Perhaps more insidious was the lost momentum, and the loss of what could have been achieved in terms of infant and maternal deaths prevented, in terms of increased longevity, and in terms of the wealth and happiness that could have come with better health, in the absence of war" (25).

However, despite lost years of progress, the war did not eliminate Sri Lanka's culture of community-based, population-level, multisectoral public health practice. Nor did it alter a basic expectation that people should do their part to ensure the health of themselves and communities. The professional cadres to staff health units around the country remain and have been doing their jobs. The NGO community remains vibrant and is seeking to restore a sense of national solidarity around a shared health destiny.

Since the end of the war in 2009, the government has taken urgent measures to rebuild the destroyed health infrastructure, and today almost all hospitals and clinics have been rehabilitated and staffed, and are being made functional. The MOH units are also functioning, providing preventive health services.

Current Challenges and Responses

Several challenges remain for the future of public health in Sri Lanka. The country must face its epidemiological transition to noncommunicable diseases (NCDs), it needs to ensure quality of care, and it needs to grapple with rising costs of financing health care and protecting vulnerable groups from catastrophic costs. Sri Lanka's past achievements in building comprehensive PHC platforms around the country is a cause for optimism. To explore each of these challenges in further detail:

> *Changing epidemiological profile to NCDs.* Sri Lanka has brought down morbidity and mortality due to maternal and perinatal causes and has made great strides in controlling infectious diseases. Sri Lanka was declared malaria-free by the World Health Organization on September 5, 2016 (World Health Organization 2016). However, the burden of NCDs is rising and will continue to expand in the years to come.
>
> *Quality of care.* Though "access to care" for the entire population seems to be satisfactory, the quality of care in terms of availability of medical personnel in remote areas, availability of medicines, long waiting times, and so forth are not optimal. Further attention to these matters will be needed moving forward.
>
> *Health financing.* High out-of-pocket expenditures and high utilization of private sector services even by those in the lowest income quintile remain concerns. There is also an issue of an emerging "third tier,"* where some individuals accessing state health care that is free at the point of delivery actually bear some of the costs of drugs, investigations, and surgery (de Silva et al. 2016). This cost sharing with patients is resulting in catastrophic health expenditures for individuals as well as delays in and noncompliance with treatment.

The Role of Primary Health Care in Responding to Twenty-First-Century Health Challenges

First and foremost, Sri Lankans are served by a network of effective health units, and many if not most Sri Lankan communities have NGO-based health

---

*Third tier is defined broadly as payment to a private party for obtaining goods or services, as part of accessing state-sector services.

organizations such as the local Sarvodaya Movement chapters. These are important resources to cope with each emerging and ongoing challenge. The control of NCDs requires a multisectoral response that can emerge when community groups and public health professionals gather to understand and counteract root causes. Responses to tobacco, alcohol, injuries, and climate change can require the coordination of representatives from education, industry, commerce, transport, and energy at all levels of society. Sri Lanka's legacy of coordinated social action for health is well poised to spread the necessary political will to gather and deploy evidence-based solutions. For example, local chapters of the Sarvodaya Movement have played an important role in organizing measures to prepare for the natural disasters due to climate change.

Political will for health is essential because NCD control measures and progress to mitigate climate change typically generate vociferous opposition from industries that profit from the status quo. Restrictions on tobacco, alcohol, and unhealthy food are always difficult to launch and sustain.

Networks of concerned citizens have been an important component of social accountability approaches to health care quality. Having well-trained public health officers present in every part of the country gives Sri Lanka a platform from which to launch cycles of supportive supervision and provider education to improve medical care practices. Citizen-based social accountability systems are yet to be introduced in Sri Lanka. However, the recently introduced National Health Performance Framework (Ministry of Health 2018) and the citizen engagement mechanism proposed in the new strategy for reorganization of PHC in Sri Lanka provide promise (Ministry of Health 2017).

Finally, the efforts to engage the community in responding to their concerns about their growing NCD burden and health care quality naturally lead to a groundswell of interest in achieving better health care financing and coverage. An important part of the political solutions to create fiscal space for health care for all is a sense of social solidarity regarding health that enables pooling public finances.

Toward the end of 2017, the Ministry of Health, Nutrition and Indigenous Medicine initiated a major process to restructure PHC in Sri Lanka. (Ministry of Health 2017). There has been a keen interest to review the health system, particularly primary care systems (World Health Organization 2017).

The Ministry of Health, with technical assistance from the World Bank, initiated a process to develop a new strategy for the health sector based on a PHC approach. This is very timely as Sri Lanka is experiencing a demographic and epidemiological transition. There has been a resurging interest

Table 11.2. Action and thematic areas of Sri Lanka's new primary health care approach

Action Area	Thematic Areas
#1: Restructuring primary health care	Reorientation of primary health care (including Ministry of Health and primary medical care unit integration, human resources, specific measures to tackle noncommunicable diseases, referral and transportation system, and health life centers)
#2: Using information and data	Reorientation of primary health care (especially: monitoring and evaluation)
	Health information and IT systems
#3: Strengthening the health sector	Procurement systems Health financing The private sector Beneficiary engagement and citizen voice

in strengthening the PHC approach with comprehensive community-based and family-focused care to address the existing health issues in Sri Lanka (Senanayake 2017; World Health Organization 2017).

The proposed strategy adopts three general areas of action: (1) reorganizing PHC to meet Sri Lanka's future needs; (2) using data and information to improve health care; and (3) strengthening the health sector. The table 11.2 gives the details of thematic areas identified under each action area.

This new initiative is aimed at enhancing citizen engagement in PHC institutions. As of now, the citizens' engagement at the PHC level has been limited to the status of passive receivers (patients); PHC institutions have also lacked a proper system to address public grievances. In response, the new initiative aims to

- engage "the people" in people-centered PHC to ensure meaningful citizen participation in oversight of the PHC system;
- build health staff capacity to understand the importance of and to provide respectful and effective communication and care for patients;
- develop, adopt, and promote the use of a Patients' Rights Charter at all PHC facilities;
- foster patients' engagement in managing their own health through health cards, health awareness training, and health education;
- solicit input from the community and clients through suggestion boxes at all government health facilities, conducting regular patient

satisfaction surveys, strengthening community advisory and oversight committees for health services, and facilitating citizen participation in monitoring and evaluation assessments of health services;

- create mechanisms for submission and independent investigation of grievances against public and private sector health services; and
- enable representatives from health centers to participate in other community processes.

Open Government Partnership

The Open Government Partnership (OGP) was launched in 2011 to provide an international platform for domestic reformers committed to making their governments more open, accountable, and responsive to citizens. The Government of Sri Lanka committed to the OGP in 2015. More information can be found at: https://www.opengovpartnership.org/countries/sri-lanka. One of the twelve commitments of the OGP is on health. Under the OGP health component, the Government of Sri Lanka subscribed to three commitments:

1. improving public access to preventive and curative strategies to combat chronic kidney disease of unknown etiology,
2. transparent policy to provide safe and affordable medicines for all, and the
3. National Health Performance Framework.

There has been some progress on all three commitments since 2015. The Sarvodaya Movement and the People's Health Movement in Sri Lanka are jointly driving the OGP civil society partnership to pressure the government to implement the commitments. The Right to Information legislation is also giving an opportunity for the citizens to address their grievances by demanding information related to service delivery.

Way Forward

Dr. Ruviaz Haniffa, the newly elected president of the Sri Lanka Medical Association, posed the question of Sri Lanka's future as follows: "Has Sri Lanka got health system mechanisms in place to provide services to match the current and future health care consumption needs of our population?" (Haniffa 2018, 6). He observes that while the country's health system has been successful in delivering satisfactory curative and preventive care in the state sector, the primary curative care services vary in terms of quality and quantity between state and private sectors. He calls for "a shift from diseases to patients" (14).

In recent years, particularly since the change of the government in 2015, there have been several important initiatives to critically look at current health care delivery services and make necessary policy changes. In 2016, the Ministry of Health took the lead to prepare a new national health policy and called for public input (Ministry of Health, Nutrition and Indigenous Medicine 2016). It is unclear as to the extent of the response, but it is encouraging to note that the views from the public were sought by the government. Civil society organizations such as the Sri Lanka Chapter of the People's Health Movement convened consultations to discuss the draft policy and submitted its recommendations to the ministry. The new Sri Lanka National Health Policy, 2016–2025, was finalized and cabinet approval obtained on July 18, 2017. The policy is claimed to be a "patient- and people-centered policy, considering the concept of Universal Health Coverage, assuring the patient's rights and social justice" (Ministry of Health, Nutrition and Indigenous Medicine 2017).

Sri Lanka counts its ability to extensively pursue PHC as one of its greatest historical assets. Factors that enabled Sri Lanka to implement comprehensive PHC combine both gifts from history and deliberate choices. Sri Lanka inherited a sociocultural milieu based on Buddhist philosophy, which created a positive public consciousness reinforcing health-promoting behavior patterns. They also inherited a conducive environment for both indigenous medical systems and allopathic systems to take root. However, the Sri Lankan people also made choices to pursue progressive policies based on democratic governance. As a result, politicians were receptive to initiatives that provided universally free education and health services with equitable access, and provision of food subsidies to vulnerable communities.

Having realized the importance of strengthening PHC, Sri Lanka's most recent efforts can be interpreted as serious steps by the government to restructure the PHC system, building on historical gains while adapting to face new challenges. However, as it has been proven in the past, the success and the sustainability of a reformed health care system in Sri Lanka continues to depend on the effective performance of the health workforce, particularly at the community level. It will also depend on the degree of people's involvement through community-based organizations and NGOs. These organizations help perpetuate the maintenance of the culture of positive health behavior, and they facilitate the mechanisms by which the citizens hold service providers (mainly the state) accountable.

REFERENCES (SEE PAGE 341 FOR FULL CITATIONS FOR BOXED TEXT)

Caldwell, J. C. 1986. "Routes to low mortality in poor countries." *Popul Dev Rev* 12 (2): 171–220.

de Jong, K., M. F. Mulhern, I. Simpson, A. Swan, and S. van der Kam. 2002. "Psychological trauma of the civil war in Sri Lanka." *Lancet* 359 (9316): 1517–1518.

de Silva, A., T. Ranasinghe, and P. Abeykoon. 2016. "Universal health coverage and the health Sustainable Development Goal: Achievements and challenges for Sri Lanka." *WHO South-East Asia J Public Health* 5 (2): 82–88.

Department of Census and Statistics. 2016. *Demographic and Health Survey.*

Election Commission of Sri Lanka. n.d. "Our history—establishment of the Department of Elections." Accessed September 11, 2019. http://elections.gov.lk/web/index.php/en/about-us/our-history.

Ellepola, Y., and G. Dayaratne. 2016. *Historical review of disease burden in Sri Lanka.* Colombo: Institute of Policy Studies of Sri Lanka.

Family Health Bureau. 2010. *Health status of people exposed to war in Sri Lanka.* Colombo: Ministry of Health, Nutrition and Indigenous Medicine.

Fernando, L. 2010. *An introduction to the local government system in Sri Lanka: Changes and key issues.* Colombo: University of Colombo.

Gunatilleke, G. 1985. "Health and development in Sri Lanka—An overview." In *Good health at low cost*, 111–125. New York: Rockefeller Foundation.

Halstead, S. B. 1985. "Good health at low cost." In *Good health at low cost, conference report*. New York: Rockefeller Foundation.

Haniffa, R. 2018. *Shifting focus from diseases to patients: Today's vision, tomorrow's reality—SLMA presidential address.* Colombo: Sri Lanka Medical Association.

Hewa, S. 2011. "Sri Lanka's Health Unit Program: A model of 'selective' primary health care." *Hygiea Inter* 10 (2): 7–33.

Johnson, S. 2017. "The cost of war on public health: An exploratory method for understanding the impact of conflict on public health in Sri Lanka." *PLoS One* 12 (1): e0166674.

Marga Institute. 1984. *Intersectoral action for health: Sri Lanka study.* Colombo: Marga Institute.

———. 2006. "Burden of disease and equity." *Marga J.*

Ministry of Health. 2015. *Health performance monitoring indicators.*

Ministry of Health. 2016. *Annual health statistics: Sri Lanka.* Colombo: Ministry of Health. http://www.health.gov.lk/moh_final/english/public/elfinder/files/publications/AHB/2017/AHS%202016.pdf.

———. 2017. *Preserving our progress, preparing our future—restructuring primary health care in Sri Lanka.* Colombo: Ministry of Health. http://www.health.gov.lk/moh_final/english/public/elfinder/files/publications/2018/ReorgPrimaryHealthCare.pdf.

Ministry of Health, Nutrition and Indigenous Medicine. 2016. *Daily News.* June 19.

Ministry of Health, Nutrition and Indigenous Medicine. 2017. *Sri Lanka national health policy 2016–2025.* Colombo: Ministry of Health, Nutrition and Indigenous Medicine. http://www.health.gov.lk/moh_final/english/public/elfinder/files/publications/policiesUpto2016/policiesForPublicOpinion/NHP2016-2025draft.pdf.

Ministry of Health, Nutrition and Indigenous Medicine. 2018. *Reorganizing primary health care in Sri Lanka, preserving our progress, preparing for the future.* http://www.health.gov.lk/moh_final/english/public/elfinder/files/publications/2018/ReorgPrimaryHealthCare.pdf.

Pieris, I. 1999. *Disease, treatment and health behaviour in Sri Lanka.* New Delhi: Oxford University Press.

Rannan-Eliya, R., and L. Sikurajapathy. 2009. *Sri Lanka: "good practice" in expanding health care coverage.* Colombo: Institute of Health Policy. http://www.ihp.lk/publications/docs/RSS0903.pdf.

Senanayake, S. B. 2017. "How to strengthen primary health care services in Sri Lanka to meet the future challenges." *J Coll Community Physicians Sri Lanka* 23 (1): 43–49.

Siriwardhana, C., and C. Wickramage. 2014. "Conflict, forced displacement and health in Sri Lanka: A review of research landscape." *Confl Health* 8 (22): 1–9.

Szreter, S. 1988. "The importance of social intervention in Britain's mortality decline: A reinterpretation of the role of public health. *Soc Hist Med* 1 (1): 1–38.

Uragoda, C. 1987. *A history of medicine in Sri Lanka: From the earliest times to 1948.* Colombo: Sri Lanka Medical Association.

World Health Organization. 2016. "World Health Organization certifies Sri Lanka malaria free. SEAR/PR/1631." https://www.who.int/southeastasia/news/detail/05-09-2016-who-certifies-sri-lanka-malaria-free.

———. 2017. *Primary Health Care Systems (PRIMASYS): Case study from Sri Lanka.* Geneva: World Health Organization: Alliance for Health Policy and Systems Research. https://www.who.int/alliance-hpsr/projects/alliancehpsr_srilankaprimasys.pdf?ua=1.

CHAPTER TWELVE

How Vietnam's Doi Moi Reforms Achieved Rapid Gains in Health with Comprehensive Primary Health Care

Nguyen Thanh Huong and Hoang Khanh Chi

Vietnam has made great strides in socioeconomic development in the transition from a central planning economy to a market-oriented one. *Doi Moi* (literally "renovation") is the term used for a large set of 1986 reforms to create a socialist-oriented market economy. Economic and political reforms begun under Doi Moi in 1986 have spurred rapid economic growth and development and have transformed Vietnam from one of the world's poorest nations to a lower-middle-income country (World Bank 2017). There has been dramatic progress in health, economics, and demography. The integration of health policies into many other aspects of development was critical to this progress and owes inspiration to the vision of comprehensive, multisectoral, community engagement enshrined in the 1978 Alma-Ata Declaration. This chapter briefly reviews Vietnam's achievements in health and then supplies the historical context for how these gains were achieved through a primary health care (PHC) approach.

Vietnam's Recent Progress in Health, Economic Growth, and Demography

Vietnam's life expectancy at birth reached 75.6 in 2016, which is the second highest in Southeast Asia according to the Human Development Report 2016 (UNDP Vietnam 2016) (figure 12.1). Since 1990, Vietnam's gross domestic product (GDP) per capita growth has been among the fastest in the world, averaging 6.4% a year in the 2000s. Stable economic growth has resulted in steadily increasing GDP per capita, to its current level of $6,290.50 (in pur-

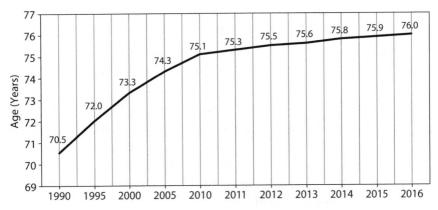

Figure 12.1. Trends of life expectancy in Vietnam, 1990–2016. Source: UNESCO 2017; UNDP Vietnam 2018

chasing power parity–adjusted dollars). According to the World Bank, the proportion of the population living below the line reached 13.5% in 2014, down from close to 60% in 1993. More than forty million people escaped poverty over the course of these two decades (World Bank and Ministry of Planning and Investment of Vietnam 2016). Fertility decline has allowed Vietnam to start reaping a demographic dividend. Vietnam had a population of more than ninety-three million in 2017 (GSO of Vietnam 2017). Young people aged 10 to 24 constitute the largest age group, accounting for approximately 30% of the total population. These youth are the most highly educated generation ever, with a 99% primary school completion rate as of 2014 (GSO of Vietnam and United Nations Children's Fund 2015). However, Vietnamese demography includes a growth in aging—the population over 65 has risen to 11.1% (General Statistics Office of Vietnam 2016). Development policy in Vietnam has needed a life course perspective to simultaneously address the health and welfare needs of both young and old. The PHC approach has been an ideal way to embrace a complex variety of concerns.

Historical Context

Colonial Legacy and Health System in 1950s and 1960s

After it declared independence in 1945, the government of the Democratic Republic of Vietnam inherited a health system from the previous colonial government, who was incapable of meeting the needs of its population, with a physician-to-population ratio of 1 to 180,000 (Nguyen 1972; Cima

1987; Lahmeyer 2003). In the years following independence in 1954 and the development of its health policy, the Vietnamese health system remained underdeveloped. In noncombat zones, the health system was based on the Soviet model, in which all health care facilities were owned by the state and made services available to the public. All citizens were entitled to free access to the health care system (Democratic Republic of Vietnam 1959; Socialist Republic of Vietnam 1980). Built on a four-layer system of care, from central to commune levels, the system operated on centrally top-down planning and management processes with no competition in providing health care services. It focused on achieving specific quantitative health systems outputs (e.g., number of medical doctors and hospital beds) rather than on outcome measures indicating changes in health status (Le 2013).

Effect of War on the Health System

During the Vietnam War (1945–1975), a state-socialist health system was implemented based on collectivist and centrally planned economic management. Health care facilities received an operating budget and resources from both central and local governments. Agricultural collectives provided a community contribution (agricultural benefits) as payment for commune health workers, while medicine, equipment, and labor were allocated by the central government as planned (Nguyen 1972). Although health care services were provided free of charge, the Vietnamese health system experienced uneven spatial development due to the wartime economy. Commune health centers in rural areas and district health centers in urban areas were designed to oversee basic preventive and curative services (Nguyen 1972). Numbers grew from only 500 commune health centers and 800 private maternity homes in 1959 (Ministry of Health 1959) to 5,764 commune health centers associated with agricultural collectives in the early of 1970s (Nguyen 1972). The sick were served by a group of trained individuals: family health workers and barefoot doctors (Nguyen 1972; Bryant 1998). Although family health workers no longer exist, barefoot doctors are still prevalent and are now known as village health workers (VHWs). Due to wartime scarcity, commune health centers were bare bones with obsolete equipment and no way to perform medical tests, hence diagnoses were based on clinical symptoms only. Relatives of the sick pitched in to offer patient care due to labor shortages (Nguyen 1972; Ladinsky and Levine 1985).

Postwar Influence from Communist Bloc Countries

During postwar recovery, public expenditure for health was severely reduced. Health expenditure was low compared with other sectors, because the government considered health an unproductive sector (Hanoi Medical University 2002). Around 30% to 40% of the national health budget was committed to financing drugs, health equipment, training, and buildings, but this was insufficient to meet estimated medical needs. The remaining 60% to 70% of the health expenditure was for salaries (Hanoi Medical University 2002). Vietnam's pharmaceutical industry had produced only about 30% of its domestic needs for medicines (Council of Ministers 1982). Health care facilities, especially health care centers at commune and district levels, were paralyzed because of limited public funds and the lack of local health personnel (Gellert 1995; Witter 1996).

The 1980 Constitution of Vietnam was committed to free health care for all citizens; however, the constitutional promise was not adequately financed. Only 2% of the total government budget was spent on health during the 1980s (Valdelin et al. 1992). The political report at the Seventh Communist Congress noted that the health system faced many challenges in the period from 1986 to 1991 based on insufficient state funding for health care needs (Communist Party of Vietnam 1991). Despite limited resources, state-funded health services and the PHC network at the grassroots level still played a vital role in the bright picture of health systems in Vietnam. Remarkably, the health outcomes achieved have been higher than those of other countries with similar incomes (Ensor 1995; Bloom 1998; Ladinsky et al. 2000; Ministry of Health 2001; World Bank 2001; Carrin 2002).

One-Party Communist Rule

Established in 1930, the Communist Party of Vietnam (CPV) plays a unique role in the country's political scene (National Assembly of Vietnam 2013). The 2013 Constitution of Vietnam affirms the CPV as the only ruling political party (National Assembly of Vietnam 2013). The Doi Moi progress with economic reform is a dynamic illustration of the CPV's leadership in every sector, including the health sector (Communist Party of Vietnam 1986). The CPV's views on health as a priority and its commitment to applying strong PHC delivery systems by developing a health care network at the grassroots level and combining preventive and curative health care have been reflected

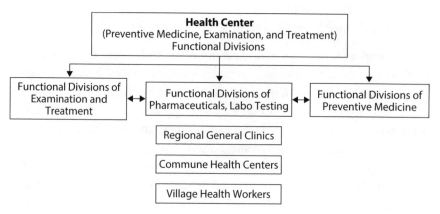

Figure 12.2. Grassroots health network in Vietnam.

in all resolutions related to health care and protection for the people (Communist Party of Vietnam 1993b; Communist Party of Vietnam 2017).

Doi Moi Effect on Health System

The guidance of the CPV at the Doi Moi Congress (1986) regarding the health system required that health facilities at the grassroots level (figure 12.2) be enhanced and developed. The key issue was amending essential policies to ensure the rights and benefits for health workers at all levels, especially at the commune level, which aimed at improving the attitudes and behaviors of health workers. The policies also ensured increasing the stock of inpatient beds at the PHC level and gradually renovating and changing health equipment at national hospitals (Communist Party of Vietnam 1986).

Private health care services began booming after the Doi Moi introduction. In the early 1990s, there were no private health facilities, but in the 2010s, the private sector had grown to 212 hospitals (Hanoi Department of Health 2017) and about 35,000 private clinics and 40,000 drug stores (Ministry of Health 2019). The private sector now plays a significant role in health systems in Vietnam (Ministry of Health 2017a). Importantly, the private sector in Vietnam has been used to mobilize private finances for PHC services that people value, helping the public sector conserve resources for VHWs and more essential public health operations.

At the grassroots level, VHWs continue to be focal points of PHC programs. From 1999 to 2009, they were paid only a small amount of money for their health-related work at the community level, offering PHC services such as health education, some epidemiology activities, health care for mothers and children, and family planning, first aid, and general health care (Ministry of Health 1999, 2010, 2013). In 2009, the monthly allowance for VHWs was increased from about VND40,000 a month (equivalent to US$1.72)to VND402,500 a month (equivalent to US$17.30) for delta/mountainous areas and VND632,500 a month (equivalent to US$27.20) for especially difficult areas (Prime Minister 2009). This more generous financial support policy helped to reform the PHC system, with a focus on the first point of contact. In 2017, approximately 97.5% of villages had VHWs (Ministry of Health 2017a). VHWs play a crucial role in improving population health by supporting the implementation of national targeted programs in their local areas, such as malaria prevention, vaccination, malnutrition prevention for children, safe motherhood, and among others, as well as other disease prevention programs in the mountainous, remote, and island areas (Ministry of Health 2017b).

PHC has been a key strategy for health system development in Vietnam as part of Doi Moi (National Assembly of Vietnam 1989; Vietnam Government 1996; Prime Minister 2001, 2013). PHC policies aim at ensuring that all people receive quality primary care. Comprehensive strategies focus on human resource development for health, universal health insurance coverage, and upgrading regional polyclinics and hospitals (Ministry of Health and Health Partnership Group 2015). By the end of 2015, 86.9% of commune health centers had at least one physician, 96.4% of commune health centers had a midwife, 97.2% of children under 1 year had been fully vaccinated, and only 14.1% of children under 5 years had had stunting (Ministry of Health 2017a).

Health as Part of the Social Economic Development Strategy
Integration of Health with Development

Policies of the CPV, the National Assembly, and the government continue to stress the important role of people's health in achieving social advancement and equity, improving people's lives and meeting requirements of industrialization and modernization in the country. Leaders see investment in health as a direct investment in sustainable development. Vietnam's top leaders see health objectives as development policy objectives (Ministry of Health 2016b).

The success of Doi Moi shifted the state's focus from a narrow focus on GDP growth to sustainable socioeconomic development of Vietnam's capability to improve all aspects of human thriving. The Social Economic

Development Strategy (SEDS) plans for 2001 to 2010 focused on efficiency and equity. There was special attention to improving access for the poor, ethnic minorities, people in remote areas, and war-affected people. Maternal and child health were made high priorities (Vietnam Government 2000a). The government's Socio-Economic Development Plan (2006–2010) increased investment in PHC, with an explicit focus on education in reproductive health, nutrition, traffic safety, and tobacco control (National Assembly of Vietnam 2006).

In Vietnam's SEDS plans for the period of 2011–2020, health was identified as one of twelve pillars for growth and restructuring of the economy. The plan stated, "Strongly develop health . . . and improve the quality of healthcare work for the people." The government is concentrating on strengthening the capability of commune health centers, completing the construction of hospitals at the district level, and guaranteeing quality health service accessibility, especially for the poor, children, and the elderly (Vietnam Government 2010).

How Vietnamese Traditional Culture Accords with Primary Health Care

According to traditional Vietnamese health beliefs, the notion of prevention is very important (Jansson, 2012). Traditional medicine informs the health beliefs of many (Schirmer et al. 2004). The relationship between culture and health care therefore helps to explain why health was given priority in Vietnam's development plans. Traditional cultural respect for women has ensured that women are engaged and reached by community health programs. A flexible combination of traditional and modern medicine is one of the mainstays of the health strategies. The term *integration/hybrid medicine* has come to be widely used to express the official incorporation of traditional medicine

---

Vietnamese Proverbs

Suc khoe la vang
Health is gold.

Co suc khoe la co tat ca
Good health is everything.

–Vietnamese proverbs

---

into national health systems and services (Raffin 2008). The government has strengthened audits of quality of care of traditional medicine and integrated traditional medicine from the central level to local levels. Integration of traditional medicine offers greater equity and cultural sensitivity, and makes health services more acceptable to all people (Ministry of Health and Health Partnership Group 2017).

Community Participation

Community participation along with equity, intersectoral coordination, and appropriate technology are pillars of PHC. In Vietnam, community participation was traditionally seen by the medical establishment as mobilizing people to adopt an intervention such as mass immunization or nutrition campaigns. Above and beyond this, community participation in Vietnam has attempted to address the wider social and structural determinants of health, such as access to clean water and safe sanitation conditions (Vietnam Government 2000), as well as housing and infrastructure upgrading (Ngo 2016). For example, Vietnam's Participatory Hygiene and Sanitation Transformation is a method to encourage community management of water and sanitation facilities, improve hygiene behaviors, and prevent diarrheal diseases. It consists of preparing trainers to assist villagers in identifying and analyzing of problems, selecting among different types of water supply and sanitation facilities as well as different hygiene practices, planning, and monitoring and evaluation through a standard set of participatory activities (Mai et al. 2004).

Community participation has embraced many forms of citizen action for community problem-solving, including self-help, and social support groups such as those for tuberculosis and HIV/AIDS prevention and treatment. Formal and informal activities are voluntarily undertaken by organized individuals who share interests and goals in programs that aim to bring about a planned change or improvement in community life and services. Community participation has always been supported by national policies that promote bottom-up planning and decision-making. For example, the 2007 Grassroots Democracy Ordinance (National Assembly of Vietnam 2007) called for extensive public involvement at the commune level in decisions related to the use of public resources. According to the ordinance, people have the right to be informed, to participate in discussions, and to make decisions on local socioeconomic development activities, especially when these activities require community resources. Ultimately, most community-based projects have not been initiated and conducted by the communities themselves; thus, community participation requires support from the local government for its activities (Ngo 2016).

High-Placed Support for Population-Level Prevention

Vietnam has focused on disease prevention and health promotion. Resolution number 4 of the Central Communist Party Session VII (1993) clearly states: "Health care and dealing with health problems should be done from the perspective of positive and active disease prevention, promotion of hygienic movement, physical practices and effective treatment" (Communist Party of Vietnam, 1993a, n.p.). Resolution 46 (2005) of the Standing Committee of the Politburo reaffirmed this by stating: "Practice overall health care: integration of prevention and treatment, rehabilitation and physical training so as to promote health" (Politbureau of the Communist Party, 2005, n.p.). More recently, Resolution 46 also specified some major tasks: (1) develop and effectively operate national target programs on health and health promotion; (2) develop hygienic, preventive, and physical practice activities; (3) apply preventive measures and limit negative impacts to people's health caused by changes in lifestyle, environment, and working conditions; (4) speed up preventive activities on occupational diseases; (5) strengthen and develop school health; (6) emphasize health for mothers, children, and older persons, and rehabilitation; and (7) effectively strengthen intersectoral cooperation in health protection, caring, and promotion for the people. This direction has continued to be emphasized in the recent Resolution number 20 of the Central Communist Party Session XII (2017) as it relates to strengthening health protection, care, and promotion in new context (Politbureau of the Communist Party 2017). Health promotion and strengthening capacity on epidemic prevention and control together with reforming grassroots engagement in health are some essential strategies mentioned in this resolution.

A system of national health target programs (NHTPs) must be credited with helping Vietnam realize the goals of government leadership. Priority setting and concentration of available resources to address key problems of population health through NHTPs has been an effective approach, positively contributing to equity and efficiency in people's health care and protection. The NHTPs started in 1991, with an initial five-year program from 1991 to 1995, and have been conducted up to now under a new name: "Health and Population Target Program in the 2016–2020 Period" (Vietnam Government 2017).

Multisectoral Collaboration for Health

At the central level, the Ministry of Health has carried out a series of programs that involved a joint effort between and among different ministries and other stakeholders. All other line ministries, such as the Ministry of Planning and Investment, the Ministry of Finance, the Ministry of Labor, Invalids and Social Affairs, the Ministry of Education and Training, the Ministry of Home Affairs, the Ministry of Public Security, the Ministry of Transport, and the Ministry of Defense, have important roles in collaborating and supporting the Ministry of Health in providing health care and protection as well as promotion for the population as indicated in various national strategies over time, such as the National Strategy for People's Health Care, Protection and Promotion in the Period 2011–2020 and Vision to 2030 (Vietnam Government 2011). At the provincial and district levels, and especially at the commune level, the coordination among education, health, and social welfare sectors is also emphasized.

The Ministry of Health has also taken the lead in mobilizing and broadening participation of a variety of other stakeholders, such as international agencies, states, and nongovernmental organizations and communities (Health Partnership Group 2013). The government has a high degree of coordination with civil society organizations (CSOs) (Ministry of Health 2015) who act as a bridge toward improved implementation of health and development plans (Association Batick International and Centre for Development and Integration 2013). CSOs have been generating evidence on best practices in dialogues and contributing to support policy advocacy and program intervention, especially in remote areas (Ministry of Health et al. 2015).

The Vietnamese media have played an active role in disseminating information about health issues and have received considerable support from various national bodies in this process. Mass organizations including the Viet Nam Fatherland Front, the Women's Union, and the Youth Union usually have a four-layered organizational structure—central, provincial, district, and commune levels—and have implemented many development-oriented activities. Mass organizations have provided supplemental public services that the government does not provide (e.g., childcare, HIV/AIDS clubs, nutritional awareness classes for parents, microcredit for the poor, intervenience in the case of domestic violence disputes). This four-level structure has distinct advantages, including helping the health sector identify households in need of PHC based on locally contextualized knowledge (Jones et al. 2014). Vietnam's experience has shown the value of developing task force units for coordination and investing in capacity-building in planning, budgeting, and management (ADB 2016). Engagement with the business sector has helped the government start sustainable public-private partnerships (UNFPA 2011).

Priority Given to Those in Need

The social protection system in Vietnam currently comprises four basic policy groups: (1) minimum income and poverty reduction, (2) social insurance, (3) social assistance, and (4) basic social service. Social services include education, health care, accommodation, clean water, and information (National Bureau of Asian Research and Institute of Social and Medical Studies 2009; Dao 2017). Targeted groups span the life course, from infants (the law on child protection and care, adjusted in 2016) to seniors (the law on the elderly, 2009) as well as disabled people (the law on people with disabilities, 2010).

Resources for social assistance come from diversified sources, combining the central budget with local budgets and other social resources. Assistance forms, including health care, education, accommodation, and clean water, continue to be diversified.

In Vietnam, a government-led health insurance system was introduced in the early 1990s, and by the end of 2018 about 89% of the population (Financial News 2019) covered by health insurance in which all children under 6, the poor, the near-poor, ethnic minorities, and other people living in border or difficult areas received full or partial premium subsidization (National Assembly of Vietnam 2014) (figure 12.3).

Recent Challenges and Solutions to Overcome Health System Bottlenecks
Challenges for the Health System

The organizational structure and management mechanism of the grassroots health network have changed three times within ten years, creating instability in the system nationwide. This has affected the efficiency of the health workforce and decreased the ability to deliver integrated, comprehensive, and continuous health services (Ministry of Health and Health Partnership Group 2015).

An aging population and increasing burden of noncommunicable diseases (NCDs) requires more comprehensive and continuous integration of care. At the same time, the appearance and unpredictable evolution of some emerging diseases have resulted in the increase in health care needs and costs. The

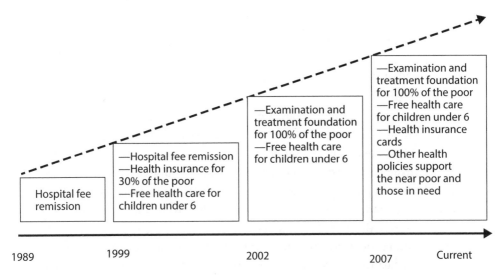

Figure 12.3. Health policies support for those in need. Sources: Council of Ministers 1989; MOLISA et al. 1999; Prime Minister of Vietnam 2002; National Assembly of Vietnam 2014

epidemiologic transition is continuing, and the magnitude of NCDs is sure to increase further. The epidemiological disease structure is changing, with NCDs accounting for an increasing share of death and morbidity (Ministry of Health and Health Partnership Group 2015). Recently, Vietnam was ranked twelfth in terms of tuberculosis burden and fourteenth in terms of multi-drug-resistant tuberculosis burden worldwide, and the country continues to be a hot spot for emerging diseases such as influenza A (H7N9 and H5N6) and reemerging diseases like dengue hemorrhagic fever and influenza A (H5N1 and H1N1). The country faces an increasing number of risk factors due to industrialization, urbanization, unhealthy lifestyles, and environmental pollution. Within the region, Vietnam is among the nations with a comparatively high smoking prevalence and high consumption of alcohol. It is also dealing with health issues related to climate change and is considered to be one of the ten countries most heavily affected by the rise in sea levels (Ministry of Health and Health Partnership Group 2014, 2015).

Rapid increases in health care costs are confronting limited health resources. The foremost challenge is to ensure universal access to quality health care at an affordable cost for the country and with manageable out-of-pocket expenses for families. Regarding total social expenditure on health, although Vietnam spends up to 6% of its GDP on health care, health spending per capita in Vietnam is only ranked 127 out of 191 countries (World

Health Organization 2015). Nevertheless, health insurance coverage reached 87.62% by the end of 2018 (Social Insurance Magazine 2018). By law, insured patients are entitled to 80% to 100% coverage (National Assembly of Vietnam 2014). However, in practice the reimbursement from the pool is less than 50% of patients' actual expenditures (figure in 2017; see Pekerti et al. 2017). The share of out-of-pocket payments has not decreased much over the years; this figure was 48.8% in 2012 (Ministry of Health 2016a).

The organization of health service delivery is fragmented, leading to inability to provide integrated, comprehensive, and continuous care. Linkages are limited between preventive and curative care, between levels of care, and between public and private health facilities, leading to low levels of cooperation. Moreover, there are few mechanisms for integrating activities of different NHTPs, particularly programs for the prevention and control of NCDs. Quality of health services at the grassroots level, especially at commune health centers, is limited. Commune health centers currently can perform only 52.2% of the technical services according to the national classification of technical services by level of facility (Medical Services Administration 2011). Apart from the inadequate facilities, equipment, and medicine, the limited expertise of health workers at commune health centers is considered a critical factor for commune health centers' service quality, especially at commune health centers in mountainous areas (Trần 2011). While the number of human resources for health at the grassroots level is insufficient, health workers at commune health centers are also faced with a number of difficulties and shortcomings such as limited knowledge and poor practical skills due to inadequate links between training and required competencies of health workers (Ministry of Health 2016a).

Solutions to Overcoming Health System Bottlenecks

According to the Ministry of Health, strengthening the health system and professional capacity are a high priority for ensuring better service delivery (in both preventive and curative care) at the grassroots level (Ministry of Health 2016a). The ministry's plan for people's health protection, care, and promotion for 2016–2020 proposes restructuring community services to respond to the rise in NCDs (Ministry of Health and Health Partnership Group 2015). Additionally, the Viet Nam Health Financing Strategy for 2016–2025 sets out financing reforms including new payment mechanisms for PHC services, reallocation of funds for community health care, and prioritization of PHC services and NCD care in a cost-effective health service package (Ministry of

Orientation for Solutions toward Health Priorities at the Grassroots Level

- Implement strategies for comprehensive access including management and prevention of risk factors, screening for early detection of disease in the community for noncommunicable diseases, and intervention measures appropriate for each locality.
- Reform grassroots organizational models and primary health care (PHC) service delivery following an orientation toward comprehensiveness, continuity, and strengthened linkages between treatment and prevention and between the grassroots- and higher-level facilities.
- Continue to strengthen coherent and sustainable grassroots-level investments in physical facilities and human resources, particularly in disadvantaged regions.

- Strengthen surveillance systems for epidemics, ensure preparedness in terms of equipment and human resources to actively respond and control outbreaks, and continue to effectively implement the Expanded Program on Immunization.
- Strengthen capacity of the health sector and intersectoral collaboration for control of climate change, and master planning for industrial production, evaluating, and monitoring effects of pollution due to industrialization and urbanization.
- Implement Sustainable Development Goals, paying special attention to mothers, children, and the elderly. Study the mechanism and road map appropriate for integrating national health target programs into the routine PHC activities at the grassroots level.

Health and World Health Organization 2016). Importantly, in 2017, the Resolution 20-NQ/TW was issued, focusing on strengthening health protection, health care, and health promotion. This resolution emphasizes that health prevention and PHC will be covered by the government budget (Party Central Committee 2017). These reforms will improve grassroots infrastructure and staff availability as well as quality, which will indirectly strengthen the quality of PHC services (World Health Organization 2018) (see box on this page).

Conclusion

There is a striking concordance between the principles defining PHC in Article VII of the Alma-Ata Declaration and the principles that guided Vietnam's post–civil war health system evolution. Vietnamese traditional culture and postwar politics resonated with the core principles announced in Alma-Ata. During the 1978 Alma-Ata Conference, Vietnam was preoccupied with postwar recovery. The Communist Party was ideologically predisposed to include health in its multisectoral development strategies, to build up preventive population-level strategies, and to embrace community involvement and consultation on local strategies. However, real progress on Vietnam's PHC strategy occurred after the Doi Moi reforms of 1986.

From the Law on People's Health Protection and Care in 1989 through a series of national health-related strategies and policies, the CPV has been consistently committed to improving population health, strengthening grassroots health care networks, and advancing PHC availability for all.

Vietnam's comprehensive approach to health in development is part of why there has been simultaneous progress on literacy, life expectancy, and the reduction of poverty across the life course and across urban and rural settings. Vietnam's health achievements were not the result of a small set of selective health interventions, and they were achieved with a health budget that was quite modest. Private sector health providers helped to provide services to those who could pay, freeing the public system to pursue a public health and PHC approach that could focus on those most in need. In an ironic refutation of Walsh and Warren's (1979) thesis that good health at low cost can be had through selective interventions and without comprehensive PHC, Vietnam's comprehensive PHC approach has led to the construction of a low-cost and sustainable system that has achieved great strides toward health for all.

Vietnam's tremendous efforts to meet the complex health and development challenges of the twenty-first century require stronger focus on comprehensive PHC. Support for strong PHC has also expanded far beyond the group of early universal health coverage advocates, presenting a historic opportunity for action.

REFERENCES

Asian Development Bank. 2016. *Country partnership strategy: Viet Nam, 2012–2015. Sector assessment (summary): Health sector*. Hanoi, Vietnam. http://www.adb.org /sites/default/files/linked-documents/cps-vie-2012-2015-ssa-07.pdf.

Association Batick International and Centre for Development and Integration. 2013. *Civil society and corporate social responsibility in Vietnam: Bridging the gap*. Hanoi, Vietnam. http://www.batik-international.org/data/batik/media/site/pdf/BATIK-EN -etude-OSC-CSR-14-09.pdf.

Bloom, G. 1998. "Primary health care meets the market in China and Vietnam." *Health Policy* 44 (3): 233–252.

Bryant, J. 1998. "Communism, poverty, and demographic change in North Vietnam." *Popul Dev Rev* 24 (2): 235–269.

Carrin, G. 2002. "Social health insurance in developing countries: A continuing challenge." *Int Soc Sec Rev* 55 (2): 57–69.

Cima, R. 1987. "Government and politics." In *Vietnam: A country study*. Washington, DC: Library of Congress.

Communist Party of Vietnam. 1986. "Orientation and objectives of socio-economic development in 5 years from 1986 to 1990." Ha Noi. http://chinhphu.vn/portal/page /portal/chinhphu/kehoachphattrienkinhtexahoi?categoryId=865&articleId=3117.

———. 1993a. Resolution 4 on 14 January 1993 of the Central Committee of the 7th Party Congress on Continuing Reform of Education and Training.

———. 1993b. *Resolution No. 4-NQ/HNTW on urgent issues of healthcare and protection.* http://dangcongsan.vn/tu-lieu-van-kien/ban-chap-hanh-trung-uong/cac -uy-vien-trung-uong-dang/books-11520162411956/index-3152016245085620 .html.

———. 2017. *Resolution No. 20-NQ/TQ on enhancing the care for and improvement of people's health in the new situation.* Hanoi.

Council of Ministers. 1982. Directive on meeting the need of medicine for prevention and treatment. Hanoi.

CPV Online News. 2018. "The establishment of Communist Party of Vietnam 3-2-1930." *Communist Party of Vietnam Online Newspaper*, January 26.

Dao, Q. V. 2017. *Social protection in Vietnam: Achievements, challenges and development orientation.* http://ilssa.org.vn/en/news/social-protection-in-vietnam -achievements-challenges-and-development-orientation-213.

Democratic Republic of Vietnam. 1959. *The 1959 Vietnam Constitution.* Hanoi.

Ensor, T. 1995. "Introducing health insurance in Vietnam." *Health Policy Plan* 10 (2): 154–163.

Financial News. 2019. *Health insurance coverage achieved 89% of whole population* [*Tỷ lệ bao phủ bảo hiểm y tế đã đạt 89% dân số*]. http://thoibaotaichinhvietnam.vn /pages/tien-te-bao-hiem/2019-06-05/ty-le-bao-phu-bao-hiem-y-te-da-dat-89-dan-so -72302.aspx.

Gellert, G. A. 1995. "The influence of market economics on primary health care in Vietnam." *J Am Med Assoc* 273 (19): 1498–1502.

GSO of Vietnam. 2016. *The 1/4/2015 time-point population change and family planning survey: Major findings.* Hanoi, Vietnam.

———. 2017. *Press release: Socio-economic statistics of 2017* [*Thông cáo báo chí tình hình kinh tế - xã hội năm 2017*]. Hanoi, Vietnam. https://www.gso.gov.vn/Default .aspx?tabid=382&ItemID=18667.

GSO of Vietnam and United Nations Children's Fund. 2015. Viet Nam Multiple Indicator Cluster Survey (MICS) 2014. Hanoi, Vietnam.

Hanoi Department of Health. 2017. *Private hospitals continue to provide health care and treatment for health insurers in 2018.* http://soyte.hanoi.gov.vn/vi/news/chuong -trinh-y-te/cac-benh-vien-tu-nhan-tiep-tuc-duoc-kham-chua-benh-bao-hiem-y-te -trong-nam-2018-2871.html.

Hanoi Medical University. 2002. "The unification time (1975–2002)." *The history of Hanoi Medical University.* Hanoi: Medical Publishing House.

Health Partnership Group. 2013. *Improving the effectiveness and efficiency of development co-operation in the health sector.* Hanoi, Vietnam. http://www.wpro .who.int/vietnam/one_un/vietnam_health_partnership_2013_en.pdf.

Hoang, D. C. 1972. "The rural health network in the Democratic Republic of Viet Nam." In *Vietnamese studies: Rural health work and disease prevention*, edited by K. Nguyen. Hanoi: Xuhasaba.

Jansson, M. 2012. "Physical activity gives health benefits, but is this new to the Vietnamese? An analysis of articles from Vietnamese newspapers." Bachelor's thesis, Linnaeus University, Kalmar.

Jones, N., E. Presler-Marshall, and T. V. A. Tran. 2014. *Early marriage among Viet Nam's Hmong: How unevenly changing gender norms limit Hmong adolescent girls' options in marriage and life.* Hanoi, Vietnam: Overseas Development Institute.

Ladinsky, J. L., and R. E. Levine. 1985. "The organization of health services in Vietnam." *J Public Health Policy* 6 (2): 255–268.

Ladinsky, J. L., H. T. Nguyen, and N. D. Volk. 2000. "Changes in the health care system of Vietnam in response to the emerging market economy." *J Public Health Policy* 21 (1): 82–98.

Lahmeyer, J. 2003. Vietnam. *Historical demographical data of the whole country.* http://www.populstat.info/Asia/vietnamc.htm.

Le, V. T. 2013. *Soviet Union's support for Vietnam in combating with the American (1954–1975).* http://khoalichsu.edu.vn/bai-nghien-cu/509-s-chi-vin-giup-ca-lien-xo-vi -vit-nam-trong-cuc-khang-chin-chng-m-cu-nc-1954-1975-pgsts-le-vn-thnh.html.

Mai, V. H., N. Ksor, and H. Stoltz. "Experiences from a Rural Water Supply and Sanitation Programme, Vietnam." People-centred approaches to water and environmental sanitation, 2004 Vientiane, Lao PDR. https://wedc-knowledge.lboro .ac.uk/resources/conference/30/Danida.pdf.

Medical Services Administration. 2011. *Báo cáo kết quả công tác khám, chữa bệnh năm 2011.* Hanoi, Vietnam.

Ministry of Health. 1959. Circular No. 21-BYT/TT on establishing private commune health center. Hanoi, Vietnam.

———. 1999. Regulating on functions and duties of village health workers. Hanoi, Vietnam. https://thuvienphapluat.vn/van-ban/the-thao-y-te/Quyet-dinh-3653-1999 -QD-BYT-chuc-nang-nhiem-vu-nhan-vien-y-te-thon-ban-45982.aspx.

———. 2001. *55 years—the development of Vietnam Health Sector (1945–2000).* Hanoi: Medical Publishing House.

———. 2010. Regulating on functions and duties of village health workers. Hanoi, Vietnam. https://thuvienphapluat.vn/van-ban/the-thao-y-te/Thong-tu-39-2010-TT-BYT -tieu-chuan-chuc-nang-nhiem-vu-nhan-vien-y-te-111650.aspx.

———. 2013. Regulating on functions and duties of village health workers. Hanoi, Vietnam.

———. 2015. Plan on prevention and control of infectious diseases in 2015. Hanoi, Vietnam.

———. 2016a. *JAHR 2015: Strengthening primary health care at the grassroots towards universal health coverage.* Hanoi, Vietnam.

———. 2016b. *Plan for people's health protection, care and promotion 2016–2020.* http://www.euhf.vn/upload/Strategic%20documents/82.%20MOH%205-year%20 plan%20(Eng).pdf.

———. 2017a. *Health statistics yearbook 2016.* Hanoi, Vietnam. https://moh.gov.vn /documents/20182/244466/Ni%C3%AAn+gi%C3%A1m+th%E1%BB%91ng+k% C3%AA+y+t%E1%BA%BF+2016/d7c56421-fdfa-45d7-8468-8fdd8e5537de.

———. 2017b. *Village health workers play an important role in healthcare services of mountainous areas.* https://www.moh.gov.vn/hoat-dong-cua-lanh-dao-bo/-/asset

_publisher/vZJbYmQh1lGZ/content/y-te-thon-ban-co-vai-tro-quan-trong-trong-cong
-tac-y-te-o-mien-nui?inheritRedirect=false.

———. 2019. *The Ministry of Health summarizes nne years of implementation of the law on examination and treatment* [Bộ Y tế tổng kết 9 năm thi hành Luật khám bệnh, chửa bệnh]. https://moh.gov.vn/web/guest/hoat-dong-cua-lanh-dao-bo/-/asset _publisher/vZJbYmQh1lGZ/content/bo-y-te-tong-ket-9-nam-thi-hanh-luat-kham -benh-chua-benh.

Ministry of Health and Health Partnership Group. 2014. *Joint annual health review 2014: Strengthening prevention and control of NCDs.* Hanoi, Vietnam. http://jahr .org.vn/downloads/JAHR2014/JAHR%202014_EN_full.pdf.

———. 2015. *Joint annual health review 2015: Strengthening grassroots health care towards universal health care.* Hanoi. http://jahr.org.vn/downloads/JAHR2015 /JAHR2015_full_EN.pdf.

———. 2017. *Joint annual health review 2016: Towards healthy aging in Vietnam.* Hanoi, Vietnam. http://jahr.org.vn/downloads/JAHR2016/JAHR2016_full _EN.pdf.

Ministry of Health, Partnership for Maternal, NCH, World Health Organization, World Bank, and Alliance for Health Policy and Systems Research. 2015. *Success factors for women's and children's health: Vietnam.* Switzerland. http://www.who.int/pmnch /knowledge/publications/vietnam_country_report.pdf.

Ministry of Health and World Health Organization. 2016. *Viet Nam Health Financing Strategy for the period 2016–2025.* Hanoi, Vietnam. http://www.euhf.vn/activities/on -going-activities/heath-financing/viet-nam-health-financing-strategy-for-the-period -2016-2025.

National Assembly of Vietnam. 1989. Law on Protection of People's Health. Hanoi, Vietnam. https://thuvienphapluat.vn/van-ban/the-thao-y-te/Luat-Bao-ve-suc-khoe -nhan-dan-1989-21-LCT-HDNN8-37690.aspx.

———. 2007. Ordinance on the grass-root democracy in communes and wards. Hanoi, Vietnam. http://vanban.chinhphu.vn/portal/page/portal/chinhphu/hethongvanban?class _id=1&mode=detail&document_id=55805.

———. 2013. *The constitution of Vietnam.* Hanoi, Vietnam.

———. 2014. *Law on health insurance.* Hanoi, Vietnam.

Ngo, H. V. 2016. "Community participation in urban housing and infrastructure upgrading projects in Vietnam." PhD dissertation, Erasmus University, Rotterdam.

Pekerti, A., Q.-H. Vuong, T. M. Ho, and T.-T. Vuong. 2017. "Health care payments in Vietnam: Patients' quagmire of caring for health versus economic destitution." *Int J Environ Res Public Health* 14: (10): 1118.

Politbureau of the Communist Party. 2005. Resolution No. 46-NQ/TW dated 23/2/2005 of Politbureau on "Protection, caring and promotion of people health in the new period." https://thuvienphapluat.vn/van-ban/the-thao-y-te/Nghi-quyet-46-NQ-TW -cong-tac-bao-ve-cham-soc-va-nang-cao-suc-khoe-nhan-dan-trong-tinh-hinh-moi -53277.aspx.

———. 2017. Resolution No. 20-NQ/TW dated 25/10/2017 of Politbureau on "Protection, caring and promotion of people health in the new period." https:// thuvienphapluat.vn/van-ban/the-thao-y-te/Nghi-quyet-20-NQ-TW-2017-tang-cuong -cong-tac-bao-ve-cham-soc-nang-cao-suc-khoe-nhan-dan-365599.aspx.

Prime Minister. 2001. Decision No. 35/2001/QĐ-TTg approving strategy on the protection, care and improvement of people's health for the 2001–2010 period. Hanoi, Vietnam. https://thuvienphapluat.vn/van-ban/the-thao-y-te/quyet-dinh-35-2001-qd-ttg -phe-duyet-chien-luoc-cham-soc-bao-ve-suc-khoe-nhan-dan-giai-doan-2001-2010 -47513.aspx.

———. 2009. Decision on regulating allowance for village health workers. Hanoi, Vietnam. https://thuvienphapluat.vn/van-ban/the-thao-y-te/quyet-dinh-35-2001-qd-ttg -phe-duyet-chien-luoc-cham-soc-bao-ve-suc-khoe-nhan-dan-giai-doan-2001-2010 -47513.aspx.

———. 2013. Decision No. 122/QĐ-TTg approving the national strategy for people's health protection, care and promotion 2011–2020. Hanoi, Vietnam. http://www .chinhphu.vn/portal/page/portal/chinhphu/hethongvanban?class_id=2&mode =detail&document_id=165437.

Prime Minister of Vietnam. 2002. *Decision 139 on the Health Care Fund for the Poor.* Hanoi, Vietnam.

Raffin, A. 2008. "Postcolonial Vietnam: Hybrid modernity." *Postcolonial Stud* 11 (3): 329–344.

Schirmer, J., C. Cartwright, A. K. Montegut, G. Dreher, and J. Stovall. 2004. "A collaborative needs assessment and work plan in behavioral medicine curriculum development in Vietnam." *Fam Syst Health* 22 (4): 410–418.

Social Insurance Magazine. 2018. *Tỷ lệ bao phủ BHYT đạt 87,62% dân số cả nức* [Health insurance coverage has reached 87.62%]. http://tapchibaohiemxahoi.gov.vn /tin-tuc/ty-le-bao-phu-bhyt-dat-87-62-dan-so-ca-nuoc-20189.

Socialist Republic of Vietnam. 1980. The 1980's Vietnam Constitution. Hanoi, Vietnam. https://thuvienphapluat.vn/van-ban/bo-may-hanh-chinh/Hien-phap-1980-Cong-hoa -Xa-hoi-Chu-Nghia-Viet-Nam-36948.aspx.

Stern, Lewis N. 1993. *Renovating the Vietnamese Communist Party: Nguyen Van Linh and the Programme for Organizational Reform, 1987–91.* Singapore: Institute of Southeast Asian Studies.

National Assembly of Vietnam. 2006. *Vietnam: Five Year Socio-economic Development Plan, 2006–2010.* https://paris21.org/node/1075.

National Bureau of Asian Research and Institute of Social and Medical Studies. 2009. *Maternal and newborn health: A Vietnam roundtable discussion.* https://www.nbr .org/publication/maternal-and-newborn-health-a-vietnam-roundtable-discussion/.

Party Central Committee. 2017. *Resolution 20-NQ/TW on the protection, care and improvement of people's health in the new situation.* http://unaids.org.vn/wp -content/uploads/2017/12/RESOLUTION.-En.pdf.

Trần, T. M. O. 2011. *Đánh giá việc thực hiện các chức năng, nhiệm vụ của một số trạm y tế xã khu vực miền núi* [Evaluating the implementation of commune health statitions' performance in mountain areas]. Hanoi: Health Strategy and Policy Institute.

UNDP Vietnam. 2016. Human development report 2016—Briefing note for countries on the 2016 Human Development Report. Vietnam. http://hdr.undp.org/sites/default /files/2016_human_development_report.pdf.

UNFPA. 2011. *Advocacy brief: Revitalization of voluntary family planning in Viet Nam 2011–2020.* https://vietnam.unfpa.org/sites/default/files/pub-pdf/Advocacy%20brief _Revitalization%20of%20Voluntary%20FP_Eng.pdf.

Valdelin, J., E. Michanek, H. Persson, T. Q. Tran, and B. Simonsson. 1992. *Doi moi and health: Evaluation of the health sector co-operation programme between Vietnam and Sweden*. Stockholm: SIDA Project.

Vietnam Government. 1996. Resolution No.37/CP of the government on the strategy on health care and protection for the people in the 1996–2000 period and Vietnam's national policy on medicines. Hanoi, Vietnam. https://thuvienphapluat.vn/van-ban /The-thao-Y-te/Nghi-quyet-37-CP-dinh-huong-cong-tac-cham-soc-va-bao-ve-suc -khoe-nhan-dan-trong-thoi-gian-1996-2000-va-chinh-sach-quoc-gia-ve-thuoc-Viet -Nam-39784.aspx.

———. 2000. *Strategy for socio-economic development, 2001–2010*. Hanoi, Vietnam. http://siteresources.worldbank.org/INTVIETNAM/Resources/Socio_Economic_Dev.pdf.

———. 2010. *Vietnam's socio-economic development strategy for the period of 2011–2020*. Hanoi, Vietnam. http://www.economica.vn/Portals/0/Documents/1d3f7e e0400e42152bdcaa439bf62686.pdf.

———. 2011. National strategy for people's health care, protection and promotion in the period 2011–2020 and vision to 2030. http://www.chinhphu.vn/portal/page /portal/chinhphu/hethongvanban?class_id=2&mode=detail&document_id=165437.

———. 2017. Health and population target program in the 2016–2020 period. Hanoi, Vietnam. https://thuvienphapluat.vn/van-ban/the-thao-y-te/Quyet-dinh-1125-QD-TTg -2017-phe-duyet-Chuong-trinh-muc-tieu-Y-te-Dan-so-2016-2020-357420.aspx.

Walsh, J. A., and K. S. Warren. 1979. "Selective primary health care: An interim strategy for disease control in developing countries." *N Engl J Med* 301 (18): 967–974.

Witter, S. 1996. "'Doi Moi' and health: The effect of economic reforms on health system in Vietnam." *Int J Health Plan Manage* 11 (2): 159–172.

———. 2001. *Vietnam growing healthy: A review of Vietnam's health sector*. Washington, DC: World Bank.

World Bank. 2017 (last updated 2019). *Vietnam overview*. http://www.worldbank.org /en/country/vietnam/overview.

World Bank and Ministry of Planning and Investment of Vietnam. 2016. *Vietnam 2035: Toward prosperity, creativity, equity, and democracy*. https://openknowledge .worldbank.org/handle/10986/23724.

World Health Organization. 2015. *World health statistics 2015*. https://www.who.int /gho/publications/world_health_statistics/2015/en/.

———. 2018. Viet Nam improving equity in access to primary care. https://www.who .int/docs/default-source/primary-health/case-studies/viet-nam.pdf.

CHAPTER THIRTEEN

Cuba's Progress on Primary Health Care since the Alma-Ata Conference

Sasmira Matta, David Bishai, and Pedro Más Bermejo

The Cuban government and Ministry of Public Health brought the principles of the Alma-Ata Declaration to life. The planners of the 1978 declaration were heavily influenced by Cuba because a 1975 World Health Organization publication documented both Cuba's progress and its approach to applying intense state energy to improving health in a resource-constrained environment. Margaret Chan, former director-general of the World Health Organization (WHO), noted that Cuba "provides solid evidence that factors other than national wealth can produce health outcomes that rival that in the richest nations" (Chan 2009, 1). As it turns out, Cuba did sustain both progress in health and a comprehensive system of primary health care (PHC) after the Alma-Ata Conference. Despite severe economic deprivation, the country was still able to prioritize and maintain population health during the Special Period of the 1990s.

A study of Cuba's health system can guide other countries in achieving better population health despite scarcity (Table 13.1). However, there are limits to the Cuban object lesson. Cuba's unique sociopolitical context with a revolutionary footing and populist leadership has been a principal factor in its success. It is also important to acknowledge lingering questions about the accuracy of Cuban health statistics. Despite these caveats, faith in Cuba's health statistics is not a prerequisite for curiosity about the principal features of Cuba's health system. Remarkable achievements include universal coverage of all health services, an extensive health workforce, and integration of civilian committees as participants in public health (Hirschfeld 2006; Kath 2007).

Table 13.1. Comparison of selected Cuban and American health indicators

Indicator	Year	Cuba	United States
Life expectancy at birth male/female (years)	2016	77/81	76/81
Total expenditure on health as percentage of gross domestic product (%)	2014	11.1	17.1
Number of under-5 deaths (thousands)	2015	1	27
Infant mortality rate (probability of dying between birth and one year of age per 1,000 live births)	2015	4.3 [4.1, 4.4]	5.7 [5.4–5.9]
Number of infant deaths (thousands)	2015	1	23
Under-5 mortality rate (probability of dying by age 5 per 1,000 live births)	2015	5.6 [5.4, 5.8]	6.6 [6.4–6.9]
Maternal mortality ratio (per 100,000 live births)	2015	39 [33, 47]	14 [12–16]
Hospital beds (per 10,000 population)	2014	52	29

Note: Table reflects most up-to-date data from the World Health Organization. Data are reported to WHO by each country's governmental agencies (Editor 2016).

Sociocultural, Political, and Economic Background

> What we are trying to do is to solve the problems of society the cheapest way possible. But we are not designing programs to reduce medical costs, but to improve people's health.
> —*Fidel Castro*

Developments in the health care system during two periods in Cuba's history are the focus of this chapter. The 1959 Revolution marked the inception of efforts to transition Cuba from a capitalist to a socialist country, as Fidel Castro overthrew the former president, Fulgencio Batista. In 1961, Cuba was officially declared a socialist state and became a close ally of the Soviet Union; Cuba supported the Soviet Union against the United States during the Cold War and in turn received financial, military, and technical support (Whiteford and Branch 2008). As a result of Cuba's newfound alliance, the United States imposed an embargo on Cuban trade and cut diplomatic ties with the country (Whiteford and Branch 2008). After the fall of the Soviet Union, Cuba fell into a deep economic crisis otherwise known as the Special Period (1990s), which was further exacerbated by the US embargo because it limited potential trading partners—particularly among its immediate neighbors (Andaya 2009).

Health care was not a prominent platform of the revolution—Castro only mentions "health care" once in his famous "History Will Absolve Me" speech of 1954. Yet in the 1960s, the revolutionary government took several steps to address the population's health and education needs. Cuba was faced with a mass emigration of professionals—the majority of the medical faculty and half of the island's physicians fled following the revolution (Shapiro 2012). At this time, the health care system was also organized such that medical care outside of the major cities was practically nonexistent (Lambe 2012). With good reason to be discontented with the inequity and questionable quality of health care on the island, Fidel and the Cuban government focused on health as a defining characteristic of its socioeconomic and political reform (Brotherton 2012). The revolution's health principles were as follows (*Editorial* 1976):

1. the health of the population is a government responsibility,
2. health services should be available to everyone in the population,
3. the community should actively participate in health, and
4. preventive and curative health services must be integrated.

Government commitment to improving health was reflected in national budgets. A larger than average portion of the Cuban gross domestic product is spent on health, especially when compared to that of developing and developed countries (Kuntz 1994; Marrero 2000; Garrett 2010; Shapiro 2012). Moreover, this allocation was maintained even when the country was financially challenged during the Special Period of the 1990s. For example, in 1982, 7.8% of the national budget was invested in health (Perez-Stable 1985). During the height of the Special Period in 1994, 7.5% of the budget was allocated to health and in 2000 11% was invested in health; between 1994 and 2000, this percentage steadily increased (Erikson et al. 2002).

These budgetary allocations emerged from Cuba's exceptional politics. But the Cuban social context also bears on its health system. As a result of being a resource-limited country, informal practices among citizens have emerged in order to meet the basic needs of everyday life (Brotherton 2008; Jenkins 2008). Black market, family, and social networks have become commonplace vehicles for finding resources and making life work with limited incomes. Despite being a socialist state for the past fifty years, there are distinct class differences, which cultivate hierarchal power relations within communities (De Vos 2009; Garrett 2010). Even though having a health care degree in

Cuba does not offer a high income by international standards, enrollment in health professions offers advancement in social class. Individual physicians embrace an ethos of service to their community and their country that reinforces the honor and respect afforded to their station in society. Their social position also helps them cope with life in Cuba despite physician salaries hovering between $12 and $25 dollars per month in 2002 (Thomas 2016).

Finally, a specifically Cuban trait is the extent to which the government exerts social control. As a socialist state, the government maintains a broad consensus that the state is responsible for the well-being of the Cuban citizens. The consensus includes the understanding that sacrifices of individual freedoms and suppression of private initiative are an acceptable and even expected price of social provision. Other countries that lack this social understanding of the state's role simply cannot contemplate some of the policies that Cuba has established. This is not to say that individuals in Cuba willingly sacrifice all of their freedoms and privacy. For instance, patients censor their discourse with doctors to avoid any mention of political and social dissent because they recognize that doctors are agents of the state (Hirschfeld 2006). Additionally, social groups such as the Comités de Defensa de la Revolución (Committees in the Defense of the Revolution, or CDR) or Federación de Mujeres Cubanas (Federation of Cuban Women, or FMC) lend themselves tremendously to community-based strategies in developing the health system but also serve as the eyes and ears of the government in the local communities. This surveillance in neighborhoods would be unacceptably intrusive in other societies but was made possible in Cuba by the revolutionary principles that privilege the state's objectives over individual rights (Whiteford and Branch 2008). The Cuban government is able to circumscribe actions of their more prominent figures in the interest of public health and safety. Even though Castro incorporated a lit cigar into his persona, other role models have been prohibited from smoking publicly (Guttmacher 1987).

With the caveat that Cuba's socialist society is exceptional, the remainder of this chapter systematically examines how Cuba put the basic principles of PHC announced in the Alma-Ata Declaration into practice. The discussion aims at revealing both the universal principles of implementation as well as attention to Cuba's particular enabling features.

Panel: Medical Diplomacy

Castro's firm belief in "salud para todos," or health for all, is not limited to the Cuban island. Cuba's medical education model is interesting because tuition is free for both Cuban students and their foreign underprivileged counterparts (Chan 2009; Feinsilver 2011; Keck 2012). In return for free education, foreign students are expected to work with the most vulnerable populations in their respective countries upon graduation. Similarly, Cuban students work in remote areas of the island or get deployed to another country to support or even help build medical infrastructure (Huish 2008). As a result, Cuba has aided approximately 107 other countries in both short-term and long-term emergencies, built medical schools in the Middle East and Africa, and trained doctors from around the world (Feinsilver 2011). While it is evident that Castro's belief of health as a human right was a pillar of these foreign expeditions, medical diplomacy was also a huge asset for the Cubans. Though lacking medical supplies and money, Cuba was able to provide other countries with human capital since the island was graduating a growing number of health professionals following the revolution (Huish 2008). As a result, medical diplomacy helped Cuba garner support from the majority of United Nations countries in condemning the United States embargo (Feinsilver 2011). Additionally, it proved to be economically beneficial since wealthier nations such as Venezuela provided Cuba with oil priced significantly lower than the market rate (Feinsilver 2011).

Integrated Systems Giving Priority to Those in Need

> The needs of the collective significantly outweigh the needs of the few.
> —*Fidel Castro*

Following the 1959 Cuban Revolution, Castro was tasked with reconciling the disparity between the urban and rural areas with regard to accessibility of health services (Keck 2012). Before the Cuban Revolution in 1959, the majority of those living in remote areas had little or no access to basic health services (Newell 1975; *Editorial* 1976). To illustrate this disparity, the average life expectancy in 1953 in Havana was 62.7 years, whereas that of more rural provinces was 58.8 years (Lambe 2012). Similarly, Havana had 9.6 hospital beds per 1,000 people, while other provinces had between 1.9 and 2.7 beds per 1,000 (Lambe 2012). Thus, the revolution brought about the greatest impact in rural areas (Newell 1975; Younge 1982; Whiteford and Branch 2008).

Today, Cuban doctors and clinics can be found in the most remote areas on the island, which can be attributed to two facets of the Cuban medical education (Erwin 2015). First, the Cuban medical curriculum teaches stu-

Table 13.2. Differentials in mortality and contraceptive use in Cuba

	Urban	Rural
Proportion of mothers reporting child ever died[1]	2.22%	2.07%
Proportion of women reporting use of oral contraception[2]	71.92%	75.10%

Note: Tabulation based on MICS data (United Nations Children's Fund 2014).

[1] Urban versus rural child mortality experience was not statistically significantly different in age-adjusted comparison using a weighted logistic regression and five-year age dummies.

[2] Urban contraceptive prevalence was not statistically significant in an age-adjusted comparison using a weighted logistic regression and five-year age dummies.

dents that the duty of the doctor is to help others, especially those who are financially disadvantaged (Kirk 2011). Second, Cuban medical students are required to spend two years working in primary care community clinics, otherwise known as *consultorios*, before they are allowed to further pursue their medical specialties (Souers 2012; Erwin 2015) (table 13.2).

Consultorios and Home Visits

All health-related services in Cuba are free, which allows even the most impoverished residents access to care (Newell 1975). Cuban consultorios have changed the way in which populations receive continuous care. They are the gateway to medical care in Cuba and are essentially small clinics that are staffed by a doctor and a nurse. This team is required to live in close proximity, often above or next to the clinic, so that they can provide medical attention at any time. Living in the community provides a significant advantage for the doctor and nurse team, as they are able to better understand the larger problems challenging the community. The Ministry of Public Health has placed consultorios such that they each serve about 500 to 700 individuals or 120 to 150 families (Hirschfeld 2006). The lack of bureaucratic intermediaries such as a secretary or billing specialist within the consultorios allows for direct communication between the patients and their providers, creating a more informal environment of direct access. Patients stop by to clarify paperwork, check prescriptions, and even to say hello (Hirschfeld 2006). In addition to creating a relaxed atmosphere, this direct communication helps the provider team to foster strong relationships with the families they care for. Consultorios' social aspect makes them the basis of surveillance for illnesses as well as the social determinants of illness. Providers' extensive interactions with families allow them to see how social and environmental stressors are contributing to and affecting health.

Typically, the doctor and nurse team are in the consultorio during the earlier half of the day. In the afternoon, the team conducts visits *a terreno*, meaning home visits. The provider team is required to make two home visits to each family home in their respective area each year (Brotherton 2012). However, if a family member in a particular household is suffering from a chronic disease or is hindered from physically coming in to the clinic, the provider team will visit that person more frequently in his or her home (Keck and Reed 2012). In addition to patient comfort, home visits are also economically advantageous in that in-home care frees up hospital beds and diminishes the cost of admitting patients (Brotherton 2012).

Bottom-Up, Community-Engaged Planning, Organization, and Control

Following the revolution, social groups were formed to target different populations including women, men, and schoolchildren (Brotherton 2012). Most of the population belongs to the committees for the CDR and the FMC (Swanson et al. 1995). These social groups are an extension of the government in the citizen community, and they are all under the direction of the state (Donate-Armada 1996).

Each CDR zone, often defined by an apartment building or a neighborhood block, has its own CDR group. The CDR group has five people in charge: a president, a public health officer, a cultural officer, a vigilance officer, and the secretary/treasurer. The president orchestrates all of the different activities, maintains responsibility for the functioning of the entire CDR chapter, and works closely with other leadership team members. The public health officer is specifically involved in mobilizing the CDR for different health promotion activities. The cultural officer coordinates birthday celebrations, holidays, and other social gathering activities within the zone to cultivate strong relationships among members. The vigilance officer is tasked with making sure that everything is functioning appropriately and that rules are not being broken. The leadership team of the CDR is elected by the people in that CDR (Donate-Armada 1996). If a new person is appointed to one of these positions, there is a communal effort by the more seasoned CDR leaders to help orient the newer leader. CDR presidents from neighboring zones also meet approximately once a month and collaborate by sharing their experiences. In order to join a CDR, one must be 18 years old and pay a nominal fee of three Cuban pesos. Approximately 8 million out of the 11.5 million Cubans on the island participate in their local CDR (Granma 2017).

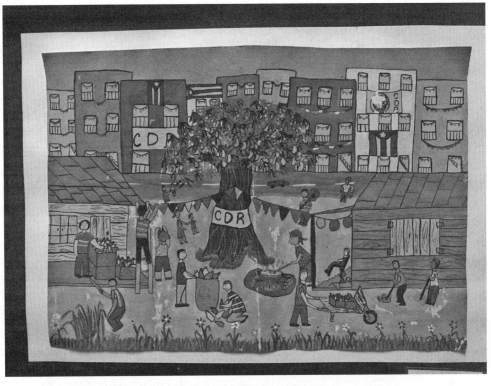

Figure 13.1. Artwork from the National Museum of the Committee for the Defense of the Revolution in Havana depicting the role of CDR in a neighborhood.

While it is not mandated, members are encouraged to attend monthly meetings and participate in the CDR's programming. Figure 13.1 shows a child's drawing of the multiple things the CDR volunteers do to control litter and maintain public spaces.

At inception, the CDRs were implemented in neighborhoods to detect dissidence, project state control into residential areas, and consolidate power by controlling the local rationing of state food provision programs (Donate-Armada 1996). The role and purpose of the CDR has evolved and softened since the revolutionary period; it now works as a mobilizing group to address the community's needs. Today's CDRs play a role in local public health, education, volunteer work, defense, citizen security, and other social activities (Guttmacher 1987; Hernandez et al. 1991). Since CDR leadership teams live and conduct CDR programming in their respective zones, they get to know the different families. This heightened familiarity and trust between the CDR leadership team and their member families helps CDR leaders across the island encourage participation in programming and to carry out the tasks mandated by the government.

The CDR's first foray into health was a large-scale immunization campaign (Newell 1975). Polio was eliminated in Cuba in the early 1960s by conducting a seventy-two-hour vaccination campaign as CDR members worked with physicians to ensure that everyone in their zone was vaccinated (Brotherton 2012). This coordinated effort helped Cuba eliminate polio long before the United States. Similarly, CDR leaders have been critical in facilitating public health campaigns such as blood drives since they maintain registries of blood donors (Guttmacher 1987; Younge 1982). In 1962, during the missile crisis, the Ministry of Public Health wanted to organize blood drives to have blood on supply in case of an emergency. CDR chapters were mobilized, and the leadership team succeeded in getting eight thousand Cubans to give blood within a ten-day period (Brotherton 2012). These blood drives and immunization campaigns required the CDR leaders to accompany the doctors who were carrying out the campaigns in order to gather baseline and epidemiological data to track participation (Swanson et al. 1995). The CDR leaders are able to work closely with health care workers since the Ministry of Public Health trains CDR chapters to work with staff in polyclinics for disease surveillance purposes (Keck and Reed 2012). This surveillance is twofold because in addition to routine disease surveillance, CDR chapters are also required to evaluate the competence of the medical teams that they work with (Keck and Reed 2012).

CDRs also promote sanitation by cleaning up neighborhoods, transforming empty lots into vegetable gardens, repairing broken water pipelines, and removing animals and other disease-carrying vectors (Newell 1975; Terris 1989; Almaguer et al. 2005). For mosquito control, CDRs encourage members to clean standing water from their neighborhoods, take garbage directly to the dumps, and recycle local materials (Kuntz 1994; Stewart 2006; Spiegel et al. 2008). Following an outbreak of dengue fever, CDR chapters combed gardens and yards to remove water-holding plants to eliminate potential breeding sites for dengue fever vectors following a government edict, which outlawed such plants (Whiteford and Branch 2008). In addition, CDRs can coordinate with specialist vector control teams who might be better able to detect breeding grounds for mosquitoes. Consistent with their role as quasi-public health districts, CDR chapters lead disaster preparedness training and organize evacuation plans for emergencies (De Vos et al. 2009).

It is also worth mentioning that the CDR is supported and works closely with the National Assembly of People's Power, which is the legislative parliament of Cuba. Specifically, the National Assembly of People's Power relies on the People's Councils, which are extensions of the People's Power at the municipal and provincial levels. Those on the People's Councils are called *delegados*, and there are at least five delegados elected by those in their municipality. According to Article 75 of the Cuban Constitution, delegados are required to coordinate and ensure cooperation among existing entities within municipalities. Deemed an organ of the People's Power, delegados are supposed to exercise their power order to satisfy the economic, health, cultural, and other needs of their area (Government of Cuba 2018).

In summary, the CDR, with the help of delegados, works in bridging the citizenry to the health care providers and enables participation in addressing and assessing the health needs of the community (De Vos et al. 2009). Each local CDR agenda is set in part by national authorities, but there is substantial leeway for local community initiative and priority-setting (Thomas 2016).

Epidemiologically Relevant, Community-Based Strategy

The doctor and nurse home visits to every patient in their area transcends the typical role of the health care provider (Franco et al. 2013). When the provider team visits a household, they take the form in table 13.3 with them. In the first part of the chart, under the heading "Dirección," the provider team records each household member's name, sex, age, date of birth, level of education, and occupation. In addition to the demographics, the provider team also must record the category of risk (Group I-IV) they believe the family member falls into depending on the status of that person's health. Group I individuals are thought to be healthy and free of concerning risk factors; Group II individuals have risk factors but are not sick; Group III individuals have been diagnosed as sick; and Group IV individuals are disabled or handicapped (Suárez et al. 2014). Finally, the physician has a space at the bottom of the document to record any other notes pertaining to the consultation. The next portion of the chart allows the provider team to record when they had visited the family to make sure that each family has been visited the requisite number of times.

In the next portion of the chart, titled "Característica Higiénicas," the provider team records the day of the visit and assesses the hygiene of the family home. The provider team inspects the water supply and notes the presence of pools of still water, garbage, prevalent disease vectors, animals, and the general condition of the household and the area surrounding the dwelling. The team then also assesses the social and economic factors of the household, including the financial situation of the family and the dynamics of the family both inside and outside of the household. If the provider team notices

Table 13.3. Home visit sheet (MOD 54-50)

MOD 54-50
Ministry of Public Health

Family Clinical History

Address:

	Demographics						Health Problems					
ID	Name	Sex	Age	Date of Birth	Education Level	Occupation	Group I	Group II	Group III	Group IV	Risk Factors	Treatment Plan
1												
2												
3												
4												
5												
6												
7												
8												
9												

Month	Jan	Feb	Mar	Apr	May	Jun	Jul	Aug	Sept	Oct	Nov	Dec

Hygienic Characteristics

Date	Water Supply	Residual Liquids	Garbage	Vectors	Domestic Animals	Condition of Housing	Environmental Factors	IND HAH

Socioeconomic Factors

Date	Sanitary Culture	Social Integrations	Family Function	Economic Situation

Observations

anything that may not be delineated on this sheet but is likely complicit in risking or harming the health of the family, the team records it in the comments section. Following the assessment, the provider team then counsels the family on how to improve their health by improving their built environment and behaviors. For example, if a family has garbage strewn all over the household, the family would be counseled on how garbage can be a breeding ground for disease, which can be deleterious to their health.

When necessary, the physician and nurse team may involve the local government representative delegado and CDR chapters. For example, if the doctor and nurse notice that there are many potential breeding spots for mosquitoes while they are on a home visit, they will ask the local government representative delegado and the CDR chapter to coordinate a fumigation of that housing unit. Likewise, if they notice that many people in their area are coming in to the consultorio with mosquito-borne disease, they will also contact the delegado and CDR chapters to organize fumigations.

Population-Level Responses

As defined in the Alma-Ata Declaration, PHC was far more than clinical primary care, since it required that population-level threats to health be addressed. Cuba's health system has maintained attention to macro-level health policies in response to crises. Following the revolution, the population was severely malnourished, which led the country to develop the dairy, beef, and egg industries to introduce more animal protein–rich foods to the population (Guttmacher 1987). In order to establish new dietary habits and support the newly flourishing dairy system, for example, all school-age children were receiving a liter of milk per day (Younge 1982). The Cuban agricultural industry faced setbacks in the 1990s, when there was a shortage of imported petroleum and replacement parts for outdated Soviet agricultural technology (Brotherton 2012). Decreased food production drastically altered the levels of nutrition (especially intake of folic acid and vitamin B12). This came to light in the form of an epidemic of nutrition-related neuropathy (Kuntz 1994). Public health officials responded in 1993 by distributing a multivitamin supplement to all Cubans (Kuntz 1994). Milk rations were also reallocated during this time to focus scarce dairy products on children up to 5 years of age, pregnant women, and the elderly (Swanson et al. 1995). More recently, in 2009, Cuba worked with United Nations Children's Fund to combat high rates of iron deficiency, by increasing the fortification of different foods and administering iron supplements to women of reproductive age and young children (Perez 2009).

There have been other population-level interventions to better lifestyle habits as well. In order to encourage heightened physical activity in communities, most secondary schools built after the revolution are equipped with athletic facilities that are open to the whole community (Marrero et al. 2000). In addition to increased physical culture for youth, these public resources allow physicians to manage hypertension by prescribing exercise and thus preventing complications and sparing scarce resources and costly medications (Whiteford and Branch 2008). Population-level interventions extend to social capital creation as well. Grandparent Circles were created to provide health promotion activities to reduce the need for medications among the elderly (Swanson et al. 1995). Grandparent Circles provide the elderly with peer social interaction, daily exercise activities, and hypertension management assistance.

Multisectoral Approach and Development

Dr. Juan Piedra, Cuba's former director of public health, acknowledged that the roles of the sectors outside of public health are critical to achieving health outcomes and that intersectoral cooperation would not be as effective if the government as a whole was not as keen on improving health (Kath 2007). This chapter has already covered how schools were used for exercise promotion and how the agricultural sector responded to malnutrition; this section delineates how additional sectors coordinate their efforts to improve health outcomes.

The largest portion of the Cuban budget is allocated toward the education system (Garrett 2010). Education in Cuba is mandatory up until ninth grade, and all levels of education (primary, secondary, university, postgraduate) are free. Free medical education allows students to learn medicine without experiencing the financial burden of tuition. Thus, with decreased barriers to entry to medical school, Cuba protects against a physician shortage and ensures a constant flow into the health care workforce (Huish and Kirk 2007; Keck 2016). Free and mandatory education has helped Cuba achieve universal literacy, which has simultaneously advanced health literacy since Cuba's school systems are integrated with a health approach (Newell 1975; *Editorial* 1976; Kuntz 1994; Almaguer et al. 2005). In other words, the Cuban educational program integrates health education into the curriculum to teach students about health risk factors and how to avoid them (Almaguer et al. 2005). Many textbooks, for example, convey anti-smoking messages through anti-smoking imagery (Guttmacher 1987). The high levels of literacy, but more specifically health literacy, facilitate the population's understanding and

Table 13.4. Zika indicators in Cuba and neighboring countries

Country	Incidence Rate	Autochthonous Cases		Number of Imported Cases
		Suspected	Confirmed	
Cuba	1.64	0	187	58
USA	.06	0	227	5,885
Cayman Islands	460.34	237	30	11
Jamaica	284.01	7,772	203	0
Haiti	27.12	2,995	5	0

Note: Data as of January 1, 2018 (Pan American Health Organization and the World Health Organization 2018).

interpretation of different health messages and campaigns (*Editorial* 1976). Unlike other countries, what is interesting about the transmission of such messages and campaigns in Cuba is that billboards, newspapers, television, and radio are all government controlled (Whiteford and Branch 2008). In other words, health promotion advertisements do not compete for airtime with other commercial advertisements. Therefore, these are all vehicles for the government to promote health and reach different populations on the island. In fact, it is quite common to find billboards on the island that encourage people to wash their hands, save water, breastfeed, and participate in community groups (Whiteford and Branch 2008). It is also common to see didactic advertisements on television that teach people how to effectively sanitize drinking water and how to detect infant dehydration.

Recently, Cuba implemented very strong Zika prevention efforts. In response to the high prevalence of Zika cases in neighboring countries, the national alert for Zika was declared in December 2015 before any cases had actually been detected (Castro et al. 2017). Following the WHO guideline for Zika control, Cuba magnified vector control, surveillance, and training of health professionals, risk communication, and resource mobilization. As a result of strong preventive efforts, Cuba has fared better with Zika than some of its neighboring countries and the United States (table 13.4).

Panel: Vector Control

Mosquito control in Cuba is methodical and well staffed. There are about thirty thousand field workers throughout the country who conduct entomological surveillance, larval source reduction, adult mosquito control, health education, and enforcement of mosquito control legislation (Perez et al. 2013). The headquarters of these units can be found throughout the country. The number of control units in a particular area is dependent on the population density. (For example, there are more control units within the capital of Havana.) Control teams are required to inspect different areas of their assigned region every day to look for vectors and sources of possible vectors and to fumigate as needed. If the control team, local CDR chapter, or consultorio identifies a vector-borne illness outbreak, the vector control team will use thumbtacks to mark the outbreak on the paper maps in their office. Then, they will coordinate with local governments and CDR leaders to fumigate the area. As proactive as these units are, the fumigation machines are severely outdated and emit black fumes and harsh odors that could be detrimental to the fumigators, who lack appropriate protective gear, and the residents whose apartments are being fumigated. Figure 13.2 shows a photo of fumigation for vector control in Havana in 2018.

Auxiliary Workers

Following the revolution, polyclinics were implemented to expand outpatient care and decentralize services traditionally provided by hospitals (Brotherton 2012). They are more advanced than a consultorio but less advanced than a large hospital. Polyclinics are staffed with a doctor and nurse team as well as a social worker, epidemiologist, hygienist, and psychiatrist (Younge 1982). Distributed equally throughout the country, polyclinics are able to provide comprehensive care to the populations they serve (Guttmacher 1987). Specifically, polyclinics offer four basic kinds of services: (1) curative and preventive clinical services, (2) environmental services such as hygiene and sanitation, (3) community health services such as health campaigns, and (4) social services (Brotherton 2012). Data from the Cuban Ministry of Public Health indicate that the majority of outpatient and emergency doctors' visits take place at the polyclinics instead of in a hospital (Keck and Reed 2012) (figure 13.3).

Closing Remarks

The Cuban health model was an archetype for the PHC approach promoted at the Alma-Ata Conference. Since Alma-Ata, the Cuban government has been able to sustain this approach to health despite a serious economic crisis and the growing demand by its citizens for increasingly costly health care treatments and pharmaceuticals.

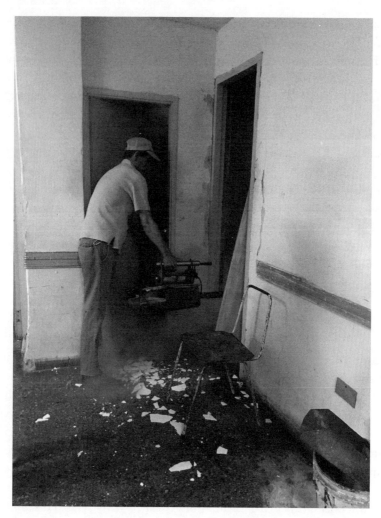

Figure 13.2. Demonstration of a fumigation.

There remains a lot of room for improvement for the Cuban public health system. To some extent, a great deal of time, energy, and resources in Cuba are invested in fortifying the primary care setting. Cuban children still succumb to acute diarrheal cases due to regions that still lack adequate sanitation (Terris 1989). Cuba's population could benefit from further improving liquid and solid waste management and implementing healthier diets. Some of the changes require substantial capital investments that have not been prioritized. Macroeconomic constraints, including the US embargo, play an important role.

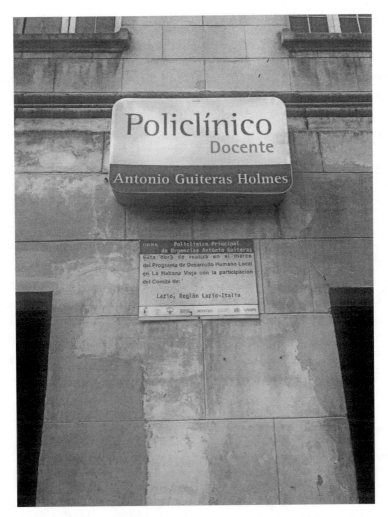

Figure 13.3. Polyclinic in Havana.

Like many other countries, Cuba is faced with an epidemiological transition from communicable to chronic diseases as well as an aging population (Hernandez et al. 1991; Shapiro 2012). Since the CDR structure is so influential within communities, its role can be further utilized to promote health. Exercise and blood pressure management are among some of the many social behaviors that could be influenced by watching one another in a CDR group. Moreover, the generation of epidemiological data in the consultorios and vector control facilities remains weak simply because the data is kept on paper records and is not yet digitized.

This chapter has refrained from endorsing Cuba's PHC approach as the cause of Cuba's exceptional health statistics. The validity of Cuba's high life expectancy and low infant mortality has been called into question by data showing that Cuba is an extreme outlier in the ratio of high fetal deaths to low infant deaths (Gonzalez 2015). Subtle pressure on attending physicians to code the demise of a live birth as a fetal death as well as promotion of abortions for high-risk pregnancies could be skewing health statistics (Hirschfeld 2006; Geloso and Gilbert 2017). Until a full set of age-specific mortality rates is released for external demographic analysis, the truth about Cuba's life expectancy remains unverified.

However, Cuba's PHC system is absolutely remarkable. Few health systems are able to provide annual home visits or to orient a medical workforce to record proximal and social determinants of ill health. Few health systems are able to achieve functional operation of a system of community-level committees that concern themselves regularly with sanitation, hygiene, and community social determinants of health. Few health systems integrate health into agricultural and education policy. Cuba has done all this and sustained it with a cultural priority for health as a civic responsibility. Cuba is testament to the viability and reality of comprehensive PHC as a path taken, which has been transformative in creating a people-centered system of health promotion and health care.

REFERENCES

Almaguer, M., R. Herrera, J. Alfonso, C. Magrans, R. Manalich, and A. Martinez. 2005. "Primary health care strategies for the prevention of end-stage renal disease in Cuba." *Kidney Int Suppl* 2005 (97): S4–S10.

Andaya, E. 2009. "The gift of health: Socialist medical practice and shifting material and moral economies in post-Soviet Cuba." *Med Anthropol Q* 23 (4): 357–374.

Brotherton, P. S. 2008. "We have to think like capitalists but continue being socialists": Medicalized subjectivities, emergent capital, and socialist entrepreneurs in post-Soviet Cuba." *Am Ethnol* 35 (2): 259–274.

———. 2011. *Health and health care: Revolutionary Period (Cuba)*. Charles Scribner's Sons.

Castro, M., D. Pérez, M. G. Guzman, and C. Barrington. 2017. "Why did Zika not explode in Cuba? The role of active community participation to sustain control of vector-borne diseases." *Am J Trop Med Hyg* 97 (2): 311–312.

Chan, M. 2009. *Remarks at the Latin American School of Medicine, Havana, Cuba*.

De Vos, P., W. De Ceukelaire, G. Malaise, D. Pérez, P. Lefèvre, and P. Van der Stuyft. 2009. "Health through people's empowerment: A rights-based approach to participation." *Health Hum Rights* 11 (1): 23–35.

Donate-Armada, M. 1996. "Sociedad Civil, Control Social y Estructura del Poder en Cuba." *Cuba in Transition*, ASCE, 283–299.

Editor. 2016. *Global health observatory country views*. Geneva: World Health Organization.

"Editorial: Alternative approaches to meeting basic health needs in developing countries." 1976. *Med J Aust* 1 (23): 857–858.

Erikson, D., A. Lord, and P. Wolf. 2002. *Cuba's social services: A review of education health, and sanitation*. Washington, DC: Inter-American Dialogue.

Erwin, P. C. 2015. "Public health and Cuba: Trading on a two-way street." *Am J Public Health* 105 (Suppl. 4): S561–S562, S559–S560.

Feinsilver, J. 2012. "Health and health care: Medical diplomacy and international medical education." In *Cuba*, edited by Alan West-Durán, 488–493. Detroit: Gale Cengage Learning.

Franco, M., et al. 2013. "Population-wide weight loss and regain in relation to diabetes burden and cardiovascular mortality in Cuba, 1980–2010: Repeated cross sectional surveys and ecological comparison of secular trends." *BMJ* 346 (7903), https://doi.org/10.1136/bmj.f1515.

Garrett, L. 2010. "Castrocare in crisis: Will lifting the embargo make things worse?" *Foreign Aff* 89 (4): 61–73.

Geloso, V., and B. Gilbert. 2017. *The paradox of good health and poverty: Assessing Cuban health outcomes under Castro*. SSRN. https://papers.ssrn.com/sol3/papers .cfm?abstract_id=2962742.

Gonzalez, R. M. 2015. "Infant mortality in Cuba: Myth and reality." *Cuban Stud* 43:19–39.

Government of Cuba. 2018. *Ley de los Consejos Populares* [Law of the Popular Councils]. Havana: Government of Cuba. http://www.parlamentocubano.gob.cu /index.php/documento/ley-de-los-consejos-populares/.

Granma. 2017. *Declaración de los Comités de Defensa de la Revolución*, in *Granma*. http://www.granma.cu/cuba/2017-06-23/declaracion-de-los-comites-de-defensa-de-la -revolucion-23-06-2017-22-06-55.

Guttmacher, S. 1987. "The prevention of health risks in Cuba." *Int J Health Serv* 17 (1): 179–189.

Hernandez, R., et al. 1991. "Political culture and popular participation in Cuba." *Latin Am Perspect* 18 (2): 38–54.

Hirschfeld, K. 2006. *Sociolismo and the underground clinic: The informal economy and health services in Cuba*. Association for the Study of the Cuban Economy. https:// www.ascecuba.org/asce_proceedings/sociolismo-and-the-underground-clinic-the -informal-economy-and-health-services-in-cuba/.

Huish, R. 2008. "Going where no doctor has gone before: The role of Cuba's Latin American School of Medicine in meeting the needs of some of the world's most vulnerable populations." *Public Health* 122 (6): 552–557.

Huish, R., and J. M. Kirk. 2007. "Cuban Medical Internationalism and the Development of the Latin American School of Medicine." *Latin Am Perspect* 34 (6): 77–92.

Jenkins, T. M. 2008. "Patients, practitioners, and paradoxes: Responses to the Cuban health crisis of the 1990s." *Qual Health Res* 18 (10): 1384–1400.

Kath, E. 2007. "Inter-sectoral cooperation, political will and health outcomes: A study of Cuba's Maternal–Infant Health Programme." *Policy Polit* 35 (1): 45–64.

Keck, C. W. 2016. "The United States and Cuba—Turning enemies into partners for health." *N Engl J Med* 375 (16): 1507–1509.

Keck, C. W., and G. A. Reed. 2012. "The curious case of Cuba." *Am J Public Health* 102 (8): e13–22.

Kirk, E. J. 2011. "Operations miracle: A new vision of public health." *Int J Cuban Stud* 3 (4): 366–381.

Kuntz, Diane. 1994. "The politics of suffering: The impact of the US embargo on the health of the Cuban people. Report to the American Public Health Association of a fact-finding trip to Cuba, June 6–11, 1993." *J Public Health Policy* 15 (1): 86–107.

Lambe, J. 2012. "Health and medical care: Pre-1959." In *Cuba*, edited by Alan West-Durán, 474–478. Detroit: Gale Cengage Learning.

Marrero, A., et al. 2000. "Towards elimination of tuberculosis in a low income country: The experience of Cuba, 1962–97." *Thorax* 55 (1): 39–45.

Newell, K. W. 1975. "Health by the people." *WHO Chron* 29 (5): 161–167.

Pan American Health Organization and World Health Organization. 2018. *Zika cases and congenital syndrome associated with Zika virus reported by countries and territories in the Americas 2015–2018 cumulative cases.* https://www.paho.org/hq /dmdocuments/2017/2017-jan-18-phe-ZIKV-cases.pdf.

Perez, R. 2009. "The public health sector and nutrition in Cuba." *MEDICC Rev* 11 (4): 6–8.

Perez, D., P. Lefèvre, M. Castro, M. E. Toledo, G. Zamora, M. Bonet, and P. Van der Stuyft. 2013. "Diffusion of community empowerment strategies for Aedes aegypti control in Cuba: A muddling through experience." *Soc Sci Med* 84:44–52.

Perez-Stable, E. J. 1985. "Community medicine in Cuba." *J Community Psychol* 13 (2): 124–137.

Shapiro, E. R. 2012. "Health and health care: Introductions." In *Cuba*, edited by Alan West-Durán. Detroit: Gale Cengage Learning.

Souers, J. M. 2012. "Cuba leads the world in lowest patient per doctor ratio: How do they do it?" Social Medicine Portal, https://www.socialmedicine.org/2012/07/30/about /cuba-leads-the-world-in-lowest-patient-per-doctor-ratio-how-do-they-do-it/.

Spiegel, J. M., et al. 2008. "Promoting health in response to global tourism expansion in Cuba." *Health Promot Int* 23 (1): 60–69.

Stewart, J. 2006. "Housing and health in Havana, Cuba." *J R Soc Promot Health* 126 (2): 69–71.

Suárez, P. E., L. Suárez Isaqui, E. Troya Borges, and J. Martínez Abreu. 2014. "La evaluación médica en la atención primaria de salud." *Rev Méd Electrón* 36 (2): http://scielo.sld.cu/scielo.php?script=sci_arttext&pid=S1684-18242014000200013.

Swanson, K. A., et al. 1995. "Primary care in Cuba: A public health approach." *Health Care Women Int* 16 (4): 299–308.

Terris, M. 1989. "The health status of Cuba: Recommendations for epidemiologic investigation and public health policy." *J Public Health Policy* 10 (1): 78–87.

Thomas, J. G. 2016. "Historical reflections on the post-Soviet Cuban health-care system, 1992–2009." *Cuban Stud* 44 (1): 189–213.

United Nations Children's Fund. 2014. *Cuba MICS.* https://mics.unicef.org/surveys.

Whiteford, L. M., and L. G. Branch. 2008. *Primary healthcare in Cuba: The other revolution.* Lanham, MD: Rowman and Littlefield.

Younge, R. G. 1982. "Health care: Lessons from China and Cuba." *J Natl Med Assoc* 74 (4): 391–395.

CHAPTER FOURTEEN

Health for All in the Twenty-First Century

Lessons for the Next Forty Years of Implementing Primary Health Care

MEIKE SCHLEIFF AND DAVID BISHAI

Since 1978, many countries have taken the comprehensive multisectoral, community-led, equity-focused primary health care (PHC) vision of Alma-Ata to heart and as a reality. The preceding chapters have described these efforts across time, across cultural and political contexts, and from different perspectives. In 2018, the Astana Conference on Primary Health Care rededicated leaders of the world's health systems to make comprehensive PHC the foundation upon which to achieve universal health coverage (UHC) (World Health Organization 2018). Participants at both Alma-Ata and Astana Conferences agreed on a vision of PHC that insisted on promotive, preventive, curative, and rehabilitative aspects of the health system—not just financing and delivering (primary) sickness care. In this final chapter, we synthesize some of the takeaway messages and suggest some priorities and opportunities for the coming years.

One of the main goals of this book has been to correct the common misimpression that the comprehensive PHC declarations of Alma-Ata and Astana have been primarily idealistic aspirations. The cases we purposively selected aim to describe different approaches in different contexts to engage communities and address health and social determinants of health within local populations as well as at scale as part of the overall health system of a country. The stories of Bangladesh, Ethiopia, Nepal, Ghana, Sri Lanka, Vietnam, and Cuba all show that the vision of Alma-Ata has been a viable strategy that has led to *sustainable, scalable* good health at low cost. This is an irony. Proponents of selective interventions met in Bellagio in 1979 under a banner of "good health at low cost" to convince global health leaders to depart from comprehensive PHC in order to be "practical." Under a premise that urgent needs mandated deferring comprehensive approaches, the selective interventions emphasis on global health was launched and labeled as "an interim strategy" (Walsh and Warren 1979) to achieve the most lives saved for the least amount of money. This is false economy.

This book shows clearly that low-income countries can marshal the resources to build functional platforms that engage citizens and local health workers in understanding and supporting the multiple policy changes that are required to alter the upstream social genesis of ill health. At the same time, selective disease control interventions are indeed effective. Programs that promote vaccinations, malaria control, human immunodeficiency virus (HIV) treatment, tuberculosis control, and so on effectively mobilize billions of dollars of global financing that has saved millions. There never should have been a perceived contest between vertical disease control and horizontal public health systems. None of the country case studies in this book refrained from implementing vertical disease control programs or deferred them because their strategy had emphasized a systems strengthening approach. As stated clearly by Svea Closser in chapter 4, comprehensive PHC makes disease control programs easier to support and operate.

Although horizontal approaches pave the way for vertical disease control programs to succeed, the reverse may not always be true. It is too easy for health policy to devolve into an alphabet soup of acronyms for all the disease control programs vying for the attention of the health ministry. An array of vertical programs staffed by narrow specialists is not comprehensive PHC and does not routinely evolve into comprehensive PHC. Sometimes, however, disease control programs can evolve this way, with leadership, a supportive context, and a clear strategy. The case of Ghana (chapter 10) shows how what was originally a regional vitamin A distribution project using community health workers (CHWs) morphed over the course of a decade into comprehensive PHC that scaled up nationally.

An exclusive focus of the health sector on delivering and paying for medical care (whether primary medical care or other) often crowds out policy attention focused on engaging other elements of society, such as schools, law enforcement, agriculture, public works, and transport, from rising to the vision of comprehensive PHC.

There is a fundamental asymmetry shown in figure 14.1.

Vertical approaches that equate health policy with the masterful allocation of funds to various disease control packages do not automatically lead to horizontal community platforms that help citizens and local health workers become the ongoing solution to arising health threats. Comprehensive PHC

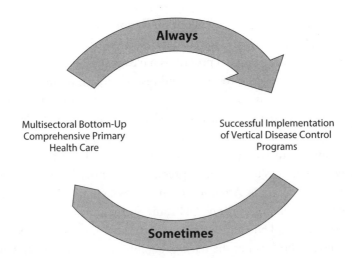

Figure 14.1. Asymmetric relationship between horizontal programs on the right supporting vertical approaches but not always vice versa.

is a deliberate choice and not a natural consequence of disease control efforts. Countries had to choose and champion strong comprehensive PHC. Their choice required political will to raise and allocate funds toward PHC activities rather than toward hospital-centric health system plans. With comprehensive PHC comes the ability to mobilize and "pull" vertical programs into the population. Comprehensive PHC programs such as those in Cuba, Nepal, and Ethiopia generated a workforce of CHWs who were trusted because they came from the community and were also trained to provide valued services to those communities. Public health leaders can implement public health cycles to engage whole communities in the genesis of shared solutions, as described in chapter 3. A public health cycle requires conducting assessments of health threats followed by participatory policy development and the assurance of solutions delivered and paid for across multiple sectors of government and private enterprise.

Chapter 1 opened with a review of the historical challenges obstructing the path to implementation of PHC approaches due to (1) lobbying and pressure for specific, vertical, and contained interventions; and (2) political and financial dynamics, nationally and globally. Critical aspects and holistic approaches to furthering the mission of health for all have emerged and matured. While having a strong PHC foundation has been a consistent feature in the health systems of countries that are able to produce improvements in population health, being able to maintain adequate resources and commitment to this unglamorous component of many health systems has been problematic (chapter 2). While there is growing appreciation for the potential of comprehensive PHC systems to complement vertical programs such as polio eradication, in practice vertical programs have repeatedly crowded out PHC systems due to their ability to reveal and resolve urgent needs for commodity delivery. If a health commodity (e.g., zinc or an antiviral) is urgently needed, then it is a demonstrable result to have delivered it regardless of how. Resources gravitate to programs that can show short-term results.

Investments in distributing drugs and products related to a single issue have appeal to donors and agencies pressed to quantify immediate progress toward targets and goals. Attention to integrated, comprehensive PHC systems will be essential to achieving UHC, the Sustainable Development Goals (SDGs), and the implementation necessary to fulfill the Astana Declaration. Attentiveness to PHC is not the natural equilibrium of a health system, and the countries discussed in this book required deliberate effort by dedicated and perceptive leaders to develop and support PHC models.

There are specific implementable strategies that countries can use to build up "muscles" in comprehensive PHC. These include: (1) developing the workforce to deliver core public health and PHC services, (2) using principles of community organizing and coalition-building to engage multiple stakeholders, (3) creating the political will as well as clear strategies to enable scale-up of PHC structures such as CHW programs and different modes of services delivery in communities, and (4) building and honing the case for how a strong PHC system supports the rest of the health system—including the goals of various vertical programs.

Chapter 3 outlined the use of workforce capacity development built around measuring the performance of essential public health functions. Report cards that are accompanied by supervisory coaching can assist workers in being mindful of their own professional development as data-driven community organizers. One of the foci for integration of PHC into the rest of health systems is the utilization and support for human resources—from CHWs to physicians—who are able to deliver integrated packages of services and mobilize and engage communities when given appropriate training, supervision, and support. CHWs in particular have a unique and essential role in this bridging or interface function. Recently, more attention has been paid to concerns about economic hardship, exploitation, and gender for CHWs, leading to advocacy for professionalization, payment, and higher status of CHW cadres (Maes et al. 2014, 2015a, 2015b). CHW cadres have diverse expectations, workloads, and competing opportunities for economic and social advancement, so supporting their professionalization remains a context-specific undertaking without a one-size-fits-all solution (Cometto et al. 2018). Nepal's female community health volunteers have been largely uncompensated. In Ghana and Ethiopia, more and more CHWs are being compensated.

Chapter 6 offered several field-based examples of the type of community organizing that is the basis of comprehensive PHC. The acronym SALT (stimulate and support; appreciate, authenticity; listen, learn, link; and transfer, team, trust, and transform) has been put into practice in many contexts to build partnerships in the health system. What is constant across contexts is the necessity of community buy-in and a widely perceived value of the CHWs and PHC tier of the health system. This requires an ongoing dialogue between communities and the health system to adapt priorities, address challenges, build trust, and celebrate successes (Rigoli and Dussault 2003; Molyneux et al. 2013).

The second half of this book relayed country experiences related to institutions and structures that helped PHC go to national scale. Government policies have been critical, but comprehensive PHC does not occur by edict. Successful governments have built social spaces and a facilitating workforce congenial to multiple stakeholder involvement in health policy. Governments have also drawn upon, included, and greatly valued the experience, resources, and collaboration of donors, implementing partners, health workers, communities, and other stakeholders. Exemplars in this kind of institution strengthening include Ethiopia, Cuba, Vietnam, and Ghana. Variations, such as Bangladesh's system that relied heavily on nongovernmental organizations for service provision parallel to a public sector framework, have also proven effective as long as there is a healthy partnership and communication process in place.

PHC continues to gain traction (Bryant and Richmond 2008; Shi 2012; Chou et al. 2012; Cometto et al. 2018). It retains relevance because it can fundamentally support all other programs and goals of a health system. Rather than being prone to duplication or siphoning off of human resources—as vertical programs have tended to be—PHC aims to establish relationships, structures, processes, evidence, and engagement that can support an ever-evolving set of programs needed to meet population demand. For example, Ghana, Vietnam, and Cuba as well as recent efforts of the Global Polio Eradication Initiative have aimed to manage communicable diseases and specific health improvement goals through investing in Integrated Management of Childhood Illness, sanitation, and other preventive and integration-oriented approaches. In addition, these investments in prevention, education, and behavior change are more and more clearly essential to improving maternal and child health outcomes (as in polio) and addressing emerging issues within the SDG targets, including noncommunicable diseases (NCDs) and other rising contributors to ill health. Further, there are increasing efforts to integrate disease-oriented programs—such as HIV, tuberculosis, and malaria as well as polio eradication—into PHC systems, though this is not yet done consistently.

The country cases in part II illustrate the diversity of social, political, and cultural environments that were receptive to the pursuit of bottom-up approaches to multisectoral, participatory, and prevention-oriented solutions. Bangladesh and Vietnam particularly emphasized self-reliant communities. Governments with a socialist perspective also facilitated the integration of these strategies. Direct engagement of communities, as was achieved in Ethiopia and Ghana, has also created social support and essential buy-in for PHC systems. The Comprehensive Rural Health Project in Jamkhed has been historically famous for doing exactly this as well, and its work has informed India's accredited social health activist and Anganwadi worker programs, though the fully developed philosophy has not consistently scaled across the country (Arole and Arole 1994).

Emerging Themes for Primary Health Care after Astana

The current social and epidemiological landscape looks quite different from that pondered by global leaders and communities in 1978 at Alma-Ata. To name a few of the health-related changes that are now central but were peripheral or largely unconsidered a few decades ago: Double burden of disease and rising chronic disease rates across the world, climate change, migration, urbanization, and changes in population demographics all present complex and pressing concerns for the health of populations. Many of the country cases described in this book are actively working to address these challenges. Bangladesh is facing imminent threats of climate change and managing migration and the needs of refugees. Ethiopia is grappling with a growing urban population and change in the disease profile. Vietnam is also facing serious climate change threats. All countries are having to look closely at their populations' knowledge and awareness level and the information they can access, largely instantly, via media and technology. Remote populations are now using data to navigate the services offered by the health system. The role of the health workforce is shifting from being a sole source of health information to being a checkpoint for accurate and appropriate information and also in building the capabilities to respond to the changing—and generally increasing—demands of a more informed, globalized clientele.

What Is Needed Going Forward in the Twenty-First Century?

As we look toward the coming decade and beyond, the challenges are daunting and awe-inspiring. The opportunities are also exciting and hope-inducing. Focusing on utilizing and channeling the tools, evidence, resources, and momentum that are available and continually being developed further to create the desired outcomes and impact is the next great phase of work. The Astana Declaration and accompanying operational framework (World Health Organization and United Nations Children's Fund 2018) both recognize diversity in the contexts that will implement PHC. This diversity requires national—and subnational—adaptation of the PHC strategy. It requires national and subnational buy-in. Political will to sustain the level of investment and attention necessary to strengthen PHC across the world can come from a growing realization that bottom-up PHC is essential for sustainable success. The polio eradication experience is testament to this. Comprehensive PHC is a philosophy and a set of strategies and criteria for building political will and engaging communities for better public health across the board. As pointed out in chapter 3, the public health cycle underlies PHC and brings data-informed community deliberation of policies and execution based on shared collective resources.

Furthermore, meaningful community engagement is critical in order to make the essential linkage within PHC between community realities that need to be understood and addressed, and the rest of the health system that is needed to support PHC. Importantly, such engagement cannot be merely a token or symbolic kind of engagement but must truly enable community voices, hear their stories, and determine possibilities for joint responses and action (Jewkes and Murcott 1998; Morgan 2001; Head 2007). Many countries have invested a great deal in these structures and processes, including Bangladesh, Cuba, Ethiopia, and Ghana. Chapter 6 outlined a stepwise approach to engage and involve community members in the understanding and solution of local health concerns.

The financing of health systems and PHC also looks quite different than it did forty years ago. Health services are becoming more sophisticated and rapidly expensive as care needs shift toward management of chronic diseases and in response to populations' rising demands for additional curative services—as has happened in Ethiopia, Bangladesh, and many other countries.

At the same time, international development assistance—at least from the United States—has stagnated in recent years (USAID 2019). Although many countries—particularly middle-income countries and those with strong government plans oriented toward health and societal well-being—have resources of their own to invest, large new investments will be needed in the coming years in order to progress toward the SDGs. As much as an additional $371 billion per year is needed to reach ambitious SDG targets (Stenberg et al. 2014, 2017). In a polarizing global political climate, building shared understanding for what resources are needed, mobilizing those resources, and then allocating them toward PHC could be a great challenge. Many are now looking to low- and middle-income countries—who have a duty to ensure the health of their populations—to set an example of establishing policies and criteria for adequate and equitable financing for health, including allocation of domestic resources (Rottingen et al. 2014). While this is necessary and appropriate, similar pressure and accountability for external financing is necessary: to ensure that high-income countries contribute to global public goods and help countries not yet able to bear the full cost of their health systems, and that they do so in a way that is transparent, coordinated, and supportive of recipient country policies and priorities (Rottingen et al. 2014).

The history of PHC is woven together by a lineage of thinkers, leaders, and inspiring personalities (captured in chapter 1) whose philosophies and actions have demonstrated what is possible and also what is required to achieve the vision of health for all. We will need future generations of leaders whose vision matches the complexity and scale of the barriers to achieving PHC goals and who dedicate themselves with equal fervor, humbleness, and compassion as those who have come before them.

Closing Thoughts

In the decades since Alma-Ata, we have accumulated vastly more experience, models, and evidence for why comprehensive PHC is important, in large part thanks to the many country- and local-level efforts to adapt and implement the definition of PHC in their own contexts. The 2018 conference in Astana, which commemorated the fortieth anniversary of the Alma-Ata Declaration, brought forward the same core themes but with additional granularity about where investment is needed and how to proceed toward health for all in the SDG era. The cases in this book described countries that are investing in the core elements of PHC in order to be able to address some of the underlying dynamics and determinants rather than just symptoms and short-term outcomes. The seven core elements were all laid out in Article VII of the original 1978 Alma-Ata Declaration:

1. pay attention to the sociocultural, political, and economic background;
2. address local epidemiology with promotive, preventive, curative, and rehabilitative services accordingly;
3. respond at the population level as well as provide individual services;
4. use a multisectoral approach;
5. maximize community and individual self-reliance in organizing and controlling the health system;
6. integrate systems, giving priority to those in need; and
7. include multiple counterparts (auxiliary workers).

(The full original text of Article VII is given as an annex in table 14.1.)

Table 14.1. ANNEX Article VII of the Alma-Ata Declaration

Primary health care:

1. reflects and evolves from the economic conditions and sociocultural and political characteristics of the country and its communities and is based on the application of the relevant results of social, biomedical, and health services research and public health experience;
2. addresses the main health problems in the community, providing promotive, preventive, curative, and rehabilitative services accordingly;
3. includes at least: education concerning prevailing health problems and the methods of preventing and controlling them; promotion of food supply and proper nutrition; an adequate supply of safe water and basic sanitation; maternal and child health care, including family planning; immunization against the major infectious diseases; prevention and control of locally endemic diseases; appropriate treatment of common diseases and injuries; and provision of essential drugs;
4. involves, in addition to the health sector, all related sectors and aspects of national and community development, in particular agriculture, animal husbandry, food, industry, education, housing, public works, communications, and other sectors, and demands the coordinated efforts of all those sectors;
5. requires and promotes maximum community and individual self-reliance and participation in the planning, organization, operation, and control of primary health care, making fullest use of local, national, and other available resources, and to this end develops through appropriate education the ability of communities to participate;
6. should be sustained by integrated, functional, and mutually supportive referral systems, leading to progressive improvement of comprehensive health care for all and giving priority to those most in need; and
7. relies, at local and referral levels, on health workers, including physicians, nurses, midwives, auxiliaries, and community workers, as applicable, as well as traditional practitioners as needed, suitably trained socially and technically to work as a health team and to respond to the expressed health needs of the community.

The authors of the Alma-Ata Declaration had experience in addressing the perpetual challenge of aligning diverse stakeholders across many different contexts with different jargon, numerous and sometimes competing priorities, and constantly shifting targets and aspirations. Some of the countries that implemented the Alma-Ata Declaration faced severe disagreements about their political order. Bangladesh, Vietnam, Nepal, and Sri Lanka all had civil wars that preceded a top-level commitment to comprehensive PHC. Cuba had a socialist revolution before embarking on this path. However, other countries, like Ethiopia and Ghana, as well as Thailand (not covered in this book), chose to endorse PHC because their initial experiences with that approach were persuasive. Thanks to the authors of the preceding chapters, more public health leaders can now know enough about what to do to make a strong argument for comprehensive PHC and strategies that work to implement the approach. In order for more people to achieve health for all and the SDGs, readers can share these chapters and write their own. It will be our own collective action that keeps making health for all a reality.

REFERENCES

Arole, M., and R. Arole. 1994. *Jamkhed: A comprehensive rural health project.* Jamkhed, India: Shri Samarth Printers.

Bryant, J., and J. Richmond. 2008. "Alma Ata and primary health care: An evolving story." In *International encyclopedia of public health*, edited by Stella Quah, 152–174. Oxford: Elsevier.

Chou, V. B., I. K. Friberg, M. Christian, N. Walker, and H. B. Perry. 2017. "Expanding the population coverage of evidence-based interventions with community health workers to save the lives of mothers and children: An analysis of potential global impact using the Lives Saved Tool (LiST)." *J Glob Health* 7 (2): 020401.

Cometto, G., N. Ford, J. Pfaffman-Zambruni, E. A. Akl, U. Lehmann, and B. McPake. 2018. "Health policy and system support to optimise community health worker programmes: An abridged WHO guideline." *Lancet Glob Health* 6 (12): e1397–e1404.

Head, B. 2007. "Community engagement: Participation on whose terms?" *Aust J Polit Sci* 42 (3): 441–454.

Jewkes, R., and A. Murcott. 1998. "Community representatives: Representing the 'Community'?" *Soc Sci Med* 46 (7): 843–858.

Maes, K., S. Closser, and I. Kalofonos. 2014. "Listening to community health workers: How ethnographic research can inform positive relationships among community health workers, health institutions, and communities." *Am J Public Health* 104 (5): e5–e9.

Maes, K., S. Closser, E. Vorel, and Y. Tesfaye. 2015a. "Using community health workers." *Ann Anthropol Pract* 39 (1): 42–57.

———. 2015b. "A women's development army: Narratives of community health worker investment and empowerment in rural Ethiopia." *Stud Comp Int Dev* 50 (4): 455–478.

Molyneux, S., D. Kamuya, P. A. Madiega, T. Chantler, V. Angwenyi, and P. W. Geissler. 2013. "Field workers at the interface." *Dev World Bioethics* 13 (1): https://doi.org/10.1111/dewb.12027.

Morgan, L. M. 2001. "Community participation in health: Perpetual allure, persist, challenge." *Health Policy Plan* 16 (3): 221–230.

Rigoli, F., and G. Dussault. 2003. "The interface between health sector reform and human resources in health." *Human Resourc Health* 1 (1): https://doi.org/10.1186/1478-4491-1-9.

Rottingen, J.-A., T. Ottersen, A. Ablo, D. Arhin-Tenkorang, C. Benn, R. Elovainio, D. Evans, L. Fonseca, J. Frenk, D. McCoy, and D. McIntyre. 2014. *Shared responsibility for health: A coherent global framework for health financing: Final report of the Centre on Global Health Security Working Group on Health Financing.* London: Royal Institute of International Affairs.

Shi, L. 2012. "The impact of primary care: A focused review." *Scientifica* 2012:432892.

Stenberg, K., J. Axelrod, P. Sheehan, I. Anderson, A. M. Gulmezoglu, and M. Temmerman. 2014. "Advancing social and economic development by investing in women's and children's health: A new global investment framework." *Lancet Health Policy* 383:1333–1354.

Stenberg, K., O. Hanssen, T. T. Edejer, M. Bertram, C. Brindley, A. Meshreky, J. E. Rosen, J. Stover, P. Verboom, and R. Sanders. 2017. "Financing transformative health systems towards achievement of the health Sustainable Development Goals: A model for projected resource needs in 67 low-income and middle-income countries." *Lancet Glob Health* 5 (9): e875–e887.

USAID. 2019. "Foreign Aid Explorer: Trends." Washington, DC. https://explorer.usaid.gov/aid-trends.html.

World Health Organization. 2018. "Declaration of Astana." Geneva, Switzerland. https://www.who.int/docs/default-source/primary-health/declaration/gcphc-declaration.pdf.

World Health Organization and United Nations Children's Fund. 2018. Primary health care: Transforming vision into action: Operational framework. https://extranet.who.int/dataform/292923?lang=en.

CONTRIBUTORS

Prior to his death in 2018, Frank K. Nyonator, MD, MPH, was a valued colleague and contributor to chapter 10.

Onaopemipo Abiodun is a PhD student at the Johns Hopkins Bloomberg School of Public Health, studying international health with a focus on health systems. Previously an analyst with Abt Associates and an intern with Jhpiego, she has several years of experience conducting program evaluations, primary health care systems research, and health financing research for the provision of health services in Nigeria, Côte d'Ivoire, and other low- and middle-income countries.

Vinya Ariyaratne, MD, is president of the Sarvodaya Shramadana Movement. Dr. Ariyaratne also serves as the director general of the newly established Sarvodaya Institute of Higher Learning and as a board member of Sarvodaya Development Finance, the economic empowerment arm of the Sarvodaya Movement. He is a past president of the College of Community Physicians of Sri Lanka. Dr. Ariyaratne obtained his MD degree from De La Salle University in the Philippines and his MPH degree from Johns Hopkins University.

John Koku Awoonor-Williams, MD, MPH, MPP, PhD, is the director of the Policy, Planning, Monitoring and Evaluation Division of the Ghana Health Service in Accra. He was formerly the Upper East regional director of health services and director of health services in the Nkwanta District of the Volta Region. Dr. Awoonor-Williams was the founding National CHPS coordinator and coprincipal investigator of GEHIP. He is currently the Ghana Health Service coprincipal investigator of CHPS+. Dr. Awoonor-Williams holds an MD degree from Minsk State University, an MPH from Leads University, an MPP from the Ghana Institute of Management and Public Administration, and a PhD in epidemiology from the University of Basel.

Kedar Prasad Baral, MBBS, MPH, is a professor at Patan Academy of Health Sciences and the director of the MPH program. He received his MBBS from Tribhuvan University Institute of Medicine, Nepal and his MPH from Royal Tropical Institute, the Netherlands. He started his career in 1979 as a health assistant, then as a primary health care worker, before attending medical school and completing his MPH. He has worked for Nepal's national health system and has been involved in policy processes, working with bilateral and multilateral agencies in different capacities. Later, he joined an academic faculty and also served as rector. He is involved in researching major public health issues of national interest, including the search for causes of and possible strategic options to reduce health disparity through the appropriate training of physicians and public health professionals, preparing them to work in rural areas and for disadvantaged populations.

Ayaga A. Bawah, MA, PhD, is a senior lecturer at the Regional Institute for Population Studies at the University of Ghana. As a scientist of the Navrongo Health Research Centre, he led the Navrongo Demographic Surveillance System. Dr. Bawah was a Population Council Bernard Berelson Fellow, an assistant professor of public health at Columbia University, and the senior research scientist at INDEPTH, an international network of demographic surveillance sites. He has an MA and PhD in demography from the University of Pennsylvania, and MA degrees in demography from the University of Ghana. Dr. Bawah was director of research for GEHIP and is coprincipal investigator of CHPS+.

Pedro Más Bermejo is a physician with dual specialties in epidemiology and public health. He is emeritus research scientist at the Tropical Medicine Institute "Pedro Kourí," emeritus member of the Cuban Academy of Sciences, and full professor of epidemiology and public health at the National School of Public Health in Cuba. He received his PhD from Charles University Prague, Czech Republic, and did postdoc training at the Liverpool School of Tropical Medicine in the United Kingdom. He has published five books and more than seventy papers, primarily dealing with epidemiology and public health. He is an editorial board member of the *Journal of Public Health Policy* and the *MEDICC Review Journal* as well as an adjunct professor of the School of Public Health and Tropical Medicine at Tulane University.

Fred N. Binka, MD, MPH, PhD, is a professor at the University of Health and Allied Sciences in Ho, Volta Region, Ghana. He was the founding vice chancellor of the University of Health and Allied Sciences, founding executive director of the INDEPTH Network, and founding director of the Navrongo Health Research Centre in Navrongo, Upper East Region, Ghana. Dr. Binka was the principal investigator of the Navrongo Community Health and Family Planning Project. He has an MD from the University of Ghana, an MPH in epidemiology from Hebrew University in Jerusalem, and a PhD in epidemiology from the University of Basel.

David Bishai, PhD, MPH, MD, is a professor at Johns Hopkins University's Bloomberg School of Public Health. He received his PhD in health economics from the Wharton School of Business at the University of Pennsylvania. He holds an MPH from UCLA and an MD from UC San Diego. He is a fellow of the American Academy of Pediatrics and a fellow of the American College of Physicians. In 2015, he was voted by students to receive the Golden Apple teaching award as well as awards for advising and mentoring. He was elected president of the International Health Economics Association in 2015. He has published more than two hundred peer-reviewed papers and keeps extensive collaborations with coauthors in China, Taiwan, Thailand, Myanmar, India, Bangladesh, Pakistan, Nepal, Sri Lanka, Egypt, Qatar, Lebanon, Iran, Uganda, Botswana, Mozambique, Ethiopia, Brazil, Russia, Mexico, Italy, Switzerland, the United Kingdom, and the United States.

Carolina Cardona is a research assistant at the Bill and Melinda Gates Institute for Population and Reproductive Health at the Johns Hopkins Bloomberg School of Public Health. Her work focuses on the economics of public health, and her main areas of research are economic demography and the economics of fertility and family planning. Prior to joining the Bloomberg School of Public Health, Ms. Cardona worked for the Bolivian Ministry of Planning and Development, conducting research related to maternal and child health. She holds a master's of health science in health economics with a focus on international health and is completing a PhD in health economics in the Department of Population, Family and Reproductive Health at the Johns Hopkins Bloomberg School of Public Health.

Dennis Carlson is a medical doctor who also studied behavioral sciences at Berkeley and was a fellow in the History of Medicine department at Johns Hopkins University. He was the dean of the Public Health College in Gondar, Ethiopia, from 1963 to 1967. In 1986, he became the director of the Save the Children Federation, assisting in famine relief and redevelopment of the primary health care program in Yifatena Timuga Awraja. Concurrently, from 1989 to 1994, he also held a faculty position in the Faculty of Medicine at Addis Ababa University. Since then, he has been a senior advisor and consultant to many projects and programs in Ethiopia, including those on public health training; perinatal, infant, and maternal health; and household nutrition.

Chala Tesfaye Chekagn is currently working at the Ministry of Health as senior health system strengthening advisor. Prior to his current position, he worked as a senior public health advisor of the Strengthening Ethiopia's Urban Health Program at John Snow, Inc. He has also served as assistant director of the Health Extension Program and primary health care at the Ministry of Health. He has extensive experience working in several health programs at different levels, ranging from program officer to team leader over the past nine years. He is a public health specialist by educational background.

Hoang Khanh Chi, BA, MPH, PhD, has been working as a lecturer and researcher in the Department of Health Policy and Integration at Hanoi University of Public Health in Vietnam since 2003. She holds an MPH from Mahidol University and a DrPH from the University of Queensland, as well as an undergraduate law degree from Phuong Dong University. Her great passion is sharing knowledge and skills with people who are going to serve the community and work in health policy and systems. She has been teaching in the area of health policy, health policy communication, and global health.

Svea Closser is an associate professor at Johns Hopkins University's Bloomberg School of Public Health. Her research focuses on the interaction between global health policy and local health systems. In her current project, funded by the Fulbright/Nehru Program, she is studying the work experiences and social relations of female community health workers in India. She is the author of *Chasing Polio in Pakistan* and has published many research articles. She is also coeditor of the textbooks *Understanding and Applying Medical Anthropology* and *Foundations of Global Health*.

Luc Barrière Constantin is one of the cofounders of the Constellation, as well as a member of the board, and was recently nominated as a voting member of the organization. Constantin's current main focus is the development of partnerships, projects, and programs for the dissemination of the SALT/CLCP approach; research and development of the approach; and training of new facilitators and coaches. Constantin is a medical doctor by training and holds an MPH in epidemiology and international public health from the Johns Hopkins Bloomberg School of Public Health. After a few years of working in private practice and with MSF France in the field, he spent most of his career with UNICEF and UNAIDS, where he had the opportunity to share and strengthen his experience in many African countries and in various situations. Before retirement, he was posted as senior planning and operation advisor at the UNAIDS headquarters in Geneva, Switzerland.

Zufan Abera Damtew is a senior policy and health systems strengthening advisor at EngenderHealth in Ethiopia. She has also worked at different levels and in various positions in the health care system of Ethiopia for more than twenty years. She has served as deputy director general for the Armauer Hansen Research Institute and as director of the Health Extension and Primary Health Service directorate at the Ministry of Health of the Federal Democratic Republic of Ethiopia. The Health Extension Program is a community-based health service that is designed to expand health service delivery to all portions of the community and to improve the health status of Ethiopians. Prior to joining the Federal Ministry of Health, she worked at the health bureau of the Amhara Region in a similar program. She has also served as a health service provider, trainer, and mentor for young health professionals and health managers. She has a BSc in nursing and an MPH. She holds a PhD from the University of Oslo. Dr. Damtew has published more than fifteen papers in different international and national journals, with her research focusing mainly on community health or the Health Extension Program of Ethiopia.

Marlou de Rouw is a cofounder of Constellation for AIDS Competence. Since 2007, she has been the manager of the Constellation Global Support Team, in charge of the daily business of the organization. As a member of the Constellation's coaching teams, she has facilitated group processes related to issues such as aging with dignity, cohousing, family life, and strength-based integration of refugees. Prior to the Constellation, she worked as a journalist at various newspapers in the Netherlands and on the Local Response Team of UNAIDS. De Rouw holds a bachelor's degree in journalism from Hogeschool voor de Journalistiek in Tilburg, Netherlands, and a master's degree in cultural anthropology (with a specialty in intercultural communication) from Universiteit Utrecht.

Nadia Diamond-Smith is an assistant professor in the Department of Epidemiology and Biostatistics and the Institute for Global Health Sciences at the University of California–San Francisco. She works primarily on issues related to women's status and empowerment as well as maternal and child health outcomes in South Asia. This includes research on newly married women and access to nutrition in Nepal, the quality of family planning and abortion services in India, and the evaluation of several interventions, including with community health workers, in India. She uses mixed methods approaches, based in a demographic perspective, and the level of focus of her work is mostly at the household level. Diamond-Smith received her PhD in the Population, Family and Reproductive Health Department at the Johns Hopkins Bloomberg School of Public Health and her master's degree from the London School of Hygiene and Tropical Medicine.

Philip Forth is currently the chair of the board of the Constellation for AIDS Competence, a nonprofit organization based in Belgium. The Constellation was formed in 2005 to respond to the AIDS pandemic. Since its founding, the Constellation has facilitated local responses in more than fifty countries, through more than one hundred partnerships with governments as well as national and international organizations. During the life of the Constellation, Dr. Forth's work has concentrated on the development and application of the Community Life Competence Process, a methodology that allows communities to take ownership of a wide variety of challenges that are frequently health related. In addition, Dr. Forth has more than thirty years of experience in the development and application of knowledge management approaches in a wide variety of sectors around the world. Dr. Forth holds a BA in physics from Oxford University and a PhD in geophysics from the Durham University.

Mignote Solomon Haile is a public health professional with a background in research and evaluation and health systems strengthening. She currently works at Abt Associates, a global research firm focusing on qualitative research methods, health finance, and program implementation, with the goal of promoting the use of evidence-based programming to improve access to quality health services at an affordable cost. Haile holds a bachelor's degree in biology from Mount Holyoke College and a MSc in public health from Johns Hopkins University.

Nguyen Thanh Huong is an associate professor at Hanoi School of Public Health and has nearly thirty years of experience in teaching, researching, and providing consultancy in the public health field. She is vice rector of the Hanoi University of Public Health. Huong has been coordinating and involved in a number of research projects at the Hanoi University of Public Health as well as in collaboration with other partners, particularly focusing on the areas of health policy and systems and health promotion interventions. She has also served as a national consultant for a number of international agencies, such as UNFPA, UNICEF, WHO, ADB, USAID, GIZ, and various INGOs, as well as for the Ministry of Health in Vietnam.

Taufique Joarder holds a DrPH from the Department of International Health at the Johns Hopkins Bloomberg School of Public Health, where he is currently serving as an associate faculty member. He is the research director of USAID's Multisectoral Nutritional Programming through Implementation Science Activity at FHI 360's Bangladesh Office. His areas of interest and expertise include health policy and systems, human resources for health, medical anthropology, mixed methods research, implementation science, and psychometrics.

Alice Kuan is an undergraduate at Johns Hopkins University pursuing degrees in public health and economics. She has gained experience through the Bloomberg American Health Initiative in community organizing around local health solutions, explored the global health landscape with the nonprofit PATH, and has collaborated internationally on various projects related to the global campaign for the fortieth anniversary of the Alma-Ata Declaration. Invested in learning about the dynamic relationship between health and economics, Kuan aspires to help countries deliver solutions more efficiently and build stronger bridges between governments and communities.

Seblewengel Lemma is a research fellow in health management information systems at the London School of Hygiene and Tropical Medicine based at the Ethiopian Public Health Institute. She has worked for more than ten years in Ethiopian health systems in different capacities. Much of her career was as a teacher and researcher at the Addis Continental Institute of Public Health, a research and training institute where she ascended to the position of assistant professor. She worked as a research officer for the International Institute for Primary Health Care for a little more than a year before assuming her current position at the London School of Hygiene and Tropical Medicine. Right after receiving her bachelor's degree in public health, she worked as a health service provider and manager at the primary health care level in Ethiopia. She received her MPH in epidemiology from Addis Ababa University's School of Public Health and holds a PhD in public health from the University of Gondar. She has published more than twenty scientific papers in international peer-reviewed journals.

Sasmira Matta graduated from Johns Hopkins University with degrees in applied mathematics and statistics, and public health. She worked as an intern and a consultant for UNICEF during her undergraduate career. At Johns Hopkins, she developed simulations for the Teaching Vaccine Economics Everywhere curriculum and analyzed performance, monitoring, and accountability datasets to assess the impact of the quality of family planning services on modern contraception prevalence in sub-Saharan Africa. She will complete her MHS degree in health economics at the Bloomberg School of Public Health in 2019 and plans to conduct more research on domestic and international health systems.

Ahmed Moen is an associate professor in the Health Sciences department at Howard University. He holds a master's in health administration from the University of Michigan and MPH and DrPH degrees from Johns Hopkins University. He has managed and directed programs in Ethiopia, including the material eradication initiatives and Medical Service Ethiopia. He also consulted with Johns Hopkins, USAID, and the World Bank. He is a founder of the Committee for Peace in Ethiopia and a member and leader of the American Public Health Association.

Rituu B. Nanda has twelve years of experience in community engagement, research, monitoring and evaluation, and knowledge management. She has a master's degree in contemporary history and a certification in public health. She is currently pursuing her second master's in evaluation from the University of Saarland. Nanda has been a long-term consultant with the Constellation, IDS (Sussex), and the Institute of Social Studies Trust. She has facilitated the SALT strength-based approach to community engagement in public health, including in immunization; HIV; and patient-centered response to NCDs, TB, WASH, aging, substance abuse, and so on. Additionally, she has incorporated the SALT approach in evaluation and participatory action research. Nanda brings a gender and equity lens into her work. This includes teaching a blended learning course on gender transformative evaluation, working as a member of the EvalGender+ Management Group, and moderating an international community of practice on gender and evaluation.

Ferdous Arfina Osman, PhD, is a professor of public administration at Dhaka University. She received her PhD in public policy and administration from the University of Manchester under the Commonwealth Scholarship Plan. She did her postdoctoral research at Johns Hopkins University under the Fulbright Visiting Scholar Program. Dr. Osman has published extensively in academic journals at home and abroad on issues and areas relevant to public policy and governance. Her book *Policy Making in Bangladesh: A Study of the Health Policy Process* was published in 2004. Her major research focus includes public policy, health policy, governance, and public management.

Claudia Pereira, PhD, MS, is an associate professor at Fundação Oswaldo Cruz (Fiocruz), National School of Public Health, Department of Health Administration and Planning, Brazil. Prior to joining Fiocruz, she was a postdoctoral fellow at the Johns Hopkins Bloomberg School of Public Health, in the Department of Population, Family and Reproductive Health, working on health economics research. She has worked as a consultant for the Inter-American Development Bank, Jhpiego, Johns Hopkins University, the Minas Gerais state government, and the Pan American Health Organization, and has experience in population health and health systems strengthening in Angola, Mozambique, Botswana, Suriname, and Peru. Pereira holds a PhD in population health with an emphasis in health economics from the University of Wisconsin–Madison; an MS in demography from CEDEPLAR, Universidade Federal de Minas Gerais, Brazil; and a BA in economics from the same university.

Henry B. Perry, MD, PhD, MPH, has almost five decades of engagement in global community health work that has covered a broad range of activities, including program implementation, program leadership, and collaborations with government officials, nongovernmental organizations, academics, donors, and international organizations. He is the author of more than two hundred publications— articles in scientific journals, book chapters, books, and other documents that have been distributed widely. His teaching and mentoring of students has been widely acclaimed, resulting in numerous awards. His massive open online course on Coursera, Health for All through Primary Health Care, has reached more than sixty thousand people around the world.

James F. Phillips, MS, PhD, is a professor in the Heilbrunn Department of Population and Family Health at the Columbia University Mailman School of Public Health. Prior to joining the Columbia faculty, he was a senior associate of the Population Council with collaborative support responsibilities for implementation research directed toward health systems development initiatives in the

Philippines, Bangladesh, Ghana, Nigeria, and Tanzania. He has served as an advisor to the CHPS Initiative and is currently principal investigator for CHPS+. Dr. Phillips has a PhD in demography from the University of Michigan and an MS in population studies from the University of Hawaii.

Meike Schleiff is an assistant scientist in the health systems program of the International Health Department at the Johns Hopkins Bloomberg School of Public Health. She has worked extensively with communities and young leaders in Haiti through the GROW project, the nonprofit that she cofounded with Haitian colleagues, and has also been engaged in community development planning, implementation, evaluation, and training in Guyana, Ugandan India, and the Appalachian Region of the United States. She has experience working in a variety of settings on projects ranging from disaster response to entrepreneurial loan programs to building primary health care infrastructure in collaboration with local governments and communities. She conducted her doctoral dissertation research in West Virginia, USA, assessing the rural health workforce's history, current capacity, and remaining gaps and opportunities for improving community-based health in the state. She is committed to building capacity and motivation globally for community health issues, mentoring young health and community development professionals, and advancing systems thinking and health systems research training opportunities.

Melissa Sherry, MPH, CPH, is the director of population health innovation and transformation at Johns Hopkins HealthCare in Baltimore, Maryland, and works both internationally and domestically to design effective and evidence-driven population health management strategies. In this role, Ms. Sherry specializes in building population health programs that engage communities and address the social determinants of health through improved alignment between communities, health care payers, and the health care delivery system, with a goal of improving health outcomes while managing health care costs. Ms. Sherry has more than ten years of experience working on population health and public health strengthening initiatives, including work in Africa, the Middle East, and Europe. Ms. Sherry holds an MPH degree with a focus on international health systems and a certificate in global health, and is completing a PhD in the Department of Health Policy and Management at the Johns Hopkins Bloomberg School of Public Health.

Rita Thapa is an alumnus of the Johns Hopkins Bloomberg School of Public Health. She represented Nepal in Alma-Ata and is pioneer chief of Nepal's Family Planning Maternal Child Health, & Primary Health Care Project and a former WHO first woman director of health systems and community health for the Southeast Asia Region. She currently serves as founding chairperson of the Bhaskar Memorial Foundation and is engaged in research influencing primary cardiovascular disease and noncommunicable disease risk behaviors among school adolescents. Upon her return from WHO, she served as policy advisor to the Minister of Health in Nepal. She is a recipient of Life Time Awards from the Nepal Public Health Foundation and Perinatal Society of Nepal, including several national and international decorations.

Kebede Worku is a physician by profession with two decades of service in public health. He has served as a state minister of health of the Federal Democratic Republic of Ethiopia for thirteen years. As state minister, he was responsible for leading the implementation of the health sector to achieve the vision, mission, and goals set by the country. He was particularly responsible for leading the overall health sector to achieve national priorities and international commitments; mobilizing resources from donor communities (domestic and international); coordination and alignment of donor and implementing partners and other stakeholders toward achieving the mission of the health sector; setting policies and implementation strategies, and leading the development of procedures, guidelines, and manuals; overseeing the implementation of the health sector missions given to agencies accountable to the Ministry of Health, such as operational and basic researches, pharmaceutical supply chain management, human resource development and management, regulatory functions (food and medicine), public health emergency management, and medical services; and monitoring and evaluation of policies, strategic plans and guidelines, and annual plans of the health sector (comprehensive and programmatic plans). He has represented the country in international and national fora and shared experiences.

REFERENCES FOR BOXES

Chapter 1

Pages 29–31

Arole M. 2002. "The Comprehensive Rural Health Project in Jamkhed, India." In *Community-based health care: Lessons from Bangladesh to Boston*, edited by J. E. Rohde and J. Wyon, 47–60. Boston: Management Sciences for Health.

Bang, A. T., R. A. Bang, and H. M. Reddy. 2005. "Home-based neonatal care: Summary and applications of the field trial in rural Gadchiroli, India (1993 to 2003)." *J Perinatol* 25 (Suppl. 1): S108–S122.

Bang, A. T., R. A. Bang, 0. Tale, P. Sontakke, J. Solanki, R. Wargantiwar, and P. Kelzarkar. 1990. "Reduction in pneumonia mortality and total childhood mortality by means of community-based intervention trial in Gadchiroli, India." *Lancet* 336 (8709): 201–206.

Bornstein, D. 2007. *How to change the world: Social entrepreneurs and the power of new ideas*, 247–61. Oxford: Oxford University Press.

Jolly, Richard, ed. 2001. Jim Grant: UNICEF visionary. Florence, Italy: UNICEF Office of Research-Innocenti.

Rohde, Jon E., and John Wyon, eds. 2002. *Community-based health care: Lessons from Bangladesh to Boston*. Boston: Management Sciences for Health (in collaboration with the Harvard School of Public Health).

SEARCH (Society for Education, Action and Research in Community Health). 2013. Accessed 10, 2020. https://searchsociety.org/.

Werner, D., and D. Sanders. 1997. *Questioning the solution: The politics of primary health care and child survival*. Palo Alto, CA: HealthWrights.

Pages 32–35

Admasu, K., T. Balcha, and H. Getahun. 2016. "Model villages: A platform for community-based primary health care." *Lancet* 4 (2): e7–e79.

Admasu, K., T. Balcha, and T. A. Ghebreyesus. 2016. "Pro-poor pathway towards universal health coverage: Lessons from Ethiopia." *J Global Health* 6 (1): 010305.

Assefa, Y., Y. A. Gelaw, P. S. Hill, B. W. Taye, and W. Van Damme. 2019. "Community health extension program of Ethiopia, 2003–2018: Successes and challenges toward universal coverage for primary healthcare services." *Globalization and Health* 15 (1): 24.

Assefa, Y., D. Tesfaye, W. V. Damme, and P. S. 2018. "Effectiveness and sustainability of a diagonal investment approach to strengthen the primary health-care system in Ethiopia." *Lancet* 392 (10156): 1473–1481.

BASICS II, The MOST Project, USAID. 2004. *Nepal Child Survival Case Study: Technical Report*. Arlington, VA: Basic Support for Institutionalizing Child Survival Project (BASICS II) for the United States Agency for International Development.

CORE Group. 2013. *History of CORE Group*. Washington, DC: The CORE Group, 2013.

———. 2019. "About the CORE Group." Accessed April 18, 2020. https://coregroup .org/about-core-group/#who-we-are.

Chowdhury, A. M. R., and H. Perry. Forthcoming. NGO *contributions to community health and primary health care, with case studies from Bangladesh and India*. New York: Oxford University Press.

El Arifeen, S., A. Christou, L. Reichenbach, et al. 2013. "Community-based approaches and partnerships: Innovations in health-service delivery in Bangladesh." *Lancet* 382 (9909): 2012–2026.

Gottlieb, J. 2007. "Reducing child mortality with vitamin A in Nepal." In *Case studies in global health: Millions saved*, edited by R. Levine, 25-31. Washington, DC: Center for Global Development.

IIfPHC-E (International Institute for Primary Health Care-Ethiopia). 2020. Accessed 25, 2020. https://iifphc.org/.

Jurberg, C., and G. Humphreys. 2010. "Brazil's march towards universal coverage." *Bull World Health Organ* 88 (9): 646–647.

Kleinert, S., and R. Horton. 1979. "Brazil: Towards sustainability and equity in health." *Lancet* 377 (9779): 1721–1722.

Loosey, L., E. Ogden, F. Bisrat, et al. 2019. "The CORE Group Polio Project: An overview of its history and its contributions to the Global Polio Eradication Initiative." *Am J Trop Med Hyg* 101 (4): 4–14.

Patcharanarumol, W., V. Tangcharoensathien, S. Limwattananon, et al. 2011. "Why and how did Thailand achieve good health at low cost?" In *"Good health at low cost" 25 years on: What makes a successful health system?*, edited by D. Balabanova, M. McKee, and A. Mills, 193–234. London: London School of Hygiene and Tropical Medicine.

Perry H. 2000. *Heath for all in Bangladesh: Lessons in primary health care for the twenty-first century*. Dhaka: Bangladesh University Press.

———. 2016. "A comprehensive description of three national community health worker programs and their contributions to maternal and child health and primary health care: Case studies from Latin America (Brazil), Africa (Ethiopia) and Asia (Nepal)." Accessed June 24, 2019. http://www.financingalliance.org/resources/.

Perry, H. B., and J. Rohde. 2019. "The Jamkhed Comprehensive Rural Health Project and the Alma-Ata vision of primary health care." *Am J Public Health* 109 (1): 699–704.

Perry, H. B., V. Solomon, F. Bisrat, et al. Lessons learned from community engagement, community-based programming for polio eradication, and the CORE Group Polio Project: Their relevance for ending preventable child and maternal deaths. *Am J Trop Med Hyg* 101 (4): 107–112.

Rice-Marquez, N., T. D. Baker, and C. Fischer. 1988. "The community health worker: Forty years of experience of an integrated primary rural health care system in Brazil." *J Rural Health* 1988: 87–100.

Rohde, J., S. Cousens, M. Chopra, et al. 2008. "30 years after Alma-Ata: Has primary health care worked in countries?" *Lancet* 372 (9642): 950–961.

Standing, H., and Chowdhury, A. M. 2008. "Producing effective knowledge agents in a pluralistic environment: What future for community health workers?" *Soc Sci Med* 66 (10): 2096–2107.

Chapter 3

Pages 77–78

Barzilay, E. J., H. Vandi, S. Binder, I. Udo, M. L. Ospina, C. Ihekweazu, and S. Bratton. 2018. "Use of the Staged Development Tool for assessing, planning, and measuring progress in the development of National Public Health Institutes." *Health Secur* 16 (S1): S18–S24. doi:10.1089/hs.2018.0044.

Bettcher, D. W., S. Sapirie, and E. H. Goon. 1998. "Essential public health functions: Results of the international Delphi study." *World Health Stat Q* 51 (1): 44–54.

Corso, L. C., P. J. Wiesner, P. K. Halverson, and C. K. Brown. 2000. "Using the essential services as a foundation for performance measurement and assessment of local public health systems." *J Public Health Manag Pract* 6 (5): 1–18.

Derose, Stephen F., Mark A. Schuster, Jonathan E. Fielding, and Steven M. Asch. 2002. "Public health quality measurement: Concepts and challenges 1." *Annu Rev Public Health* 23 (1): 1–21.

Dyal, W. W. 1995. "Ten organizational practices of public health: a historical perspective." *Am J Prev Med* 11 (6 Suppl): 6–8.

Forster, A. J., and C. van Walraven. 2012. "The use of quality indicators to promote accountability in health care: The good, the bad, and the ugly." *Open Med* 6 (2): e75–e79.

Martin-Moreno, Jose M., Meggan Harris, Elke Jakubowski, and Hans Kluge. 2016. "Defining and assessing public health functions: A global analysis." *Annu Rev Public Health* 37: 335–355.

Schwartz, R., A. Price, R. B. Deber, H. Manson, and F. Scott. 2014. "Hopes and realities of public health accountability policies." *Healthc Policy* 10 (SP): 79–89.

Upshaw, V. 2000. "The National Public Health Performance Standards Program: Will it strengthen governance of local public health?" *J Public Health Manag Pract* 6 (5): 88–92.

Veillard, J., K. Cowling, A. Bitton, et al. 2017. "Better measurement for performance improvement in low- and middle-income countries: The Primary Health Care Performance Initiative (PHCPI) experience of conceptual framework development and indicator selection." *Milbank Q* 95 (4): 835–883.

WHO Regional Office for the Eastern Mediterranean. 2017. *Assessment of essential public health functions in countries of the Eastern Mediterranean Region: Assessment tool.* Cairo, Egypt: WHO.

Winslow, C. E. 1925. "Municipal health department practice." *Am J Public Health (N Y)* 15 (1): 39–44.

Chapter 5

Page 108

Durbur Mahila Samanwaya Committee Theory and Action for Health Research Team. 2007. *Meeting community needs for HIV prevention and more: Intersectoral action for health in the Sonagachi red light area of Kolkata.* https://www.who.int/social _determinants/resources/isa_sonagachi_ind.pdf.

Page 110

Pan American Health Organization 2015. *Health in all policies: Case studies from the region of the Americas.* Washington, DC: Pan American Health Organization.
World Health Organization. 2011. *Social determinants approaches to public health: From concept to practice.* Geneva, Switzerland: WHO.
———. 2014. *Health in all policies: Helsinki Statement.* Framework for Public Action. Geneva, Switzerland: WHO.

Page 111

Blass, E., Lucy Gilson, Michael P. Kelly, Ronald Labonté, Jostacio Lapitan, Carles Muntaner, Piroska Östlin, Jennie Popay, Ritu Sadana, Gita Sen, Ted Schrecker, and Ziba Vaghri. 2008. "Addressing social determinants of health inequities: What can the state and civil society do?" *Lancet* 372 (9650): 1684–1689.
Commission on Social Determinants of Health. 2008. *Closing the gap in a generation: Health equity through action on the social determinants of health.* Geneva, Switzerland: World Health Organization.
Nugroho, Jati, and Dwi Sriyantini. 2016. "Political Reconstruction Law Society building policy action alert healthy prosperous and dignified in making healthy generation of gold in the district Lumajang." *IOSR Journal of Humanities and Social Science* 21 (11): 10–14.
Siswanto, E. S. 2009. "Community empowerment through intersectoral action: A case study of Gerbangmas in Lumajang District." *Jurnal Manajemen Pelayanan Kesehatan* 12 (1). https://journal.ugm.ac.id/jmpk/article/view/2563/2296.
Sururi, N. R., Heru Ribawanto, and Mochammad Rozikin. "Movement of building healthy communities as innovation in health care in villages Citrodiwangsan Lumajang Subdistrict." *J Public Adm* 1 (2): 238–247.

Chapter 7

Page 164

Ahmed, Syed Masud, Bushra Binte Alam, Iqbal Anwar, Tahmina Begum, Rumana Huque, Jahangir A. Khan, Herfina Nababan, and Ferdous Arfina Osman. 2015. *Health systems in transition,* Vol. 5, No. 3. Asia Pacific Observatory on Health Systems and Policies. Switzerland: World Health Organization.
National Institute of Population Research and Training, International Center for Diarrheal Disease Research Bangladesh, and MEASURE Evaluation. 2012.

Bangladesh Maternal Mortality and Health Care Survey 2010. Dhaka, Bangladesh: NIPORT, MEASURE Evaluation. measureevaluation.org/resources/publications/tr -12-87.

USAID. 2015. *Audit of USAID/Bangladesh's NGO Health Service Delivery Project*. Manila: USAID, Office of Inspector General.

Chapter 11

Page 268

United Nations Childrens' Fund. 1977. *Children in Asia 1977*. Bangkok, Thailand: United Nations Childrens' Fund, Regional Office of East Asia and Pakistan.

INDEX

Afghanistan, 88–89, 95, 98
Africa: immunization rates, 88, 89; progress on MDGs, 20. See also *specific countries*
Agape Health Clinic, 145
agriculture, 5, 6, 97, 111, 117, 118
aid, foreign, 10, 12, 326
AIDS, *See* HIV/AIDS
alcohol use, 135, 136, 137, 147, 272, 289
Alliance for Health Systems and Policy Research, 7, 8–9
All India Institute of Hygiene and Public Health, 23, 29, 108
Alma-Ata Conference: anniversary, 19, 47–48; consensus at, 3–7; divergence in approaches, 7–12; as event, 3–5, 25; influence of, 2–3, 12–13, 47–48; location of, 25
Alma-Ata Declaration: as consensus, 4–7; defining PHC, 25–26; influence of, 2–3, 19; influence of Cuba on, 298; People's Charter for Health, 33; principles of PHC, 5–7, 87, 97–98, 327; role of PHC, 118–19; and Taylor, 29
American Public Health Association, 77
Andean Rural Health Project, 36
Anganwadi centers, 92, 140, 324
Angola, 34, 70, 80–81, 90, 94, 95
antenatal care: Bangladesh, 159, 172; as core service, 44; Ethiopia, 190, 191; Ghana, 229; Liberia/Guinea, 143, 145; Nepal, 208, 217, 221, 229
appreciation in SALT approach, 129–31, 132, 133, 135, 136, 141, 146–47
Arnstein's ladder of participation, 129, 130
Arole, Mabelle, 30, 32, 42
Arole, Rajanikant, 30, 32, 42
Asia: immunization rates, 88. See also *specific countries*
assessment, *See* performance

assurance, 73, 74, 75, 82, 105, 106, 114–15
Astana Conference 2018, 12, 14, 19, 48, 319, 325, 326
Ayurvedic medicine, 261, 263

Bang, Abhay, 30–31, 32, 42
Bang, Rani, 30–31, 32, 42
Bangladesh: background and history, 153–59; BRAC, 32–33, 166; challenges, 163–64, 167, 172–74, 175, 324, 328; community study, 168–74; current program, 160–68; life expectancy, 57, 66, 67, 68, 153, 154, 158, 159; as success, 10, 14, 34, 38, 153–79, 328
Bangladesh Rural Advancement Committee (BRAC), 32–33, 166
barefoot doctors, 4, 22–23, 24, 280. *See also* health workers
Behdar Training Project, 23
Bellagio Conferences, 7, 8, 56–57, 96–98
Berggren, Gretchen, 42
Berggren, Warren, 42
Bhore Committee, 23, 29, 155, 156, 174
bidirectional learning, 110
Bill and Melinda Gates Foundation, 32, 96
billboards, 134, 137, 147, 312
Bolivia, 36, 67
Botswana, 70, 131, 132–38, 147
Brazil, 35, 38, 109
breastfeeding: as core service, 20, 44; Ethiopia, 190, 191; Ghana, 246; GOBI-FFF, 8, 27; Nepal, 221–22; vertical approaches, 7, 8
Bryant, John, 24
Burma, 57

Caldwell, John, 56–57
cancer, 78
CARE, 167

Foege, William, 24
food: Bangladesh, 170, 175; Cuba, 314; food safety, 78, 266; food SDGs, 112, 115, 117; GOBI-FFF, 8, 27n§; India, 78; Nepal, 203. *See also* malnutrition; nutrition
Ford Foundation, 7–8
funding: child survival, 33; Cuba, 300; curative focus, 71, 72; future of, 325–26; Ghana, 237, 238, 242, 244, 245, 247; health workers, 38, 46; lack of enthusiasm for PHC, 96; Nepal, 216, 219; and performance, 71, 74–75, 76, 80–81; polio, 91; public health, 82; and recession, 28; SDGs, 326; Sri Lanka, 271, 272, 273; success at low costs, 319–20; Thailand, 35; for Universal Health Coverage, 41; and vertical approaches, 96, 320–21; Vietnam, 280, 281, 282, 288, 290–91, 292

GAVI, 12, 86–87
GDP (gross domestic product), 56–57, 59–69
Gebreyesus, Tedros Adhanom, 48
gender equality: Bangladesh, 171; Nepal, 201, 203–4, 219; SDGs, 104, 112–13, 115, 117; Sri Lanka, 259
Gerbangmas movement, 111
Ghana: background and history, 225–28; development of program, 229–37; GEHIP, 244–48; life expectancy, 66, 68, 69; organization and structure, 227, 228, 243; reforms, 240–49; scaling program, 237–40, 249–50; as success, 225–57, 320, 328
Gillin, John, 8
global health education, 8, 9, 29
global health transitions, 41
Global Health Watch, 33
Global Polio Eradication Initiative (GPEI), 9, 85–99
GOBI/GOBI-FFF, 8, 27
Good Health at Low Cost 25 Years On (1985), 57, 68
Grant, James P., 8, 26–27, 29
Grant, John B., 22, 23, 27, 29
growth monitoring, 8, 27, 259, 283
Guinea, 66, 131, 142–46, 147
guinea worm, 96

Haiti, 36, 42, 312
Haniffa, Ruviaz, 274–75
Health by the People (WHO), 25, 35, 36
health education: Bangladesh, 158, 169, 170–71; as core service, 5, 44, 97, 104; Cuba, 311, 313; Ethiopia, 186; India, 108; Nepal, 222; SDGs, 107–8; Sri Lanka, 273; Vietnam, 282, 286
health expenditures: in aggregate, 11; Bangladesh, 153, 163, 172, 175; Cuba, 299; Ethiopia, 180, 195, 196; foreign aid for, 10, 12, 326; Ghana, 233; India, 153; and life expectancy, 57; Nepal, 153, 218–19; South, 10; Sri Lanka, 153, 271; US, 299; Vietnam, 281, 289–90
Health by The People (Newell), 30
Health in All Policies (HiAP), 82, 109, 110, 111, 119
Health System Performance Assessment, 169
Health Systems Global, 9
health workers: Bangladesh, 32, 158, 159, 161, 165–66, 171, 172, 173–74, 175; Bolivia, 36; Brazil, 35; and child outcomes, 39; Cuba, 321; development of, 22–23, 35–38; Ethiopia, 34, 181, 184–94, 321; funding, 38, 46; Ghana, 225, 227, 229, 231–34, 236, 245, 246, 247, 320; Haiti, 36; incentives, 46; India, 30, 32, 36, 78, 139–41, 148; monitoring of, 49; Nepal, 34, 46, 205–6, 207–13, 217, 218, 220, 321; performance and number of, 71, 73; as principle of PHC, 5, 6, 37–38, 110; qualifications of, 45, 186, 192, 210, 225, 245, 290; South Africa, 35; Sri Lanka, 265–66, 267, 270; and Universal Health Coverage, 42; Vietnam, 280, 282–83, 290; World Health Assembly on, 49. *See also* compensation; medical personnel; trust
HEP (health extension program) (Ethiopia), 182, 183–94, 196
HiAP (Health in All Policies), 82, 109, 110, 111, 119
HIV/AIDS: Botswana, 131, 132–38, 147; Brazil, 35; as core service, 44; deaths, 20; Ethiopia, 34, 183, 190; India, 108; Nepal, 210, 217; SALT approach, 131, 132–38, 147; Sri Lanka, 267; vertical approaches, 28, 320; Vietnam, 285, 287

literacy: Bangladesh, 163; Cuba, 311; Ethiopia, 181, 192; Ghana, 228; India, 108; Nepal, 200, 201, 220; Sri Lanka, 260; Vietnam, 292

Lives Saved Tool (LiST), 10

location and access to health care, 37, 38–39

Mahler, Halfdan, 25, 29, 33

malaria: as core service, 44, 97; Ethiopia, 34, 183, 187, 190; Ghana, 229, 246; mortality from, 20, 38; Nepal, 200, 202, 206, 207, 208, 222; as spur for Conference, 3, 8, 14; Sri Lanka, 266–67, 271; vertical approaches, 28, 320; Vietnam, 283

Mali, 65, 66, 68

malnutrition, 157, 187, 222, 283, 310

Manoshi Project, 32–33

maternal and child health: Bangladesh, 156, 157, 159, 171, 174; as core service, 44, 87, 97, 327; Ethiopia, 183, 187, 190, 191, 192, 196; Ghana, 246, 247; India, 31, 36, 78; MDGs, 9–10, 20; Nepal, 202, 206, 207–13, 216, 217, 220–22; NGOs, 33–34; SDGs, 117; Sri Lanka, 265, 267; Vietnam, 283, 284, 286. See also child survival

maternal mortality. See mortality, maternal

MDGs (Millennium Development Goals): Ethiopia, 34, 183, 190; Ghana, 233; health goals, 9–10, 20; Nepal, 204; vs. SDGs, 103; Thailand, 35

measles, 92, 96, 187, 219, 221, 229

medical diplomacy, 301–2

medical education: Cuba, 301–3, 311; Ethiopia, 190; Nepal, 205. See also training

medical personnel: Cuba, 300–301, 306, 311; Ethiopia, 190; Ghana, 227, 231–34; numbers who have never seen, 20; Vietnam, 279, 283, 290. See also health workers

medications: Bangladesh, 162–63, 165; as core service, 97; Cuba, 311; Sri Lanka, 271, 274; Vietnam, 281

mental health, 44, 107, 113, 172, 173, 192, 262, 270

mentoring, 75

midwives. See under deliveries

Millennium Development Goals. See MDGs (Millennium Development Goals)

Millennium Summit 2000, 7

missionaries, 21–22, 24

monitoring: Bangladesh, 163, 167; Ethiopia, 184, 187; Ghana, 239; need for, 49; Nepal, 213; in SALT approach, 137; SDGs, 103, 106, 114; Sri Lanka, 273, 274; Vietnam, 285

mortality: Bangladesh, 153; China, 22; and demographic transition, 41; Ghana, 228, 233, 245; from NCDs, 120; Sri Lanka, 260, 263, 270, 271. See also mortality, child; mortality, infant; mortality, maternal; mortality, under-5

mortality, child: Bangladesh, 38; Brazil, 35, 38; Cuba, 303; Ethiopia, 34, 38, 183; Ghana, 248; India, 36; MDGs, 20; Nepal, 38, 213, 220, 222; Sri Lanka, 259. See also mortality, infant; mortality, under-5

mortality, infant: Bangladesh, 154, 159; Caldwell study, 56–57; Care Group model, 37; China, 22, 56; Cuba, 299, 316; Ghana, 248; India, 36, 56, 57; Sri Lanka, 56, 259, 260, 271; US, 299

mortality, maternal: Bangladesh, 154, 159; Care Group model, 37; Cuba, 299; Ethiopia, 34, 189, 190; MDGs, 9–10, 20; Nepal, 200–201, 213, 220; Sri Lanka, 259, 260, 271; US, 299

mortality, under-5: Bangladesh, 154; Brazil, 35; and Care Group model, 37; Cuba, 299; Ethiopia, 190, 191; health workers and, 37, 38; and IMCI, 38–39; MDGs, 9–10; Nepal, 201; Sri Lanka, 260; US, 299

mosquito control, 143, 229, 306, 310, 312–13, 314

Mozambique, 66, 70

Narangwal Project, 30, 36

Narsingdi Model, 167

National Public Health Performance Standards Program (US), 77

National Rural Mission (India), 30

Navrongo Health Research Centre, 228, 231–34

NCDs. *See* noncommunicable diseases (NCDs)

neonatal care: Bangladesh, 159; Ethiopia, 187, 191; Ghana, 246, 247, 248; and health workers, 37, 38, 45; India, 31, 32, 36; Nepal, 210

Nepal: background and history, 199–207, 208, 213–16; challenges, 199–200, 218–20; health expenditures, 153, 218–19; life expectancy, 65, 66, 68, 201, 204, 213; organization and structure, 207–13, 216–17; polio, 90, 93n, 94; as success, 10, 14, 34, 38, 199–224, 321, 328

Newell, Kenneth, 25, 30

NGO Health Service Development Program, 164

NGOs (nongovernmental organizations): Bangladesh, 160, 163–68, 166, 169; child survival, 37, 38–39, 46, 163; funding, 33–34; GO-NGO partnerships, 164–69; lack of coordination, 11; Nepal, 209, 218; Sri Lanka, 267, 268–69, 270, 271–72; Vietnam, 287

Nigeria, 34, 66, 88–90, 92–95, 98

noncommunicable diseases (NCDs): Bangladesh, 172, 173, 175; and EPHFs, 78; Ethiopia, 192; India, 78; and relevance of PHC, 12, 21, 324; and SDGs, 119, 120; Sri Lanka, 271, 272; vertical approaches, 12; Vietnam, 288–89, 290, 291

nurses. *See* medical personnel

nutrition: Bangladesh, 32, 157, 170, 171, 175; and Care Group model, 37; as core service, 44, 97; Cuba, 310; Ethiopia, 34, 187; and IMCI, 38; India, 36; Nepal, 210, 222; SDGs, 112, 117; Sri Lanka, 259, 267, 268; Vietnam, 284, 287. *See also* iron supplementation; Vitamin A supplementation

One Health, 82, 113, 117, 118

Ontario Public Health Standards, 78

oral rehydration, 8, 27, 34, 156, 164–65, 171, 222, 229

ownership: and community engagement, 127–34, 137, 138, 140–43, 146–48; Ethiopia, 189, 194; Ghana, 234, 240; Nepal, 216, 219, 222–23

Pakistan, 85n*, 88–89, 90, 92–95, 98, 155–56

Pan American Health Organization, 47, 85–86

pandemics. *See* epidemics and pandemics

participatory learning and action, 37

partnerships: collaborative, 110; GO-NGO, 164–69; public-private, 160, 288; SDGs, 113, 115, 118

peace SDGs, 113, 115, 118

People's Charter for Health, 33

People's Health Movement, 33, 269, 274, 275

performance: Bellagio Conference 2017, 96–98; checklists, 72; coaches, 75–76, 80–81; Health System Performance Assessment, 169; improvement plans, 75–81; need for measurement, 71–72; role of public health, 70, 73, 75–78, 82; self-assessments, 70, 131; strategies, 70–84; supportive supervision, 70, 74–81. *See also* EPHFs (essential public health functions)

Perry, Henry, 42

Peru, 66, 87

PHC. *See* primary health care

plague, 1–2, 22

pneumonia, 31, 32, 36, 187, 190, 191, 210, 229, 246

polio: CORE Group, 34; Cuba, 306; Ghana, 236; GPEI, 9, 85–99; overuse of resources, 91–95; role of PHC, 85–101, 325

polyclinics, 306, 313, 315

poverty SDGs, 104, 115, 117

pregnancy. *See* antenatal care

Preston Curve, 57, 58–69

prevention as principle of PHC, 5, 6, 44, 87, 97, 327

primary health care: challenges, 42–46; consensus on, 3–7; definitions of, 3, 5, 25–26, 47, 87, 104; future of, 47–49, 324–26; history of, 21–42; key individuals and organizations, 29–35; overview of, 1–15; preconditions for, 72–73; principles and core services, 5–7, 42–43, 44, 87, 97–98, 327; renewed interest in, 19–21, 47–49; as term, 5, 21, 24, 71, 102, 119. *See also* Alma-Ata Conference; case studies; community engagement; performance; SALT approach